The Essential Guide to Native American Herbal Remedies

Natural Remedies to the Most Common Ailments

Citali Galwen

D1710854

TABLE OF CONTENT

BOOK 1

NATIVE AMERICAN HEALING HERBS

Start Your Journey into Healing Herbs and Discover
the Secrets of Native American Healing Practices

Citali Galwen

INTRODUCTION

The indigenous peoples of the United States are referred to as Native Americans. They are divided into tribal groups including the Apache, Chippewa, Cherokee, Dakota, Finnish, Haida, Iroquois, Kalispel, Lakota Sioux Nation, Lummi Nation, Mandan, Mohawk, Nez Perce, Northern Athabaskan, Ojibwe IDA), Pueblo (Hopi), Pima County/Mohawk), Salish (Shoshone), Seneca, Shawnee/Lenape), Yakama) and Yupik peoples.

Native American traditional healing practices have been passed down for thousands of years, including ceremonies, dances (the Sun Dance and Green Corn Dance), and rituals. Spiritual leaders did not only prescribe healing practices themselves but also passed them along to their people.

Many of these traditional practices are still passed on through oral tradition. They vary from tribe to tribe and from region to region. All traditional Native American healing ceremonies "recognized a fundamental belief in a spiritual order—an order they called "Wayse-aohc" (pronounced 'way-sho-ahw'), meaning "the right way" or "the good way."

It is said that Native American spiritual leaders "must have been people of deep wisdom because their knowledge was passed from one generation to the next. They not only told us where to go and what to do to obtain what we needed but also how to get there. In several cases, they lived their lives in a manner so that whatever they did became a metaphor for what we should be doing."

Native American traditional healing was given different names depending on the region. It used many different methods, but all followed a common belief system.

Through a powerful oral tradition, Native American generations have obtained medical information over the past 40,000 years. The interconnection between humanity, ecology, and the spiritual realm is emphasized by indigenous medical philosophy. A person of medicine studies the relationships of the patient with other individuals, the experiences are used to treat and cure the patient. These may include herbs, ceremonies, music, prayer, and sweating.

Native American medicine relates to over 500 nations' combined clinical practices. Native medicine is almost forty thousand years old. The particular activities differed between tribes, but everything is based on the universal idea that man is an integral part of nature and that a matter of balance is health. When interrelationships are valued, nurtured, and sustained in harmony, the natural world then moves as a consequence. The natural world cannot be seen by the mind and does not engage in science directly and intuitively. Much like a human being's inner life cannot be determined, nature has persuasive forces that need to be incorporated for balance. Just now has reporting started and has been limited to findings, so it is incomplete. Native medicine values all life and is not just a body of science or methodology that is scholarly. For fear of exploitation, Native American elders typically do not disclose their knowledge.

The balance between the inner life and open actions is tackled in Native American medicine. They all take into account the body, mind, soul, thoughts, social circle, and lifestyle. The choice and desires of a patient are often respected to establish harmony. Bodywork, naturopathy, bone setting, midwifery, hydrotherapy, botanical, and nutritional medicine can be included in every Native American healer's strategy. Often used are ceremonial and ritual medicines. Many of these have been forgotten as only by living practitioners has this undocumented living practice survived. More Native Americans have been involved in protecting their culture, and Native American medicine today is as fluid as ever with this effort.

CHAPTER 1:

NATIVE AMERICAN HEALING HERBS OVERVIEW

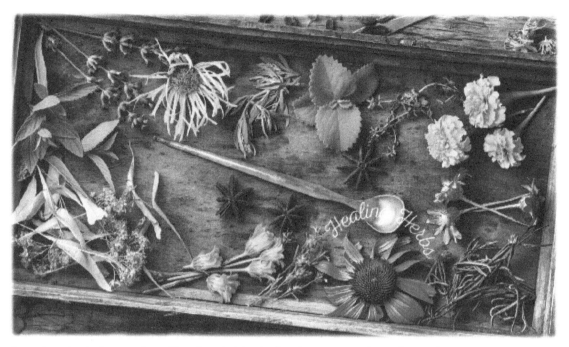

Native American herbal expertise offered a vital basis for the construction of a modern country in an age before antibiotics and awareness of the origins of infectious diseases. Every schoolchild in America knows that they were saved from starvation by the native food provided by Indians given to early colonists; it is less well established that Indians often gave native herbs to colonists that helped them withstand disease, injuries, dietary shortages, fertility problems, and other illnesses. Native plant remedies, originally established by Indians, were used quite early by United States doctors for illnesses such as constipation, respiratory disorders, snakebites, burns, & rheumatism. Witch hazel (Hamamelis virginiana) for calming sore muscles, balsamroot salve (Balsamorhiza sagittata) for curing wounds of the flesh, red trillium (Trillium erectum) root to alleviate labor pain, blue cohosh as antispasmodic, and black cohosh (Actaea racemosa) mostly as female and maternity medicine are only a few of the plants the colonists and pioneers were provided with by the Indians.

Brief History of Herbalism

When western colonization introduced Americans of European origin to new worlds as well as the eventual accidents and diseases in the 1800s, indigenous communities also offered medicinal remedies to the colonists and settlers that proved essential for their survival. Some of our great adventurers, fur trappers, physicians, and naturalists' writings, such as Meriwether Lewis and William Clark, Jedediah Strong Smith, Peter Kalm, Leonard McPhail, and William Bartram, contain references to the awareness and usage of these plants to treat disease and disability by native food and medicinal plants acquired from American Indians.

Miners subsisted on meals of bacon, beans, and coffee throughout the California Gold Rush. Thus, exhibiting signs of scurvy, they were introduced to Claytonia perfoliata by the foothill tribes (Sierra Nevada), an edible herb that restores health. Local plants like dogwood (Cornus spp.), sassafras (Sassafras albidum), leaves and bark of white oaks (Quercus alba), partridgeberry (Mitchella repens), and Liriodendron tulipifera (tulip trees) provided surgeons of the fields with a repertoire of medicines to treat injured soldiers during the Civil War. This plant was eventually discovered to be high in Vitamin C and was dubbed 'miner's lettuce.'

Immigrants of Europe to the Modern World were not solely relying on herbal Medicine from Native Americans. They took with them seeds and cuttings of favorite medicinal plants, beneficiaries of a wealthy herbalist heritage in Europe, and inexperienced with the qualities of plants native to the Modern World. They used Euphrasia officinalis (eyebright) to cure inflamed eyes, treated colds and coughs through Marrubium vulgare (horehound), and used

Hypericum perforatum (St. John's wort) as an anti-inflammatory. It was this understanding of the medicinal features of plants that prompted them to pursue herbal information from Indians and too readily introduced the native plants they heard about into their cabinets of medicine.

Much like the species of the Old World introduced to the coasts of America, both purposely and unintentionally, quickly dispersed to produce different biological mixtures across Modern World habitats, so did medicinal herbs of both local and European origins fuse together in the young nation's pharmacopeias. In the first Pharmacopeia (U.S.) issued in 1820, almost half of the compounds were local plants in use by American Indians, like Canadian fleabane (Leptilon canadense now Conyza canadensis) and American senna (Cassia marilandica and Senna marilandica). Non-native plants taken from homelands of old European or other continents became the equilibrium.

Therefore, in the early years of our country, Americans had exposure to a very large variety of medicinal herbs originating from the flora of two continents, one dating back centuries, reflecting the collective experience of two distinct herbal cultures. This mixing method, however, had one unfortunate feature for American Indians: their contributions to this substantial array of medicines were mostly neglected and overlooked. To the current day, this situation remains. More than 200 medicines that were used by American Indians have been or are now listed in the U.S. Pharmacopeia or National Type, but no guide accepts this reality. The vast advantages that we have obtained from the traditional experience of natural plant medicines are still mostly uncredited.

Native American Herbal Medicines

Many natural medicinal plants have been so essential that for decades and, in certain instances, generations, they have been subject to unnecessary agricultural cultivation. Many of these natural medicinal plants, like cascara, slippery elm (Ulmus rubra), Panax quinquefolius (American ginseng), and Goldenseal, are becoming endangered with the added stresses of habitat loss, fire suppression, and climate change. Efforts to protect these organisms and guarantee that they remain accessible in the future pose a range of challenges, not least the inherent lack of scientific understanding of the species concerned, the biological consequences of their harvesting, and the management methods that will ensure the long-term survival of the goods.

We still know very little about the specific criteria of most of these organisms for reproductive biology, ecology, and environment and have little quantitative evidence on phenology, distribution and population growth. It is no surprise that the rise in popularity of and demand for some medicinal plants results in population reduction without basic ecological awareness of these plants and no coordinated scheme of sustain-yield management.

We should look to the very same people who brought us knowledge of the uses and importance of these species in the first place to figure a way forward from this impasse. In addition to curating considerable awareness regarding the usage of natural herbal medicine, American Indians established continuous yield practices following the plants' reproductive biology and established management practices that protect their ecosystems. Both harvest and management is centered on a restraint-based ethical framework, a long-term outlook on time, as well as a body of ecological experience generated from near scientific study. We will learn a lot from these original practices, incorporate them into conservation programs and, when suitable for the local environment, combine them with Western science-based techniques.

How To Use Native Management And Harvest Practices

A particular example serves to explain how in the conservation of an endangered medicinal plant, native management and harvest practices may be utilized. For centuries, the bark of cascara sagrada was used in the U.S. (northwestern) to cure constipation, and its usage has expanded across the globe after people of European descent knew of its characteristics around 125 years ago. It has been named "the world's most commonly used cathartically."

Cascara sagrada grows in British Columbia, east to Idaho and south to Arizona and California, Montana, andWyoming. Cascara is a member of the Rhamnaceae, with a grey-to-deep red-brown bark that is smooth or scaly to longitudinally furrow. The elliptic-shaped, glossy green leaves have fine-toothed margins and are distinctly veined. It takes place under 2000 m. In various environments from semi-dry to wet, including coniferous woods of Sitka spruce, Douglas-fir, western hemlock, mixed evergreen trees, ponderosa pine, hardwood trees, montane chaparral, coastal scrub, creek ravines and drainages, swampy bottomlands with vine maple and red alder and ecotones between woodland and prairie or natural wetland. It can achieve tree size when developing in thick, fertile soils in low river bottoms, flats, rivers, and stream borders; it maintains a shrub-like shape on drier sites with sandy soils or gravelly.

. Among several tribes, cascara was much more than another cathartic; it apparently returned the gut to a healthy rhythm, making regular doses unnecessary.

The herb was brought by a physician from Colusa, Dr. Bundy, to western Medicine in 1877 and became legal in the Pharmacopeia of the U.S. in 1890. Early marketers reported that cascara was among the "best therapeutic herbs." Cascara was seen all over the world at the beginning of the 1900s.

There were many trees of cascara sagrada, considering its long-term local use when it was sought by the first missionaries and non-Indian settlers. Because of the manner indigenous individuals harvested it, cascara stayed plentiful. Through taking short strips by the main trunk or through removing a single branch so that it doesn't hurt or damage the tree, Native Americans obtain cascara bark.

Cascara was in high demand as the active ingredient of all kinds of industrial laxatives in the early years of the 20th century. Many non-Indian individuals were peelers of cascara wood, heading after trees that had achieved tremendous height and ignoring any that were smaller than some few inches in diameter. Some studied the Indians' sustainable farming practices, but long-term interests were always outweighed by the windfall of a massive one-time crop.

The bark is sliced all the way across the tree by most harvesters, destroying it, and regions that were sustainably grown were prone to "pirating," just as high as it could have been reached from the field, the unsustainable method of butchering trees. These trees died with their vast numbers of unsalvageable residual bark. Older and larger cascara trees have become rare after several decades of excessive production. In areas of the Northwest, the skeletons (bone-white) of deceased cascara trees still define habitats, testaments of the trees' thoughtless and destructive harvesting. Today, cascara sagrada is listed on the "To-Watch" list of United Plant Savers because it is "still in decline due to growing prominence and declining habitat and range."

In part, Cascara sagrada has not recovered due to the ongoing global mandate for its bark, but also due to the fact that the plant communities in which it develops are no longer as favorable as they once were to growth and reproduction. For optimal growth, cascara requires sunshine, and the trees are too thick in many environments, and the canopy is too restricted to allow for the required light levels. These circumstances are the outcome of the systematic suppression of fire and the termination of the frequent burning of the trees, lakes, and prairies formerly done by the Northwest tribes.

To hold the woods open and to hold the lakes and prairies from being overrun by vegetation, the Indians burned. In doing so, they preserved perfect environments, including cascara, for several valuable plant organisms. The forest was diversified through Indian fire, establishing a forest prairie or forest-wetland mosaic that hosted a richer range of animals and plants than might occur.

In rather open woods and in ecotones, or edge areas, between woods and large wetlands or prairies, cascara does especially well; these are exactly the types of ecosystems produced and preserved by frequent burning and those that vanish together with anthropogenic wildfire.

Not only does cascara grow in fire-prone environments, but it will also re-sprout from the root crown if the top is burnt in a low-intensity fire, an adaptation exhibited by many plants that grew in the sense of frequent fires.

CHAPTER 2:

NATIVE AMERICAN HERBS

When European colonists in the 16th century first came into contact with the inhabitants of the North American continent, they found indigenous people were quite different from what they had thought. They expected retrograde cultures, but they came across men and women of healthy and robust constitutions, caring about personal hygiene, and advanced in their holistic approach to disease prevention and treatment.

The epidemics that plagued and decimated the inhabitants of the Old Continent, (like smallpox, syphilis, and plague) were unknown to the native tribes. Minds free from prejudices would look with interest at these "strange" people, taking inspiration and adapting the Indian experiences to the European reality.

Unfortunately, history teaches us that the "evolved" whites had not landed in North America for a peaceful confrontation. But we should not go into the painful details of an invasion with tragic implications. I am most interested in bringing to light the far-sighted knowledge of the native Indians, who knew a lot about the therapeutic power of herbs, plants, infusions, and vital energy.

Specific men and women were entrusted with the usage of medicinal plants in Native American culture without sex discrinmination. In each different tribe, they played the delicate and respected role of healers. They were not sorcerers, as they were labeled with misconceived contempt by the European settlers, but simply people who often found the proper solution. Although sometimes the healers were also shamans, usually the two figures were represented by two different people.

The first contact with Indo-American medicine dates back to 1535 when the naval crew members led by the French explorer Jacques Cartier died of scurvy, a disease caused by a massive deficiency of vitamin C in the body and manifested in bleeding sores. Faced with the dramatic situation, the captain played the last card: he sent one of his sailors, sick but still with some strength, searching for unexpected help. After a few days, the man returned cured: the man was lucky to find a tribe of Native Americans who cured him with remedies based on pine and juniper, whose extracts of bark and leaves applied to the wounds. The sailor brought the cure to the ship, and the crew was saved. It was thus discovered, in a completely fortuitous way, that the Indians were aware of the therapeutic properties of many plant substances, which were used daily in the treatment of different symptoms. Let us see the main ones.

Native American Diet

Before resorting to herbs, the Indian healers were well aware that good health began at the table. Without bothering with Hippocrates, whose existence was unknown to them, they did not doubt that the first and most effective medicine was food. In the field of food, the Native Indians were quite advanced compared to the Europeans, and their daily diet consisted of a balanced mix of nutrients and healthy substances.

The combination of corn and beans provided a complete supply of proteins and carbohydrates. The abundant use of vegetables, oilseeds, and fresh fruit completed the picture; they added a little chili pepper and a lot of herbs and aromatic herbs to flavor their dishes and venison and animals that changed type according to latitudes. Nothing was wasted by using bones to make utensils for hunting and the home, tendons for hunting bows, and so on.

These healthy eating habits are now only a distant memory. The Indians living in the reserves have adopted a typically modern American lifestyle, and chronic diseases linked to progress, such as diabetes and heart disease, completely unknown at the time of life in the prairies, today represent 50% of the causes of death.

Many indigenous cultures attribute their survival to the bison. These imposing animals belonging to the family of bovids were a source of meat to be consumed fresh, smoked, dried, and provided the skins, bones, hooves, and entrails for various uses because nothing was wasted. The Indians had great respect for these animals that were hunted and killed exclusively for the survival of the tribe. Before the landing of the European settlers in the endless Indian prairies, there were over 25 million bison, while after a hundred years of useless massacres carried out by the whites, there were only a thousand of them.

Herbal Remedies

Herbs and other natural products were used to prepare a wide variety of remedies. These were gathered almost from the surrounding environment, and others were traded from distant areas if they were not available locally.

Native Americans recovered from many illnesses and injuries, which surprised the Europeans when they migrated to America 500 years ago because they had witnessed the same medical problems causing fatality in their countries. Indian herbal remedies were very effective. The only exemption was that they could not cure measles and smallpox, which they called the white man's diseases. These wiped away many natives, and much of the information was lost as the healers died with some of this knowledge. However, what remained has been extensively used by natives and non-natives, and many modern medicines are based on the plants, herbs, and ingredients the Indians used. Over 200 botanicals that Native Americans used have been listed in the US Pharmacopoeia, meaning pharmaceutical companies have used them to prepare modern-day medicines.

Efficacy Of Medical Herbs

Every scenario requiring Native American medicines is unique, and every person reacts differently to these herbs. However, there are certain key tips to follow to determine whether herbal therapy is a better choice than traditional medical treatment.

You should know that herbal medicine feeds the body on a cellular level. This produces strong adaptogens, which increase the body's capacity to cope with the changes that come with the surroundings and with life. Herbs also improve the immune system functions and work almost instantaneously for medical emergencies before reaching the hospital. For certain health conditions and auto-immune diseases like multiple sclerosis, cancer, and even AIDS, herbs keep the body healthy, encouraging proper functionality of organs, and giving you a chance to live life to the fullest even with these conditions.

You need to know that North American herbs and modern medicine work well together to improve the effects each one has on the body. However, we know that medical science on its own helps to restore and improve immune functions, which is why the combination of both factors is highly contemplated.

On the other hand, herbal medicine works to improve immune functions without upsetting the way you feel, and this is one of the reasons it is dubbed as one of the most stable ways to improve health. Numerous reports have surfaced on concerns about how good herbaceous plants are for health, with many herbs being blacklisted and termed as toxic. This is not because people are making use of herbs but because those making use of them are overdosing. Most of the herbal medicines found today are in capsules but found in higher doses than people would usually consume when taken in as herbs, which is why people consume more than they should.

Even with some of the most effective herbal medicines, negative results cannot be taken properly. Irrespective of how infrequent these cases of complications are with herbal remedies, one of the best things to do is make sure you take them in recommended quantities.

Used Plants By Native Americans

Below is a brief introduction to the most commonly used herbs by Native Americans. We'll see all the species in detail later in the next books.

Aloe vera.

American Indians used it to treat sunburn due to sun rays.

Hawthorn berries.

The natives used these berries not only as a heart tonic but also for managing various ailments, particularly in the female sphere.

Chapparal.

One of the favorite herbs of the Native Americans, it was used as an infusion for the treatment of infectious symptoms.

Echinacea.

According to the tradition of the American Indians, this plant was essential as an antidote for insect bites and children's ear infections.

Licorice.

This was widely used to flavor infusions and drinks, improving cases of persistent coughing.

Lobelia.

A plant similar to tobacco was valued among the American Indians, who believed it had magical properties and used it in spiritual rituals. It was successfully used to treat syphilis and gonorrhea, two diseases brought by European settlers.

Red elm.

It was a natural calming agent, appreciated by the Indians, who also used it to purify the body.

Polygala.

Called "squaw root," it was used to counteract snake venom and to manage problems related to the female cycle.

Dioscorea root.

American Indians used it at moderate dosages in children because it has a soothing effect on colic and in the elderly to relieve joint pain.

Oregon grape root.

It was one of the most popular herbs used by Native Americans to treat wounds and abrasions.

Valerian.

It was used to provide relief in cases of nerve symptoms and joint inflammation.

Herbs For Longevity

I've always been interested in living a healthy lifestyle as a happiness and wellness specialist. I have conducted a lot of research and talked to many specialists about how to live longer, better, and younger lives. One of the greatest and easiest things that I discovered is that to live longer, we all would need to use more herbs and spices. That's one of the main reasons which pushed me to write these pages. I discovered that you might bring additional seasons to your life by using herbs in your life.

Here below, I suggest the 5 herbs I have found to be effective in terms of longevity that you can simply use when preparing your meals.

Cloves

Cloves contain digestive system-supporting properties. They have also been utilized to promote a healthy immune and respiratory system due to their warming and digestion supporting qualities. The spice "cloves" is a lesser-known herb in the kitchen. However, this spice is prized in research laboratories for having the highest ORAC (Oxygen Radical Absorbance Capacity) score of any spice. What does this mean? Cloves have the most antioxidants. Cloves are also known for killing parasites, fungus, and bacteria in the intestine.

Ginger

Ginger is a shrub with yellowish-green blooms and leafy stalks. Ginger spice is obtained from the plant's roots. It is native to Asia's warmer regions, such as China, Japan, and India, but it is cultivated in South America and Africa. It is currently cultivated throughout the Middle East for medicinal and culinary purposes. Geraniol is a cancer-fighting compound found in the plant "ginger." in addition, ginger is an anti-inflammatory, making it good for your heart and avoiding blood clots. This herb is said to help strengthen the immune system and guard against atherosclerosis.

Oregano

Oregano is a purple-flowered plant with olive-green leaves. The leaves, both fresh and dried, are often used for cooking. Fresh oregano and oregano oil are great additions to any dish. On a per ounce basis, it contains four times the antioxidant activity of blueberries! A single tablespoon of fresh oregano has the same number of antioxidants as a medium-sized apple. Oregano oil also contains beta-caryophyllin, which helps to decrease inflammation.

Ginseng

This is a perennial plant that grows slowly. In certain areas, the plant is also known as Ginnsuu. The plant "ginseng" is said to have heart-protective properties. When you use it in your cooking, it increases blood flow, which helps to transport blood to the heart when oxygen levels are low. Additionally, ginseng's increased blood flow aids in the reduction of blood platelet stickiness, lowering your risk of blood clots.

Turmeric

Turmeric is a natural plant that is used as a spice in several dishes. It's an Indian plant also known as curcumin. According to research published in the American Journal of Cardiology, adding the spice turmeric extract to your meals reduces your risk of heart attack by 56%. Plus, according to a 2012 research published in the Nutrition Research journal, turmeric improves cardiovascular health as much as aerobic exercise! It has a "primary polyphenol" called "curcumin," which is crazy but real. Turmeric/curcumin is also said to protect the brain, reduce inflammation, and aid in cancer treatment.

CHAPTER 3:

HERBAL REMEDIES BENEFITS

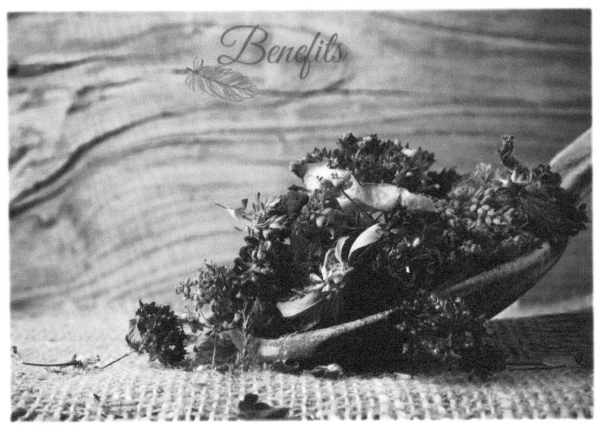

Herbal treatments are becoming very popular. More and more people choose to benefit from these natural remedies to treat their ailments and protect their health. The World Health Organization (WHO) approximates that about 80% of the entire world population includes herbal medicines as part of their health treatment.

Let's go through the best benefits when using herbal remedies.

Natural Medicines Are More Affordable

Modern medicine has been great for the overall health of humanity so far, but things are getting more expensive, and getting medical care is more complicated for numerous individuals than it is for others, and a lot of people cannot afford these things at this point.

Using herbs as natural remedies allows you to save money, which would be harder by using pharmaceutical medicines, given their typically high cost. Aside from being a more affordable solution for ailments, botanical remedies are also equally effective as drug-based medications.

Safer Treatment Than Drugs

Herbs and other natural remedies are safer treatments than drug-based medicines. Typically, herbal medicines do not carry side effects because of their natural composition. On the other hand, drugs include active chemicals that affect the body's systems; hence, the side effects. These side effects of pharmaceutical medicines often occur:

1. When you start taking the medication,
2. When we change the dosage, either to lower it or to strengthen,
3. Generally, when we stop taking medicines.

In contrast, the side effects of herbal treatments are normally attributable to the improper use of the medication.

Equal Results To Common Medicines

Apparently, herbal medicines may not be as potent as pharmaceutical medicines when comparing their dosage. For instance, a cup of willow bark tea (naturally containing aspirin and working as a pain reliever) is weaker than the standard dosage of pharmaceutical aspirin. However, rather than focusing on the dose comparison, focus on the side effects of these medicines. Why risk your general health with the typical side effects of pharmaceutical medicines? Keep in mind a general rule in medication: start taking your medicine with the lowest dosage possible.

More Efficacy For Chronic Conditions

Unless your medical condition requires immediate action or therapy, herbal remedies are usually more effective than drug-based medications. With chronic conditions, treatment may require a longer period involving repeated medication use. This could mean that the risks of side effects from pharmaceuticals are increased. Natural medicines, on the other hand, have no side effects or minimal side effects only. As mentioned earlier, the side effects typically occur only with improper use or dosage. Herbs contain natural chemicals that can sufficiently address chronic health conditions without the risk of side effects.

Available In Different Forms

Many people find it difficult to take any type of medicine, whether herbal or pharmaceutical, and many people who can't take it in one form will take it in another. Herbal medicines can be found in different herbal shops, pharmacies, and even on the internet, and this means you get your medicine close to you and in whatever form you prefer. We always advise that people should always make sure that they purchase their herbs from the right source.

Immune-Boosting Properties

Herbal medicine helps improve immune functions. It does not interfere with the body's psychological processes; rather, it supports the body and helps keep those processes going. Every aspect of the body is boosted to the point that it suddenly gets a lift and can function fully.

CHAPTER 4:

CURRENT NATIVE AMERICAN MEDICINE

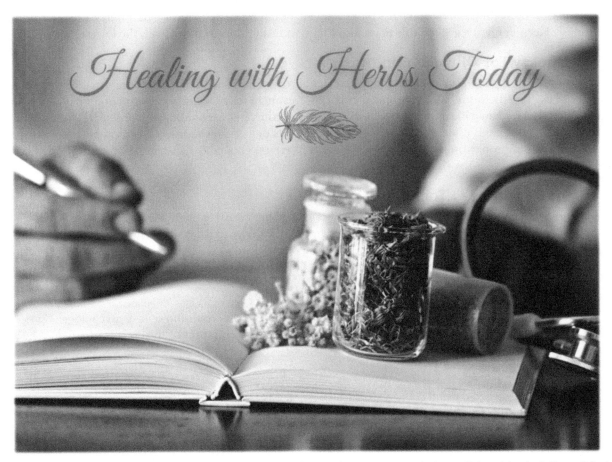

Healing with Herbs Today

Many research studies have shown that if Native American tribes return to their traditional herbal diet of fruits, wild games, and root vegetables, the adverse effects of various metabolic disorders can be reversed. But the difficulty is that different tribes have their own varying beliefs about diseases. For example, people of the Navajo tribe believe that diabetes is caused by disharmony and other influences like white people. The people of the northern Utes take diabetes as an entity taking possession of the people, compelling them to do evil things. In short, ancient native tribes in America believed illness was brought on by deviance from the traditional ways. However, it will be right to say that herbalism has been a staunch part of the medical world.

Herbal medicines are composed of active ingredients. Many of these active agents are still unknown. Still, herbal physicians believe that these active agents will be more effective as whole plants instead of using isolated versions of these active compounds. According to them, the effect of using the whole plant is greater than the sum of parts. However, critics of these herbal treatments argue that sometimes it becomes difficult to prescribe the measured dose of any specific ingredient while using herbal medicines. Herbal medicines play an important role in maintaining the natural balance of the human body. Different herbs have different effects on different body systems. Some herbs are found so commonly that they may be prescribed to cure casual diseases like cough, cold, or flu. However, there are some herbs available that require to be referred to very cautiously as their dose above the optimum quantity may cause adverse side effects. It shows that herbalism is a separate medical branch. One should be an expert on herbalism before prescribing any medicine to a patient, as the concept of taking herbal medicines completely safe is not right.

However, to emphasize the importance of herbal medicines, a few examples are quoted here. For example, the Echinacea herb stimulates the immune system, which is helpful in resisting various infections and treating ailments like fever, herpes, and boils. The Dong Quai herbs are used to cure premenstrual tensions, period pain, and symptoms of menopause. It also aids in the reduction of high blood pressure. Garlic is an abundantly used plant to deal with high cholesterol levels, thus protecting from heart diseases and is a very good antioxidant. It is also very beneficial to deal with several respiratory infections, colds, fever, and coughs. Ginger is useful for treating nausea and motion sickness. The Ginkgo biloba herb helps in maintaining the circulatory system of the body and treating tinnitus. Ginseng is used to treat fatigue, high blood pressure, and high cholesterol. Hypericum herb is a very good antidepressant. It is used by various pharmaceutical companies in their anti-depression pills. It is also very useful to deal with insomnia and anxiety.

But where herbal medicines have many benefits, some negative effects are also associated with their excessive use. One should not use any medicine without proper prescription and instruction by their physician. Always purchase medicines from the pharmacist with a good market reputation, and see the composition on the label wrap of herbal products. Be careful about the timings, dosage and consult your doctor if any irritating reaction is felt.

Traditional And Western Medicine

Today, the issue of either depending on conventional native healing practices or pursuing Western medical care is frequently confronted by Native Americans of both groups. The two cultures existed in tandem relatively until recently, with really no intersections between them. However, now, the continuum of health services can be accessed by Native Americans. Within tribal communities, most traditional healers are still practicing independently. To organize treatment for Native American patients, other healers can collaborate with Western-trained foremost care physicians. Some healthcare facilities, often at the same location, provide both conventional and Western medicine. In certain areas, patients of Native American descent receive conventional healing from the local tribal population rather than by tribal health centers or hospitals. In the Upper Plains Tribes of Lakota and Dakota, Mandan, Hidatsa, and Arikara, (MHA), a tribal member arranges for the services by directly calling nearby healers. Many Western-trained doctors often recommend patients to conventional healers and may sometimes assist a specific patient in coordinating traditional and Western medicine.

Why You Should Use Native American Medicine

There is a lot about Native American medicine that many people just don't know and certainly don't think about. Of course, Native American medicine may not be as popular as medical alternatives such as Chinese medicine, but these herbs are known to help as well. Of course, with Native American healing and medicine, it was more than just herbs, even if herbs made up a large part of what Native American medicine was.

Native Americans used leafy vegetables and mashed pumpkins or other materials as poultices. The poultice is placed on the wound or inflammation to relieve pain, increase blood circulation, and draw out pus as in case of abscess wounds.

Herbal medicine has been reintroduced in various ways in the form of alternative medicine. This includes aromatherapy, acupuncture, herbal treatment, and other forms of alternative medicine. Herbal treatment seeks to heal people of common illnesses and other health conditions using herbal remedies, which can be in the form of supplements, tea ingredients, oils, and powdered ingredients. There are clinical herbalists who supply Native American herbs that treat health conditions like arthritis, skin problems, asthma, broken bones, hormonal problems, and many other ailments. However, for the herbs to become effective, they have to be taken in the right dosage and combined as recommended. They should also be obtained from controlled sources that ensure quality.

Western medical treatments which use prescription drugs and medical procedures like surgery have been successful in treating various medical conditions. Unfortunately, the side effects are unpleasant. Some people turn to herbal remedies to relieve the side effects. Aromatherapy changes the individual's moods by smelling the scents. This enhances the body, mind, and spirit. Different materials are used, such as oils, leaves, flowers, and candles. The different scents have different effects on the individual. Take, for example, Lavender. It is known to relieve asthma, bronchitis, and other respiratory problems while also bringing peace and balance to the individual. Basil stimulates the brain. Some of the aromas used are very refreshing to the body, mind, and spirit.

Alternative medicine has awakened the Native American beliefs and practices by offering help in the form of natural remedies and is now aiming at restoring balance on the physical, mental, emotions, and spirituality as was intended in the American culture. Alternative medicine based on Native American medicine has become so popular that people are searching for it. People who have chronic ailments are looking for solutions to end their suffering, and Native American medicine is offering hope for these individuals where Western medicine has been unable to help them cope with the chronic ailments and the side effects caused by conservative treatments. Some people are even using these natural herbal remedies to prevent illnesses and diseases by becoming more proactive. American Natives and non-Natives are searching for ways to cure illnesses and diseases with fewer side-effects and less resistance and addiction with the hope of feeling better, and this lies in Native American medicine, making it gain popularity. Furthermore, some forms of conservative treatments like chemotherapy and radiotherapy are stressful and depressing to the patients and their families. Herbal remedies are not as stressful and depressing because they aim at creating a balance in the individual and harmonizing him or her with the people around him or her and with nature.

Native Americans believed that nature is the most important part of the universe, and we as humans are part of nature. That is why solutions should be sought from nature by restoring balance and harmony with nature. Native Americans believed that the reason why an individual or a community has illnesses and trauma is that there are disturbances in the balance with nature, which should be corrected. The Navajo use healing chants to repair the body, mind, and spirit. They believe that these chants attract a cure for illnesses. They aim at harmonizing the physical, mental, and spiritual to heal various illnesses and physical injuries caused by accidents and trauma.

Today, prescription drugs are expensive, and in fact, most of them are out of reach for many people who cannot afford them. The herbal remedies, which you can find in local food stores and herbal clinics, are known to be less expensive and less toxic than pharmaceutical products. Although alternative healing methods have not been tested as much as pharmaceutical products have, they have been effective in treating a range of health conditions from complicated diseases like arthritis, cancer, and tumors to common ailments like colds, coughs, headaches, sore throat, and fever. Native American Indians chewed specific plant roots to relieve colds, coughs, sore throats, and headaches, while teas were used for health problems like stomach aches and indigestion. These herbal remedies are still available, and you can prepare them at home for various ailments.

Some over-the-counter (OTC) and prescription drugs are based on natural ingredients, which are derived from Native American medicinal herbs. There is, therefore, some similarity in both approaches. Western medicine uses tested manufactured pharmaceutical products while the natives use herbs, which are in the form of food, teas, and poultices, which are extracted from leaves, roots, sap, fruits or berries, stems, flowers, and other parts of plants.

Some ingredients in modern drug products are the same as the ones used by the natives. The reason for this is that the medical profession depended and still depends to some extent on Native American natural products. Take, for example, Wild Cherry. This is a common ingredient that is found in cough syrups today. In fact, natives have contributed greatly towards health knowledge since many pharmaceutical drugs like aspirin, morphine, quinine, cough syrups, and others contain ingredients that are derived from nature, and many of these ingredients originated from Native American cultures, and these have made a break-through today.

Difference Between Native American Herbal Medicine And Mainstream Medicines

Native American herbalists love the earth, plants, and animals because they show us their plans. However, drugs are formed in laboratories by people who are not masters of nature. You have to be careful about trusting them because they are not our partners in life.

The holistic nature of Native American herbalism is an expression of interconnectedness with all things. It's based on the philosophy that all living things have a spirit or essence inside them; even stones and rocks have spirits or essences. We, humans, have an essence inside us which is called "Shen" or "Spirit"; these words can also mean energy or power. The world around us has Shen too, but it's different from ours, it's stronger. It's always there, so you don't really need to worry about what you are doing or who you are.

Native American herbalists do not use drugs because they believe they weaken the essence of a person or a plant. Drugs change a person's energy and not the spirit. When the mind is open, and will is relaxed, nothing stands in the way of your true power—your spirit. Native Americans used prayer instead of drugs to heal people because they believed that only God could help people with their Shen or Spirit as well as with their bodies.

Drinking alcohol makes it harder for people to enter into trance states where dreams, visions, and alternative healing happen because alcohol closes off channels in your body that can be used to enter into those states.

A person's essence or spirit can be damaged by a drug that has a toxic quality. Drugs interfere with a person's natural ability to change from one state of being to another. Most people have been taught that drugs are the only way to deal with their problems, but they do not really understand how drugs affect their Shen or Spirit. In ancient times tribes used herbs as medicine because they wanted people to come closer to their essence and spirit-not move further away from it. Dance medicines, music medicines, and drum medicines were used for healing. Even sacred plants were smoked in ceremonies not just for pleasure but also for healing purposes.

Mainstream Medicines are not really healing people. They are masking symptoms, so people think they are cured, but the real cause of the problem stays in them for a long time or even forever. For example, you have a headache, so you take some aspirin, but you don't know why it happens in the first place. Then you get another headache, so you take more aspirin and so on. You can get addicted to aspirin because it is a drug that covers up your problems but doesn't solve them.

Scientists don't seem to care what they do to us anymore. They are just reproducing new drugs that have the same effect on a person as the first ones. They probably think they are doing something useful for society, but actually, they are creating a new generation of drug addicts every year. Their only concern is money and fame.

Drugs have been developed to block pain, but actually, they block all feelings of being alive or well. Native Americans used herbs to remove pain-using them for ritualistic purposes was never seen as an indulgence or even as harmful; it was always considered to be very important because people needed to feel well in order for them to be able to carry out their responsibilities in life successfully.

CONCLUSION

Herbalism has been used to treat illnesses since ancient times and has always been a part of the medical world including mild fever, cold, cough, and flu to severe infections and allergies. Native Americans still believe in these traditional herbal tactics, but now most of the population incorporates modern medicines in their conventional health treatment mechanisms. Thus, their healing beliefs and health practices are diverting their attention. But it is a fact that herbal treatment has always successfully secured a very distinctive place in the medicinal world with astonishing outcomes. For this reason, the importance of herbalism is inevitable.

Modern medicines are based on individualistic and mechanistic approaches, which are very helpful in fast recovery from mild to chronic illness. Still, it is a general trend that people are more inclined towards herbal treatment, and the popularity of these natural remedies is increasing with each passing day. Because of the positive record of encouraging and the healthy benefits of herbal products, the general public trusts natural treatments more than chemically synthesized allopathic formulas. Since the past few decades, a lot of work has been done on herbalism. Several research studies and clinical trials have proved the positive and healthy impact of herbal remedies.

Herbal healing circles are now being integrated by the Native Americans into modern practices and are popular in community centers. The basic herbal treatment rules are the same; however, the discussion subjects have been changed to modern issues. A historian in California traveled to learn about the Native American tribes and composed a considerable account. According to him, although most Native American tribes have moved to urban areas still, they believe in their traditional healing system. They consider natural herbal remedies the best alternative to modern health treatment systems. They are very much concerned about their cultural heritage of herbal treatments and identity. But with the changing demands of time, health-related issues are also varying. For example, diabetes and other such chronic diseases were non-existent among Native Americans around 1000 years ago, but now such diseases are rapidly spreading. This rapidly increasing diabetes incidence may be due to the modern work schedule, less physical activity, and the consumption of highly processed food.

BOOK 2

NATIVE AMERICAN SPIRITUALITY

Healing Rituals andCeremonials: The Native American Paths to Healing Themselves

Citali Galwen

INTRODUCTION

The spirituality of the Native American tribes has been an integral part of their culture for centuries. For many Native Americans, religion was not a realm separated from daily life but rather played an active role.

Native American spirituality has been influenced by and borrows from many elements. Among these are Buddhism, Taoism, Shintoism, Christianity, Hinduism, and Islam. Influenced by these religions and the traditions and beliefs of its tribes and cultures, Native American spirituality includes many complex elements. Native Americans reflect this in their spiritual practices, including individual expressions; most revolve around participating in ceremonies or rituals to mark life passages or spiritual growth.

The spirituality of Native Americans is one that many people do not associate with the mainstream. They have unique traditions, beliefs, and spiritual practices that may be foreign to those outside their community. Given this connection to their cultures, it is not surprising that the Native American perspective on spirituality would be very personal. All of this and the associated identity can be found woven into their culture and religion.

The spirituality of the Native American tribes can be similar to Christian spirituality in that it has both beliefs and practices. In this, the Native American sees no separation between life and religion. They have a deep connection to their spiritual ways, influenced by their culture and their perspectives on life.

Connected within this is an essential concept of self-identity. Spirituality is reflected in everything from their art, music, and even social structures right down to how they act toward one another. Through this exciting mix of interconnectivity with their culture and the resulting identity, they can live with all things connected; spiritually, physically, mentally, emotionally, and intellectually.

The spiritual beliefs of Native Americans are based on traditions and the lore of their tribes. It is the basis for their faith in animism, the idea that everything is possessed of a spirit; thus, it becomes necessary to act to honor these spirits and avoid angering them. It can often be seen through rituals; such as the pow wow, sweat lodge, or purification ceremony, which are all ceremonies or rituals that Native Americans have adopted to help ensure good health, prosperity in living conditions and abundance for future generations to come.

Many Native Americans see their spirituality as a calling or how they can serve their community. As such, it is something that is both personal and communal; this results in everything from their art to their music being filled with Spirit. It has been noted that spirituality is found in all facets of Native American life. It allows people to live their lives believing and acting, following what they know to be correct according to the beliefs and traditions of their tribe. Because of this connection between spirituality and culture, life is lived with an entire focus on these beliefs, bringing them into every aspect of day-to-day living.

With this focus on everything being connected and how the spirituality of Native Americans arises from their culture, it is easy to see that there is a sizeable impacting factor between the two. It is especially true concerning identity. Thus, it is not surprising that spirituality remains one of the most defining aspects of Native American life today.

Many different views have been placed on spirituality over the past few centuries. Even though some have tried to change or even eliminate this belief system, it still influences earth-based traditions throughout the world today, particularly within Native American culture.

CHAPTER 5:

THE ROLE OF RELIGION AND SPIRITUALITY

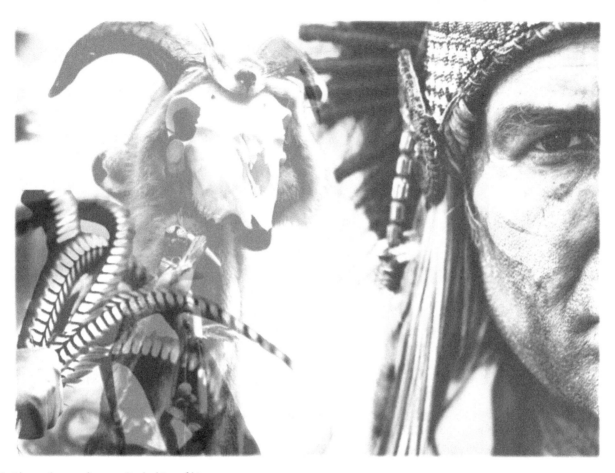

Native American Spirituality

Religious or spiritual beliefs differ widely from tribe to tribe, but certain key principles are universally shared, for example, there was a "Great Spirit" representing a great power, often called "Great Mystery" or Manitou, Wakan Tanka, Orenda, as well as in many other ways, who supported all creation.

It did not possess a personal character but every single aspect of all life existing in the universe, like the Judeo-Christian God, and could not be imagined to have a well-defined form since it had all of them because this universal "force" made everything in nature proceed according to balanced laws. Then there were the higher spirits belonging to everything that existed; that is, everything possessed a spirit that could be both good and bad in various ways: the earth that nourishes and sustains life has a particular spirit. It must be revered and respected properly because, without it, nothing can exist. All forms of life interact and depend on each other. Every individual is called to "walk in a sacred way," the sacred path to living in balance and harmony with the universe and the spirit world: people find their way, looking for signs through dreams and visions. The tribe's cultural ties and values were always passed down via just oral traditions and rituals. Thanks to this, they established a cultural connection with those who have lived before so that the tradition may be passed down to future generations.

Traditions often include sacred dances and songs, drumming for ceremonies and festivals, purification rites, fasting, and self-imposed physical tribulations. In all tribal traditions, some men or women are called in various ways but always perform various tasks for the sake of both the inner and outer good of society; they are called shamans. They look out for the spiritual growth and inner balance of the subject and the physical health of the person, helping to reconnect after periods of misfortune or particularly tough inwardly speaking. Humor is a sacred part of the culture of the American Indians because people always need to remember that we are all stupid. This leads the subject to resize the ego that can often lead a person off the sacred path of balance with the sacred mystery.

The Great Spirit energy

When the native peoples came in touch with the studies of the white people's religion, they realized, at least some of them, that there was a certain similarity between the Judeo-Christian God and the Great Mystery, only the latter was not a superior god who spoke to man but represented something more similar to the Chinese Tao, all-encompassing and permanent energy, not a jealous being morbidly attached to command like the one described in the Bible.

The words Wakan Tanka, for example, literally mean "Sacred" (Wakan) and "Buffalo" (Tanka) to identify the being who supported the life of the tribe after his death: when we talk about Wakan Tanka, we are more likely to talk about the sacred power of the universe rather than a personal god formed by human imagination. The Great Spirit cannot be seen or touched but is present in the cycles and the visible signs of nature. People can find evidence of its existence in the constant changing of the seasons, day and night, growth and death, in the movement of the Sun, Moon, and stars. Through oral tradition, people learned about the Great Spirit, or Great Mystery, tales of magical beings, and significant events. From an early age, children were taught to pay attention to the dreams they had because these dreams were messages from the Great Spirit, and they had to understand them not to disrespect the mystery that had created them. Tradition always taught that one lived close to the spirit world, which was all around them, a kind of parallel universe always at hand and with which one could communicate during dreams and where, later in the age of transition from adolescence to adulthood, they could look for the vision to understand what to do with their life. This practice was always preceded by fasting and prayer retreat mixed with the solitude that could last from 24 hours to several days, depending on the intent and age at which it was done.

In the tradition of the American Indians, there was also a sort of human prototype like Adam and Eve in the Christian-Jewish Bible. They called themselves (among the Navajo) Yakima the first man on earth and Ojiba the first woman. A key concept of Native American religion is the idea that everything in the world that can be seen or touched is alive and possesses a spirit or "breath." In many cultures, the Milky Way, that wide band with a weak light that can be seen at night in the sky, is the path of the departed souls, where everyone will go after their physical death.

The Louisiana Indian believed that the first men after they finished working on earth returned to heaven to become stars (doesn't it remind you of something? Maybe today you call it UFO), the Navajo thinks of the stars as friends because the stars help his tribe to tell the story and the legends, counting also the time and the seasons. According to the creation legends of the Pawnee tribes, their tribe would descend from the morning star (Venus?). According to legend, the Pawnees settled along the banks of rivers, while others in Nebraska, but in their stories, it is reported that the morning star has chosen suitable places for settlements, giving them names, then descended with his daughter from heaven who married the son of the Sun and the Moon (perhaps a term to recognize an earthling) and from this union was born the Pawnee people of today.

About the Great Spirit or Wakan Tanka, I also wanted to add something significant, at least for me, that I am interested in symbolism (a subject in which I specialized). Usually, this "energy" or "essence" is represented by the circle with the cross with three equal arms inside it exactly as it also appears in the sacred circle, only that they are often stated in the eight directions. Still, Wakan Tanka's sacred symbol is not the real symbol represented in sacred and mysterious ceremonies where white people cannot be admitted because only the members of the tribe can attend the original sacred rites (I'm not talking about those prepared for tourists). What follows is the generic symbol for the sacred Mystery.

Beliefs and spirituality

For centuries, Native American tribes' spirituality has been an integral part of their culture. For many Native Americans, religion was not a separate dimension from daily life but instead had an active role.

Native American spirituality has been influenced by and has borrowed from many elements. Among these are Buddhism, Taoism, Shintoism, Christianity, Hinduism, and Islam. Influenced by these religions and the traditions and beliefs of its tribes and cultures, Native American spirituality includes many complex elements. Native Americans reflect this in their spiritual practices, including individual expressions; most revolve around participating in ceremonies or rituals to mark life passages or spiritual growth. Examples of these include:

- The pow wow (a gathering where singers perform dances that tell a story),
- sweat lodge (a cleansing ritual based on American Indian traditions with participants purifying themselves through prayer),
- the purification ceremony (an initiation ceremony performed at puberty),
- vision quest.

All of these are only a few examples of traditions or rituals that Native Americans perform.

The spirituality of Native Americans is one that many people do not associate with the mainstream. They have unique traditions, beliefs, and spiritual practices that may be foreign to those outside their community. Given this connection to their cultures, it is not surprising that the Native American perspective on spirituality would be very personal. However, this does not make it any less critical. It affects everything from how they view life to what they believe and live in light of these beliefs. All of this and the associated identity can be found woven into their culture and religion.

Native Americans have a deep connection to their spiritual ways, influenced by their culture and their perspectives on life. An important concept of self-identity is intertwined with this. Spirituality is reflected in everything from their art, music, and even social structures right down to how they act toward one another. Through this exciting mix of interconnectivity with their culture and the resulting identity, they can live with all things connected; spiritually, physically, mentally, emotionally, and intellectually.

The spiritual beliefs of Native Americans are based on traditions and the lore of their tribes. It is the basis for their faith in animism. Animism is the idea that everything is possessed of a spirit; thus, it becomes necessary to act to honor these spirits and avoid angering them. It can often be seen through rituals; such as the powwow, sweat lodge, purification ceremony, vision quest, or the Ghost Dance, which are all ceremonies or rituals that Native Americans have adopted to help ensure good health, prosperity in living conditions, and abundance for future generations to come.

Many religions have influenced the spirituality of Native Americans as well as their beliefs. One such religion is Buddhism which differs from most other religions in that it emphasizes the concept of Nirvana. It can be seen in the Buddhist belief that through meditation, one can achieve Nirvana and transcend suffering, either through self-realization or by reaching enlightenment (the state of complete awareness). The Native American shaman utilizes the idea of a higher power, which corresponds to the Buddhist concept of a higher power; this higher power is believed to give them what they need for their personal spiritual growth, for example, healing abilities, visions, or psychic powers. The Native American shaman uses this in hopes of guiding his people to a better life. The spirituality of the Native Americans relies on a vast set of individual beliefs and a connection to the land. It is seen in many ways, from those that hold ceremonies or rituals, such as sweat lodges or vision quests, to those that seek guidance from their spirit guides.

While these are certain core beliefs, there are also many unique traditions and practices connected with each tribe. These may have evolved via cultural adaptation over time; others may be associated with that particular tribe's area's land and history. Many Native Americans see their spirituality as a calling or how they can serve their community. As such, it is both personal and communal. This results in everything from their art to their music being filled with spirit. It has been noted that spirituality is found in all facets of Native American life. It allows people to live their lives believing and acting, following what they know to be correct according to the beliefs and traditions of their tribe. Because of this connection between spirituality and culture, life is lived with an entire focus on these beliefs, bringing them into every aspect of day-to-day living.

With this focus on everything connected and how the spirituality of Native Americans arises from their culture, it is easy to see that there is a sizeable impacting factor between the two. It is especially true concerning identity. Native Americans' spiritual beliefs reflect everything they do, from how they live to what they eat and how they interact with others. Thus, it is not surprising that spirituality remains one of the most defining aspects of Native American life today. The spirituality that flows through every facet of Native American culture may be unique and complex, but it makes up an integral part of their being. With their core beliefs in animism, connection to the land is also found throughout their spirituality. Many Native Americans believe that there is a spiritual presence in everything, which shows in everything from their traditions to their everyday living.

The beliefs of Native Americans are also connected to the land that they live on. It is evident in their connection with the spirit of this land and in their traditional ways of living off of it. It includes things such as hunting, gathering, and farming. The entire way they live and interact with their environment is guided by a deep understanding of its spiritual value. Doing this makes it possible for Native Americans to live in the manner they feel is right. Many different views have been placed on spirituality over the past few centuries. Even though some have tried to change or even eliminate this belief system, it still influences earth-based traditions throughout the world today, particularly within Native American culture.

Healing And Spirituality

Native Americans focused mainly on natural curing techniques rather than relying on unnatural or manufactured healing procedures. Native Americans' healing practices showed their cultural evolution. These curing activities were odd in the European world, although these traditional curing methods had profound importance in Native American culture. Native Americans are always acclaimed for medicinal plant knowledge because they first observed the importance of plants or herbs in curing different diseases. However, they jumped to these conclusions when they observed that those ill animals which, when taken for grazing, consumed those plants started healing. In the same manner, they started testing numerous herbs to cure the sick among them. Those plants and herbs that proved effective were recommended for curing that specific disease. Therefore, numerous specific herbs were recommended for different diseases.

Native Americans' healing traditions were different, but different tribes selected herbs, roots, and curing knowledge. Almost 2000 plus tribes lived in North America, and almost every tribe had slightly different healing techniques and criteria. Native Americans believed that there was a strong connection between nature and human health and that it was essential to have emotional and physical well-being while maintaining harmony with nature.

Whereas in this contemporary world, where technological inventions have strengthened their roots, concepts of Native American healing techniques are not given much importance because sapiens have started relying upon knowledge and the use of different technological instruments. Nowadays, people have become more logical, so they like logical treatment rather than depending on unknown or baseless ancient healing techniques despite being quite helpful and effective.

The connection between disease and nature

As mentioned above, Native Americans always considered humans as a part of the physical aspect of nature. They have always considered that there is a strong connection between humans and natural elements such as oceans, rivers, deserts, plants, and weather conditions. They considered all of them as members of a single-family.

One of the well-known Native Americans, Robert Black Wolf, a psychotherapist, once wrote that we all share breath with everything visible. Likewise, another Native American Chief Settle, a renowned philosopher, said that a person had not weaved the web of life. Still, he is only a part of it, such that if he does anything harmful to the web, it would be equally beneficial or disadvantageous for him. Therefore, it was a widespread belief among Native Americans that any sickness brought to them was due to worsening human beings' relationship with nature. Illnesses caused by sources like dog bites or snake bites were obvious and easy to understand, whereas internal injuries caused by unknown means were quite hard to understand and cope with. For these uncertain internal illnesses caused by unknown reasons, some animals which might have been suffering through their actions were often affiliated with the angry spirits. According to their understanding, these invisible illnesses were caused by the ghost of the dead animal's vengeance for the suffering they endured at the hands of the sick community.

According to Native American traditional belief, human beings and nature are quite closely entwined. Therefore, any harm done to nature will ultimately have harmful repercussions for those who are involved in that unappreciated act. For example, if someone spits on the fire, it may displease the ghosts who will avenge this unlikeable act against them. Despite several harmful aspects of human beings' relationship with nature, there was an equal number of advantages. According to Native Americans' belief, only those people who were eligible to extract benefits from nature served nature and protected it. For those who continuously appease nature, great awards like herbs and animal organs could be of tremendous use because of their healing power. In addition to that, Native Americans used to arrange ceremonies where they called on even the spirits of dead animals to heal the subjected person. Likewise, different animals were thought to have different attributes like strength, intelligence, cunningness, hard work, and the like. Therefore, Native Americans call on the spirits of these animals to impart their attributes in favor of the one required to be healed. However, it is quite true that nowadays, people talk more about logic rather than any invisible or unrealistic thing. Still, I suppose today's doctors are unlikely to encourage calling the spirits of any animal like the fox, eagle, lion, horse, or any other animal. In that case, they still agree that there exists some connection between human beings and nature, and they still recommend keeping yourself at peace with the surrounding elements.

Notably, sunlight can also be considered a prime example to quote here in this context. On the one hand, sunlight can cause skin cancer, while on the other hand, if it is utilized properly, human beings can take numerous benefits from it (sunlight). If human beings exposed themselves to sunlight daily for 15 minutes, they would meet vitamin D requirements inside their body, which is essential for strengthening bones. In contrast, excess exposure to sunlight will cause sunburn. Likewise, we eat food that grows naturally on plants. Besides imparting our various tastes, these fruits help achieve a required balance of vitamins inside our bodies. However, it is recommended that these fruit items be consumed in excess to trigger harmful results. So, the statement counts here that excess of anything is dangerous.

The kindness of soul
Traditionally, Native Americans had an extreme love for the motherland, earth. They express their love through humility and humbleness in their relationship with nature. The standard of success and happiness among Indians was not about how rich they were or how much strength they owned. Instead, the standard of success and happiness was that those who gave away more money and donations were considered happier and more prosperous.

Kindness was deeply rooted in their traditions. For example, if Native Americans would celebrate anyone's birthday, instead of expecting any gifts from his guests and neighbors, he would give away gifts to his guests to honor his birthday and honor his guests attending the event for his sake.

According to Native Americans, a person is afflicted by any disease or illness only when he adopts immoral behavior called soul loss. According to them, soul loss is when a person loses his beliefs and depicts selfishness, cheating, evilness, disrespect, and dishonesty in his actions. As all these actions of that person go against nature, henceforth, nature will avenge all the displeasing actions inflicted on it by anyone. A person's health will deteriorate until their soul returns to his body; otherwise, it would lead to a catastrophe and even death.

Although all of these concepts seem bizarre to modern humans, there is some reality to these beliefs, evident from the number of events, research, and inventions about it. According to recent research by scientists, it has been revealed that those who hold grudges and whose minds are always overwhelmed by negative thoughts are more prone to mental and cardiac diseases. These aggressive-minded people undergo more heart attacks than those who always maintain a positive attitude and remain calm and serene. Medical scientists contend that those who undergo soul loss live unsatisfied lives, leading to a cellular breakdown. It is important to remain satisfied and humble and stay connected with our faith and nature to live a serene and healthy life.

Native American religion: the way of healing
Native Americans had a different religious culture from the Christian one that was based on a single god. The Europeans, when they first invaded their territories, called the Native Americans pagans; however, they found their supposition wrong with time. When Europeans came in close contact with Native American Traditions, they realized they did not believe in a single God but believed in the spirits of animals and plants.

In their traditions, the Native Americans propose gifts to these spirits and ask the spirits of these plants and animals to help heal those who were sick and those who were suffering at the hands of life or any other physical danger. Usually, they pray in the form of a ceremony while collectively dancing and enchanting songs in favor of these animals and plant spirits to appease them and, in some cases, to attribute them to their services towards their believers. Native American prayers were not brief, but they were quite long and more specific. In their prayers, even a single vowel had specific and different meanings.

Lewis Mehl-Madrona [1] reported the number of patients who got cured through Native American spiritual traditional belief, which he had witnessed personally. He saw a woman getting cured of cancer, a child suffering from gallbladder disease getting cured too, and likewise, a man getting cured of liver cirrhosis. All these cures were a

---

[1] The Coyote trilogy's author. His study examines healing methods from the Lakota, Cherokee, and Cree traditions, as well as how they connect with Western medicine (via a social constructionist model). Since the 1980s, Mehl-Madrona has been writing on the role of images and stories in healing. Mehl-Madrona has board certifications in psychiatry, geriatrics, and family medicine.

miracle. As a doctor, Mehl-Madrona tried to rationalize the healing techniques of Native American medicine. Still, he had always warned other people to refrain from adopting such a procedure for cure. He says that one must first develop a firm belief that he will get cured to get healed. It has been noted that whenever a healing ceremony for any patient is staged, every relative of a healing person was expected to be present in the ceremony because they thought that the more the members of the ceremony would be to pray for the healer, the more would be the strength of prayers and the relation between nature and men would get stronger, subsequently improving the rate of healing of Native American doctor. He said that all of us naturally possess the ability inside ourselves to heal.

CHAPTER 6:

NATIVE AMERICAN HEALERS

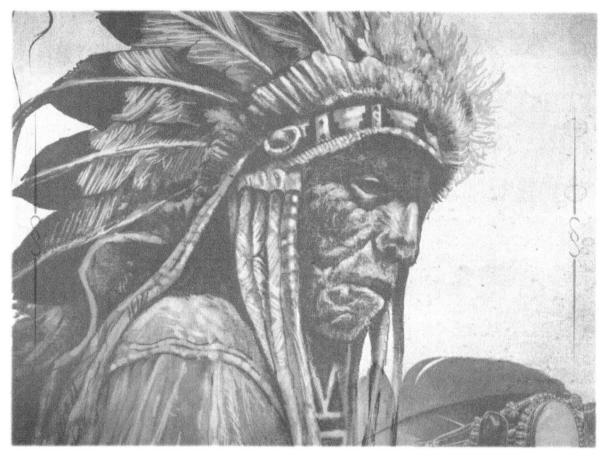

A Native healer can also be referred to as a traditional healer or a medicine man/woman. Each culture has its own vocabulary for the various roles in the healing process. Some terms used are: "shaman", "healer", "medicine-man/woman" and "spiritual leader".

Native healers incorporate ancient techniques, rituals and ingredients that have been handed down through generations of tribal knowledge into their own unique healing method. These traditional herbal techniques have been passed down from their ancestors in order to promote balance and good health.

Native healing embraces a holistic approach, recognizing that anatomy, physiology, behavior, environment and spiritual connections all influence health. Treatments are usually applied directly to the body, without surgical instruments or invasive procedures.

Native healing relies on the trust of patients who consider the medicine man/woman an extension of their family. It can be a complex process for people that is often more effective when it's approached with intention and understanding. Native healing encourages community cooperation in order to defeat illness or restore balance between the different elements in nature such as land, air, water, plants and animals as well as our own bodies. Native healing is a holistic view that prepares patients for an eventual return to their natural health.

Native healers are often traditional elders themselves, revered and well respected within their healing community. They have a keen eye for the body's energy and are proficient in the use of herbal medicine and natural materials to assist in diagnosing and treating illnesses or injuries. In order to be a Native healer you must have demonstrated mastery of ancient knowledge, practices, rituals and experiences that give you the unique ability to help others in your role as healer.

Amulets, jewelry, outfits, prayers and chants may all be involved in your healing practice. Although herbs, minerals and natural remedies may be used to assist in diagnosis, native healers often rely on their own intuition and innate wisdom to help them in the healing process. A Native healer can be a spiritual leader or even initiate new members into the tribal group. Often, native healers are revered within their local community for the spiritual gifts they have given to generations of their family or people in their tribe.

In some cultures, these positions are passed down from father to son or mother to daughter depending on the amount of influence received within that family or tribe. In others, men and women have equal roles as leaders. This is a role that can be passed down through families, from father to son or mother to daughter.

Native healing is an ancient set of practices that have been passed down through generations of tribal knowledge and wisdom. It has been used for thousands of years by tribal people throughout the world. It should not be seen as medicine in the sense that Western Medicine is practiced today.

In some native cultures it is referred to as "herbology" rather than medicine. The healer uses natural materials and plants native to their environment for diagnosis or treatment. Using herbs and natural remedies are the main methods used to treat illnesses or injuries. Native Healing relies on the intuition of healers and their inherent knowledge in herbalism, nutrition and body energetics.

Dream Catchers Among Native Americans

According to natives of America, the air gets filled by spirits, good and bad, which bring dreams to sleeping people with the fall of night. Specifically designed totems with a hook or circular shape, dreamcatcher, are hung everywhere by everyone. They believe that the center web of the dreamcatcher allows only dreams sent by good spirits to uplift the spirit of the sleeping man and hinders the path of bad dreams to reach the sleeping man, which disappears when morning light showers on it. The healers in the native community say that every person in this world has some passion, wishes, desire, whatever you call it, and some talk about them, some try their best to achieve them. However, some of the wishes also fall in the category of the person who doesn't talk; he even doesn't know about this desire because he might be afraid of even thinking about it and buries them deep in their unconscious. But these desires do find a way to come to the surface, and that path is a dream. Mostly what we dream is what we think or want. Thus, these dreams or desires need to be resolved because they result in anxiety and mental problems if left unaddressed. The common and easy method to solve the issue is to talk about it; people are motivated directly or indirectly to tell about their deepest desire and show ways to fulfill them if they are harmless or otherwise treat them accordingly.

CHAPTER 7:

NATIVE AMERICAN TRADITIONAL HEALING PRACTICE

Native American customs are varied and vibrant, reflecting the diversity of native tribal communities. The various villages did not all have the same expectations and needs, so it is very difficult to indicate common ways of doing things and believe that all peoples could use or carry on. We only need to look at how different customs are nowadays, even between small cities that are physically very close to each other.

The Treatment Approach

Native American medicine is a complete framework that balances every sphere of one's life, including lifestyle and social interactions with one inner world. Native medicine assumes that in the divine realm, the roots of every imbalance lie. In the course of every recovery procedure, spiritual approaches are vital. Including fees and rates, clinical approaches are often clearly and uniquely tailored for the patient. They require, as part of the healing method, the process of fee negotiation.

The Healing Elder is someone who is trained to use plants medicinally. A Healing Elder, or HE, specializes in the use of plants as healing agents for cleansing, strengthening, or bringing balance to the soul. Ancient healing traditions gave rise to the tradition of Alternative Medicine with its roots deeply rooted in nature's way of dealing with problems.

The Healing Elder seems to have the most healing strength, and the elder practitioner loses his prestige as a powerful healer when treatment fails. The person in need of healing makes a proposition to the doctor of medicine and waits to see if it is approved. Face-to-face, they rarely negotiate. The customer leaves the bid outside the healer's door, and if it remains there till the morning, it means that it has not been approved, and one can go somewhere else. Once they understand, therapy will, for example, start with a behavioral prescription, a pledge, a selfless act, genuine repentance, or scaling a holy mountain. Techniques include self-inquiry and discovery to ascertain whether there is a need for dietary improvement, prayer, herbs, massage, a sweat lodge ritual, or a vision quest.

Theories

The main objective is to alter the patient's comprehension of the world through a healthier self-concept, increased acceptance of others, and behavior adjustments. The healer's goal is not only to treat sickness but to change the patient's overall approach towards life and the world around him. Native American medicine combines science as well as spirit with the onset of new technology. They mostly use herbal interventions and pharmaceuticals. We can explain this by narrating a Native American story on the use of herbal medicine. Barb, a wife, mother, and lawyer, is still fighting breast cancer. She did what she could normally do, and cancer continued to spread despite all her efforts. She met with an Indian elder named Big Nose in a sweat lodge. He wanted to understand what she was doing or what hadn't changed in her life. Deep inside, as a mother-wife and lawyer, she thought she was a loser, and now she's healing herself. It was the pessimistic self-talk that needed to end, Big Nose told her. Barb decided to let go of her arrogant thought that she would be cured and started to enjoy the moment with her family due to this relationship. There is another story that talks of a woman who had had extreme arthritis. She was desperately looking for the right healer. To facilitate recovery, medicine men go further and beyond the current problem and understand radical improvement is often required. The shifts are primary, and herbs are secondary, along with massage and prayer. Right relationships, the correction of relationships with oneself, families, members of the society, and the spiritual environment are all effects of disruption of relationships and disease development.

Teaching

Native American healers teach their students through intensive apprenticeships. For preparation, several weeks of testing the purpose and dedication of a student are vital. An apprentice acquires knowledge and gains patience and respect. Native medicine is still an oral tradition. It cannot be taught in an academic setting. Students may learn the skills required only through experience, and only when the patient is ready does the older instructor encourage them to begin a medical practice.

Ceremonies, The Healing Process Scenario

The ceremony is an important part of traditional native healing. Because of the close relationship between physical and spiritual wellbeing, body and soul should heal together. Popular healing rituals encourage wellbeing by representing traditional concepts of the world, creator, and spirit. Prayer, drumming, chants, poems, legends, and the use of several religious artifacts may be a part of them. Wherever an ill person requires healing, healers perform ceremonies, and the ceremonies are sometimes performed only in sacred places. The special buildings are mostly referred to as Medicine Lodges for healing. Traditional healing rituals are considered holy wherever they occur and are only performed by the native healers and local spiritual facilitators. The Non-Natives can participate only by invitation. Native powwows, on the other hand, have grown today into social and cultural activities that include indigenous music, singing, drumming, regalia, and food. Most powwows welcome all persons.

The Medicine Wheel (Sacred Hoop)

"Medicine Wheel", has been used for health and healing by hundreds of different Native American tribes. It is also known as "Sacred Hoop". Together with Father Heaven, Spirit Tree, and Mother Earth, the Medicine Wheel represents the Four Paths, symbolizing the dimensions of well-being and life cycles. There are several shapes that Medicine Wheel could take. It could be an artwork, or an actual structure on the ground, such as an artifact or a painting. Hundreds of thousands, if not millions, of medicine wheels, have been built on tribal grounds throughout North America in recent decades. Movement is circular in the Medicine Wheel in the Native American formalities. It is typically in the direction of the clock or follows the sun's direction. It tends to sync with nature's powers, like gravity, the sun's rising and setting.

The Four Directions Sense

Various tribes have different views on the Medicine Wheel. Usually, each of the Four Directions (West, East, North, and South) is represented by a distinctive color, such as red, black, yellow, and white, representing human races for some. The Directions may also indicate:

- Stages of life: birth, youth, adulthood (or elder), and death
- Elements of nature: sun (or fire), water, earth, and air
- Animals: bear, eagle, buffalo, wolf, and many more
- Seasons of the year: winter, fall, spring, summer
- Aspects of life: spiritual, emotional, intellectual, physical
- Ceremonial plants: sweetgrass, tobacco, cedar, sage.

The Four Winds

As Native Americans are taught by their elders, there are four different winds that create the Earth.

These four winds are Good Winds, Bad Winds, Storm Winds, and Killing Winds. The Native Americans believe that Mother Earth has four hearts to balance the Four Winds.

These four hearts are the good heart of Mother Earth, the bad heart of Mother Earth, the heart of Mr. Wind, and the killing wind of Mr. Wind

Each is connected to a tribal group of Native American people by a sacred thread called "Bear's Stitch."

- The good heart of Mother Earth is connected to the "root people."
- The bad heart of Mother Earth is connected to the "rain people."
- Mr. Wind or Spirit Wind is connected to the "warriors."
- Killing wind of Mr. Wind or Spirit Wind is connected to the "witches."

These are often referred to as four races of Native Americans, but each one represents different aspects. Good Heart Root People are wise, Bad Heart Rain People are powerful, Warrior Winds are strong, and Witches are spiritual. All four must work together in order for balance in nature to take place.

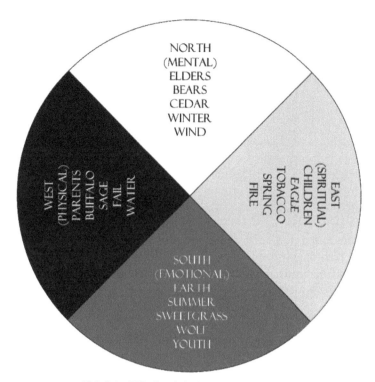

NORTH
(MENTAL)
ELDERS
BEARS
CEDAR
WINTER
WIND

EAST
(SPIRITUAL)
CHILDREN
EAGLE
TOBACCO
SPRING
FIRE

WEST
(PHYSICAL)
PARENTS
BUFFALO
SAGE
FALL
WATER

SOUTH
(EMOTIONAL)
EARTH
SUMMER
SWEETGRASS
WOLF
YOUTH

"Medicine Wheel and the four Sacred Directions"

CHAPTER 8:

NATIVE AMERICAN TRADITIONAL HEALING RITUALS AND CEREMONIES

Pow Wow

In the past, Pow-Wows referred to large gatherings of Native American communities - during which they celebrate significant events, festivals, or commemorate their history. The name of this ceremony is rooted in the Narragansett word "powwaw," which translates to either "spiritual leader" or "meeting." Nowadays, Pow-Wows often gather aboriginal people and non-Natives. They are often used to forge a connection and promote mutual acceptance. Through socializing in such an event, everyone can learn more about Native American culture. Tribes living in seclusion may organize their own specific Pow-Wow, in which only their community can participate. This only shows off their own traditions in dancing, singing, and drumming to the younger generations. Whether the gathering is smaller or all-inclusive, planning usually takes months. It often involves choreographed dancing, prayers, competitions, drumming, and featuring aboriginal crafts. The planning is done by the tribes themselves or any organization responsible for promoting Native American culture.

Music: Dance, Drum, Flute

Indigenous Native Americans first used sound therapy during their ceremonies. In their ceremonies, they used to beat drums, hand clap, sing and dance. The sound therapy spectrum is obtained by chanting (an activity used for healing long ago) and from the sounds of nature. Different sounds having different frequencies and properties are used for different kinds of healing because they differently control people's emotional and mental responses. Recent research results have shown that spine-tingling music also activates the area of the brain that is illuminated by drugs and food.

It is believed that everything vibrates at its natural frequency, and so do the human body parts. Therefore, whenever there is a disturbance in resonating frequency of the human body, it affects a person's health. There are different types of sound therapies to restore this natural frequency of body parts. Music therapy is counted as a kind of sound therapy. A person suffering from sadness or low energy is exposed to such music so that his energy level rises and he feels more comfortable than before.

In common sound wave therapy, any area of a human body suffering from pain is subjected to a sound wave of a specific frequency; this sound wave passes through that area, restoring its natural frequency and turning the body healthy again.

Let us consider the example of a church bell. It is pealed heavily for happy and joyful occasions like weddings, religious festivals and harvest festivals and it is tolled slowly to announce the death of a person.

The connection between health and sound was first noticed by an American researcher in 1986 when he observed that sounds could change the mood and improve the thought process of any human being.

Smudging

The smudging ritual is the most important of Native American rites. Smudging involves wafting a range of herbs and plants, including sage and wheatgrass, over the person, their possessions, holy and non-sacred places, and so on. Smudging is done differently by different Native Americans; some do it on a regular basis to remain healthy, while others only do it during big life events or when they are sick.

While Native American healers' motivations for smudging vary, one of the most frequent reasons, according to many sources, is to assist people to develop respect for one another and their surroundings, as well as to spend time in peaceful, constructive thought while performing this ancient ritual. Some of the same principles of reappraisal and reflection that mental healthcare experts suggest for better emotional control are offered in psychology. Native Americans have linked this to their cultural history in a manner that resonates strongly with the audience.

Smudging using a tightly wrapped bundle of herbs in a smudge-stick is a widespread technique that originated with the original Native Indian tribes of the First Nations, as well as many other tribes in North and South America.

Sacred herbs such as white sage or Palo Santo, as well as resins such as Copal, are often utilized. The herbs used to make smudge sticks vary depending on the herbs present at that time of the season, and what type of healing ceremony is there in which it will be sued.

Story-Telling

Traditionally, tribal elders tell powerful tales to the younger generations to teach them and to preserve their cultures. Each time a story is told, it breathes life into the culture and its people while imparting important teachings that bring wisdom and power to the new generation.

A good storyteller digests her experiences of the Earth walk, no matter how difficult they were at the time. From this 'digestion' comes understanding and deep soul healing, nourishment, and perspective. The more dangerous and treacherous the experience and achievement, the greater the wisdom and the story.

Through many shamanic adventures, the inner storyteller and Sage wisdom begin to emerge within the practitioner. These shamanic adventures are often misadventures, bringing challenges, sickness, and shamanic death — the spiritual death of the false personality and ego. The human self often struggles, complains, and finds herself in a limited, lower-level human experience as the ego does everything possible not to die. In this tempering process, the inner Sage shaman imbues the gift of tenacity to endure the difficult experiences. Ultimately, the practitioner emerges from the experience with the gift of wisdom and the ability to weave a wisdom story with many spiritual teachings to pass on to others.

Inipi/Sweat Lodge

For centuries, Native Americans have used sweat lodges and fasting as ways to benefit from the healing properties of detoxification. Of all the purification ceremonies in North America, the sweat lodge ceremony is the most widespread. The Lakota call the ceremony nagapie, and the Chippewa called the sweat bath ritual a Maddison. The Apache called the sweat lodge itself teach, while the Cheyenne also called it teach. Similar in action to a sauna, the sweat lodge's heat and moisture help detoxify the body—mentally, physically, and spiritually. The smoke in the lodge and the ceremonial rituals conducted there all contribute to the native healing process. Sweat lodges have several health benefits:

In the sweat lodge, healing for many physical or emotional disorders can begin. It is an opportunity to pray, speak, and ask for forgiveness from the Creator, as well as from other people who have been previously hurt.

The cleansing heat increases body temperature, thereby increasing the body's enzymatic activity. This increased activity helps the body destroy viruses and bacteria and stimulates immune function. The famous Greek physician Hippocrates once said, "Give me a fever and I can cure any disease." Increased temperatures help the body to burn away bacterial and viral agents and illnesses practically.

- Physically, sweating helps detoxify the body by opening clogged pores and eliminating internal toxins, heavy metals, excessive urea, and metabolic by-products.
- As the body's temperature rises, the endocrine glandular function is stimulated. This helps to cleanse the body and improve body function.
- The heat of the sweat lodge dilates the large blood vessels and capillaries which, in turn, stimulates increased blood flow to the skin and increases the rate at which the body's organs are flushed of toxins.
- The moist air of the sweat lodge improves lung function. Clogged respiratory passages are dilated, giving relief from minor respiratory problems and colds. Caution: Individuals with major respiratory problems and pneumonia should not use the sweat lodge.
- Hot water and steam created by pouring water over the rocks result in negative ion release. Positive ions are associated with tension, fatigue, allergies, rheumatism, arthritis, insomnia, and asthma.
- Sweat lodges can improve metabolic function. By removing toxins and other waste products and improving circulation, the digestion, absorption, and utilization of herbs and other nutrients can be improved.
- The sweat lodge can be a purifying and regenerative experience, much like a rebirth. In his book Sweat, Mikkel Aaland observes, "The warm, dark, and humid atmosphere in a sweat bath can easily be compared to the womb, or even Mother Earth's womb."

Sweat lodges can be many different sizes and shapes and are constructed using materials found in the local environment. For example, tribes of the Southwest built circular subterranean sweat lodges in which individuals descended a ladder to the underground structure, which was encased in bedrock. Other tribes used mud, wood, or animal skins to build sweat lodges. Cedar planks were used in the far Northwest; buffalo skins covered the Plains Indians' sweat lodges, while skins or birch bark might cover frames made from willow poles in the Northeast. In the Southeast, sweat lodges might be dug into a hillside or built up into earth mounds. The polar Inuit Indians even used igloos as sweat lodges.

The sweat lodge typically holds ten to fifteen people comfortably and is light-tight to ensure that they are in total darkness. Usually, hot rocks are heated on a fire and then brought into the sweat lodge. The ceremony leader then pours water onto the rocks to produce steam to encourage sweating and cleansing and to stimulate spiritual healing. Prayers are then recited, songs are sung, and the spirits are called into the lodge to purify the participants. The door is rarely opened throughout the ceremony, because the heat and dark are important to help the participants focus on what they are doing.

Pipe Ceremony

The pipe is an undeniably important sacred object for all the Native American tribes. It was used in many healing and sacred ceremonies; its presence enhanced the effect of the medicine and called to gather all the spirits of the earth.

The pipe, in all its parts, has a deep meaning: the bowl represents the female nature of life, the nurturing, the Mother Earth; the stem represents the male part, the Father Sky; the tube that connects stem and bowl, represents the connection between the visible and material world with the invisible and spiritual one.

As a complete object, it represents the thin line the man must walk to live in balance with nature. Once assembled, the pipe is the joining of all the aspects of life in one single object; it reconnects the multi-faced aspects of reality into a single entity.

The healer had the right to choose the herbs to be smoked during the ceremony (usually they were tobacco, uvaursi, sage, thyme, raspberry, and willow).

Before smoking, the healer offered small pinches of tobacco to the four directions, the plants and the animal kingdom, the sky, the earth, the mother, the sun, and the moon. With this, all the elements witnessed and were invited to the ceremony.

The one who carries the pipe is not its owner, but rather he is its keeper. He is the one who is entrusted by the whole tribe to be the intermediary with the Great Spirit, and due to this power is was taken into great consideration. Smoking was praying: each inspiration of smoke was a prayer to the Great Spirit and all its manifestation in the world.

The keeper and the pipe were deeply connected. The pipe spoke to him and created the connection between the material and the spiritual world. The more experienced the keeper, the stronger was this connection.

The Sacred Pipe Ceremony

The Sacred Pipe Ceremony is a moment of profound reconnection with the deepest nature that lies within ourselves. During the ceremony, we surpass our senses and achieve a deeper sense of meaning.

Although each tribe has its own specific rituals and peculiarities regarding the sacred pipe ceremony, the essence is very similar between all of them. Each part of the ceremony has a proper etiquette, motivated by an important, sacred meaning.

The first step of the ceremony is smudging: the bundle is lit and the participants (pipe keeper first) are smudged using a bird feather.

When all the people have been smudged, it is the turn of the parts that will be assembled to form the pipe: first the stem north to south and then west to east, then the bowl in the same way.

Smoke must penetrate all the cavities of the stem and the bowl to purify the pipe in each of its parts.

This part of the ceremony is very evocative and it gives you the possibility to concentrate on the healer and to calm your inner dialogue so you will be prepared for what comes next.

Once the smudging is completed, the bowl and stem are held up high, respectively in the left and in the right hand, and permission to smoke is requested to the Great Spirit.

Here the pipe keeper acts as an intermediary between the spiritual and the material world for the first time: he evokes the Spirit and attunes with it, looking for signs of the granted permission. It might be a light breeze rising up, or a rustling of leaves, or just the feeling that permission is granted by an experienced pipe carrier.

Granted permission, the healer joins the two parts of the pipe. As already stated, this is a very important and sacred moment because it represents the joining of all the parts of life and the reconciliation of all the dualisms. The entire universe becomes one single entity.

After the junction of the two parts, comes the filling part. The stem is laid down on the lap of the healer and the bowl on the ground.

The healer takes four pinches of the smoking mixture one at a time, he holds them up high and puts them inside the bowl with the right hand.

CHAPTER 9:

THE DANCES

A dance may look like a synchronized moving of arms and legs to rhythms and beats to some people. To Native Americans, however, dancing is so much more than meets the eye.

Sundance

The peoples of the plains primarily perform traditional Sun Dance ceremonies. There are many different versions of the sun dance ceremony, depending on the reason for the ceremony and the specific tribal belief system. The dance will usually last for 3–4 days, and it is normal for dancers to go without food or water as they commune with the Great Spirit. During the dance, the participants may receive visions. If it is part of healing, then the medicine man will perform rituals and healing on the dancers during the dance. Besides the dancing, there will also be singing, pipe ceremonies, drumming, praying, and fasting by participants and by the community during this time.

During the dance, each dancer makes a vow to their guardian spirit or the Great Spirit. The dancers are usually young men, fastened to a pole by a length of cord. They dance around the pole for the duration of the ceremony. Sometimes the participants will have their skin pierced during the ceremony, or will undergo other trials of physical endurance. Some of the participants will make a personal sacrifice on behalf of the community.

The Sun Dance is a community event, where friends and family members of the dancers will camp out near the site of the dance to pray and support the dancers.

The specific details of the ceremonies are very private and not shared with those who are not participating. Many Native American cultures, including the Lakota, wish to keep these ceremonies private and have formally asked the public to stay away from them unless specifically invited.

Other Dances:

- A stomp dance by the Chickasaw tribe is led by a ground leader holding a rattle or a shaker in his hand. As he moves toward the ceremonial fire, men and women with rattles on their ankles make a line and walk clockwise around the fire keeping the beat to the song. After the song, the leader says a prayer to the creator.
- The Ghost dance symbolizes the regeneration of the earth. It is an unstructured dance, but it allows dancers to receive closure after the death of a loved one.
- A grass dance mimics the swaying of the grass and often symbolizes victory over the enemy.

CHAPTER 10:

OTHER CEREMONIES

Painting The Body Of A Native American

The use of body paint had meanings and symbolism that depended on colors. For example, white was for peace, yellow was for death and red was for war. The use of ochre and other products of the natural environment were saved for special occasions to bring out the inner powers of a person.

Pipes Of Peace For Native Americans

When natives feel desperate to connect themselves with the spirits of another world, they arrange peace pipe smoking ceremonies to connect both worlds. They believe that the pipe and smoke coming out of it are a way of communicating with the spirits and connects the earth with the sky. They use tobacco and herbs to produce smoke because, according to them, they build a connection; their roots are underground, making a connection with the earth, and smoke produced by them goes up, connecting to the sky.

Totems And Animal Medicine In Native American Culture

Power animals are seen as bringing power to the Native Americans, which helps in their practice of shamanism. Frequently, these animals assist Native Americans in finding assistance from the spirit world, thus assisting in completing their life's journey. Some of the most common power animals seen are:

Raven

Ravens are symbols of awakening, and their presence is considered a sign that it is time for a shaman to take action and make progress on their life's journey.

Horse

The horse is an animal that is seen as powerful. That is why some Native American tribes considered the horse to be a gift from the gods, which are only given to people who need strength and healing in their lives.

Crow

Crows are generally seen as tricksters that bring messages which may not be obvious at first, but once they are discovered can help in the healing process and balance of power within an individual or a tribe.

Bear

While most bears are seen as aggressive, powerful creatures that are only present in the wild and cannot be found in captivity, certain tribes consider the bear symbols of healing and strength. The bear is also seen as a guide for shamans and their helpers regarding their life's journey.

Snake

Snakes are considered creatures that bring healing and strength, especially when they emerge from their dens on specific days of the year. Additionally, snakes are symbols of change and healing, so they are commonly seen among Native Americans in ceremonies and rituals.

Wolf

The wolf can be seen as a symbol of protection and strength while hunting for prey. This creature is also thought to be a great symbol for protecting the tribe from harm while leading them on their journey.

Spider

The spider is considered a symbol of power, strength, and wise counsel. A spider's web is seen as a symbol of energy that carries on through this life to the next.

Eagle

Eagles are considered to possess supreme powers by most Native American traditions because of their connection with the gods. This power is bestowed upon shamans to receive the information they need from the spirit world to find healing for their souls and journey forward.

Thunderbird

While this creature has many different forms, tribes that follow the religion of shamanism see thunderbirds as a symbol of power which allows their shamans to cross over into other dimensions and find wisdom in their life's journey.

Turtle

Turtles are considered a symbol of both protection and great wisdom. Because they do not move, they are seen as wise creatures who always move forward and are an example to others to follow.

Elk

While elks are strong creatures, they are also known to be gentle. This is why they are considered power animals for those who practice shamanism. The fact that elks also mate for life makes them important because this symbolizes a commitment to healing and reaching greatness in one's future.

These shamanic tools and power animals, along with the spirits and assistance from spirit helpers, help people on a life's journey to reach their full potential and heal their minds and bodies. Without these tools, many would not know what to do when faced with difficult choices or situations in life. For this reason, many consider shamanism a valuable part of their lives which helps them reach a high level of healing.

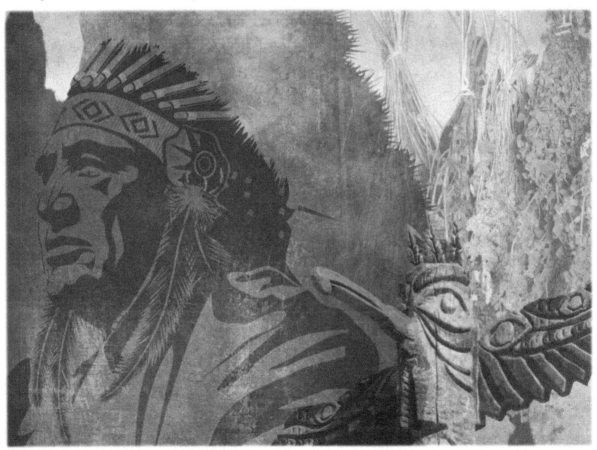

CONCLUSION

Native American herbalism has been a part of people's lives in North America for a long time. Native Americans have used various plant species for medicinal purposes to treat different health problems and illnesses. Herbalists use plants to heal and relieve some ills that might be too hard or expensive to cure with conventional medicine. Native Americans rely on herbs rather than pharmaceuticals because they are common worldwide; thus, the herbs are safer. In addition, most herbs are less expensive.

The use of herbs for medicinal purposes is an important part of the Native American culture. For centuries, herbal medicines have been used in Native American medicine. They use plants and other ingredients which are not harmful to their bodies as a source of medicine; thus, they do not need prescription drugs or other chemical medicines.

Native Americans often used to perform ceremonies and rituals that involved plants. They believed that plants would talk to them. In the tribal ceremonies, the medicine men would use some plant parts as a part of the rituals. They would use roots, berries, leaves, and bark as ingredients for the medicines. The medicine man would grind some of the ingredients to make a powder or a paste. The paste was then put into water and drank to treat health problems. Herbalists believe that plants are powerful and magical; thus, they should be handled with care. Before using the plants for medicinal purposes, Native Americans traditionally perform rituals that involve burning some sacred herbs while performing certain movements in the air. They pray to the spirits of the plants for healing.

Native Americans are very knowledgeable when it comes to herbal remedies. They have had their medicine system based on herbs and natural products from their surroundings, and they believe that these natural products are the best and safest to use because they are from their environment. Nothing from outside will harm them.

Native Americans are also very knowledgeable about how they use herbs and natural plants for medicinal purposes. They have been using herbs for a long time, and it is in their blood and daily lives.

The medicinal plants are put on the ground, and other ingredients are added. The whole mixture is then put into a basket for the sacrifice. They believe that following these rituals guarantees health and success in life.

I hope that this book has provided you with a better understanding of the Native American spirituality, rituals and ceremonies.

BOOK 3

HERBALISM ENCYCLOPEDIA VOL. 1

Learn About Native American Herbs and Their Beneficial Properties

Citali Galwen

INTRODUCTION

Native Americans possessed a variety of medicinal plants, minerals, and animal resources that they employed to cure a range of maladies known today as basic infections or the common cold. They utilized mud and plant poultices to treat wounds. They combined several roots and berries to create a pain-relieving tea for aches and pains. Indians also used the white pine tree bark's salicylic acid to cure fever of malaria, typhoid, pneumonia, diphtheria, rheumatism, or arthritis. The Indian's use of medicinal plants helped prevent many deaths due to bacterial infections during the 1800s.

Native Americans also used plants as medicine that is now used for other purposes. One of them is Tobacco, which was considered a sacred herb by many Native Americans and was an important ingredient in many ceremonies. With tobacco as a medicine, Indians slowly changed their minds about this mysterious plant that they previously rejected as an immoral substance. In 1722, the American government declared tobacco legal.

There are several legends regarding this remarkable plant: one about how an old abandoned warehouse was guarded at night by an old woman who used to smoke a pipe still exists today. The story about the Indian who found his piece of wood smoking was a legend that still exists today. Then there is the story about the man who was bitten on the leg by a rattlesnake, and his wife made it go away by smoking tobacco. Many of the Native Americans used to live in cabins made out of trees and used netting as windows, giving us a clearer idea of what the Indians were wearing at the time. With little money and no clothes to cover themselves from cold, diseases flourished. They wore reed clothing or made them out of deer hides and skins to protect themselves from these diseases. They used crude needles to make their clothes, and stitched them together with animal sinews.

Modern Native Americans continue to use medicinal plants for many ailments, and especially in some parts of North America, they still have many forms of native medicine in practice today.

CHAPTER 11:

THE TWELVE CATEGORIES OF HERBS

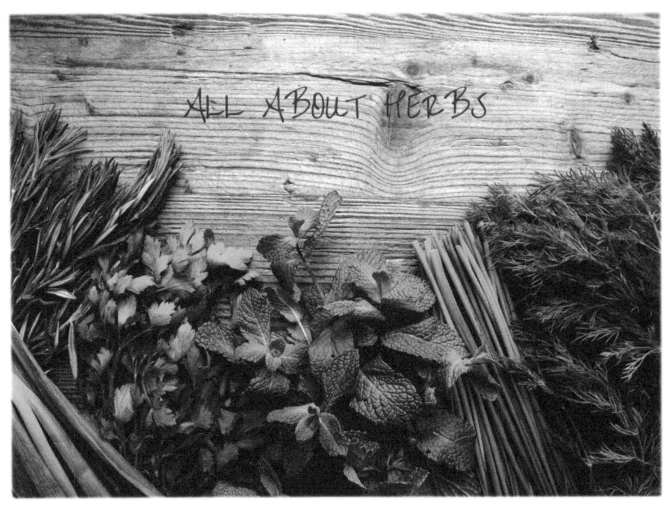

There are over three hundred different types of herbs in the world. Each kind has its own unique properties and healing benefits, and though these herbs all carry some positive power, they're are not all equal.

Here we'll explore the twelve different categories of herbs found in today's world.

1. Pungent Herbs

Pungent herbs are the most common. Pungent means "having a sharp, biting taste or smell." They're also generally hard to grow, though they produce flavorful and sometimes potent medicines. Pungent herbs include anise, caraway, cayenne, chili peppers, cloves, fennel, ginger, horseradish, lemongrass, and mustard.

2. Aromatic Herbs

Aromatic herbs like cloves, dill, mint, and rosemary are some of the most common herbs sold in stores. While not as potent as pungent herbs, they're still very tasty and fragrant. They're also easier to grow than other classes of herbs.

3. Simple Bitters

Unlike the other categories of herbs that can be used fresh or dried (though some cannot be used at all unless they're fresh), simple bitters are always used fresh and never dried out. These include plants like angelica, chicory, nasturtium, and wild bergamot.

4. Alkaloidal Bitters

Alkaloidal bitters, such as gentian root and gentian flowers, are used like simple bitters or even more frequently as tonics. They're also used in baking powder and baking soda.

5. Fragrant Herbs

Fragrant herbs include bay laurel, eucalyptus, and juniper berry. These are used fresh or dried in teas, medicines, and perfumes.

6. Acrid Herbs

Acrid herbs include basil, cayenne, and ginger. Acrid means "having an acrid taste." These are used in medicine to help with digestion or to soothe sore throats (usually eaten).

7. Astringent Herbs

Astringent herbs are used to treat problems with the skin or the mucous membrane. They include nettles, sage, and thyme.

8. Sour Herbs

Sour herbs include sorrel, wild strawberry, and yarrow, all of which can be used in teas or foods (especially salads).

9. Salty Herbs

Salty herbs help with nutrition (in small amounts) in soups and stews. They include dill weed, parsley, and sage.

10. Sweet Herbs

Sweet herbs like anise, caraway, coriander, and fennel are used to add flavor to dishes (especially meat dishes). They're also used for flavorings and seasoning. Along with being tasty, sweet herbs are generally beneficial for the stomach and belly.

11. Mucilant Herbs

Mucilant herbs include illicium verum (star anise) and peppermint, which is used as a mouthwash or to treat colds/flu symptoms.

12. Oily Herbs

Oily herbs include rosemary, thyme, and sage which are used in cooking, especially in Mediterranean cuisine. They're also used to treat sore throats and lung congestion (made into a tea). Many oil-related plants are bitter (like coffee leaves that have been roasted).

CHAPTER 12:

NATIVE AMERICAN HERBS

1) Elderberry

[Sambucus nigra]

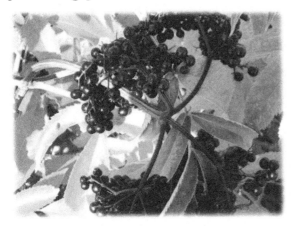

The elderberry is useful when added to the skin while treating wounds. Elderflower is used orally in many nations, including Germany, to combat respiratory illnesses such as colds and flu. Some evidence suggests that chemicals in elderflowers and elderberries may help reduce inflammation of mucous membranes, such as the sinuses, and help alleviate nasal congestion. Elderberries may have propensities to be anti-inflammatory, antiviral, and anticancer. Dosage is simple. Eat jam or wine made from elderberries only. But be mindful that the raw berries are slightly poisonous. They could have medication reactions with diuretics (water pills), diabetic medications, antibiotics, laxatives, theophylline, or immune suppressant medicines.

2) Anise

[Pimpinella anisum]

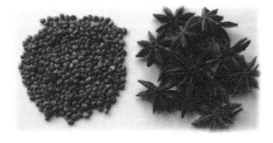

This flowering plant works out just great as an herbal antibiotic, killing most bacteria right on the spot. This herbal antibiotic also works on the urinary system, helping to clear up any incontinence that someone may be facing, and putting the whole body into a kind of detox, almost immediately. One of the best ways to administer this healing herb is to boil it into a nice and tasty tea. So, drink up, folks, because this Herbal Anise is on me!

3) Milk Thistle

[Silybum marianum]

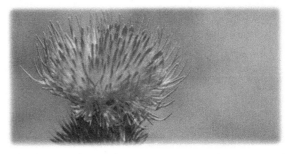

This plant is another great item to pack in your medicine chest. With its ability to reduce inflammation, this herb has been known to have some rather amazing results. Milk thistle serves to boost liver function and, in some instances, has even been seen to reverse the effects of cirrhosis. If you have any inflammation whatsoever, simply apply some Milk Thistle directly to the area afflicted, and you will see results.

4) Yarrow

[Achillea millefolium]

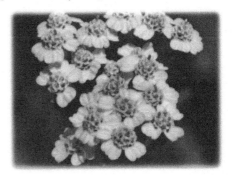

For hundreds of years, people have used yarrow as a medicine and with good reason. This herb can get to work on inflammation and congestion in the human body almost immediately. It is also a herbal antibiotic that works well against injuries, and as soon as it is applied to an injured site, it gets to work cleansing the injury and promoting the formation of blood platelets for quick and effective healing. This herb is a great antibiotic fighter, and its best work is done to reduce inflammation and boost the immune system. Just apply a small amount of this herbal antibiotic to the skin, and you will be able to enhance your body's ability to stand up to and survive all manner of airborne illnesses.

5) Red Clover

[Trifolium pretense]

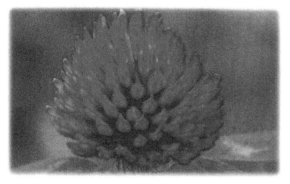

Red Clover is a powerful flowering plant antibiotic that can greatly boost the immune system. This herb has even been known to increase the red blood cell count in those that use it. Interestingly enough, Red Clover is also a natural anticoagulant and can loosen up blood clots in a rather rapid fashion. This, in turn, provides a general boost in health no matter what you may be facing.

6) Jewelweed

[Impatiens capensis]

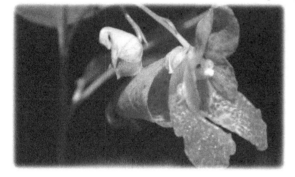

Jewelweed is well-recognized for its antipruritic properties in the treatment of poison ivy rash.
When you come in touch with poison ivy, oak, or sumac, find some jewelweed, smash the moist, purplish plant into a slimy paste, and wash it all over the affected skin. Wash the jewelweed mush away with clean water after 2 minutes of touching. If you manage to do this within 30 to 45 minutes of exposure to ivy, you will get minimal or no poison ivy response.

7) Chervil

[Anthriscus cerefolium]

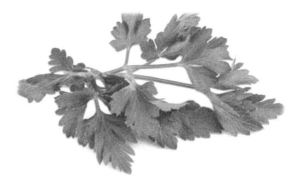

Chervil has a real proven ability when it comes to killing bacteria, getting rid of headaches, and calming upset stomachs.
It is common practice for many survivalists to simply pop a leaf of chervil into their mouth and chew it in order to relieve their upset stomach. I have tried this myself and can say that it really does wonders.

8) Cloves

[Syzygium aromaticum]

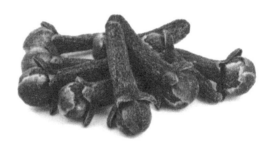

In a similar fashion to chervil, cloves have been placed directly into the mouth of many dental patients in order to kill bacteria and curb inflammatory agents. This herb also works as a mild form of pain reliever and can be used to successfully numb up a bad toothache if needed.

9) Sage

[Salvia apiana]

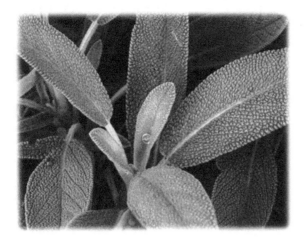

This medicinal herb takes survival medicine to a whole new level in the way that it can successfully reduce all manner of pain and kill bacterial infections on the spot. If you have fallen and sustained an injury, just a very small application of this healing herb will work to alleviate any pain that you may feel. Another great benefit of herbal sage is its ability to treat asthma.

10) Valerian
[Valerianaofficinalis]

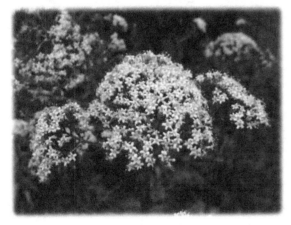

Valerian is a very popular nighttime home remedy to deal with anxiety. It contains some elements of mild tranquilizing properties that will almost guarantee you a good night's sleep, without the weird hangover feeling early in the morning that you may sometimes have to get with some other pharmaceuticals.

11) California Poppy
[Eschscholtzia californica]

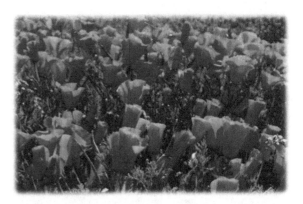

Eschscholtzia californica is a tension-relieving, anti-anxiety, sedative, and antispasmodic herb. California poppy also helps with sleeplessness and quells a headache as well as muscular spasm from stress. Some gentle and non-addictive actions are much safer for children and the elderly.

12) Lemon Balm
[Melissa officinalis]

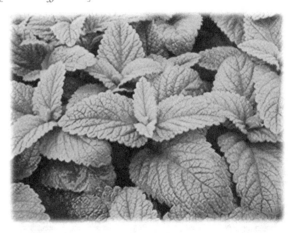

Lemon Balm, also known as "Melissa officinalis," is a herbal supplement and tea. Some studies suggest that the use of lemon balm can decrease insomnia, anxiety, hyper-excitation, and fatigue. A lemon balm extract of about 300mg should be taken at breakfast and 300mg at dinner which may help reduce insomnia mainly due to a decrease in nervousness and also to decreased agitation, guilt, hyper-excitation, and fatigue.

13) Rosemary
[Salvia Rosmarinus]

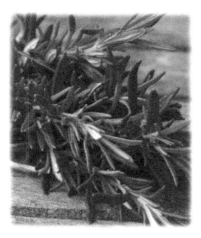

Rosemary is a Mediterranean shrub with fragrant, evergreen needle-like leaves and white, pink, purple, or blue flowers.

It helps treat headaches, nervous tension, a nervous stomach, cleanses the face, and can even help to stimulate hair growth. Great in teas, oils, and soaks.

14) Wild Lettuce

[Lactuca virosa]

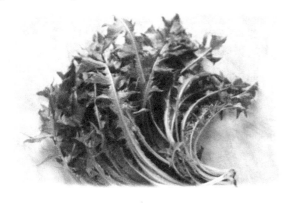

Wild Lettuce is a plant of the species of lactic vireos, which is a mild tranquilizer that may be used for calming a nervous or overactive nervous system. It is very suitable for anxious children and adolescents. It majorly helps with insomnia. It is also a general pain reliever and antispasmodic that can primarily be used for short coughs.

15) White Willow Bark

[Salicin]

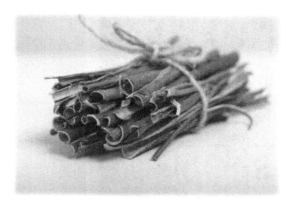

Salicin, a compound found in willow bark, is comparable to aspirin. Salicin is assumed to be responsible for the herb's pain-relieving and anti-inflammatory properties when combined with the herb's potent anti-inflammatory plant chemicals (called flavonoids).

White willow bark is completely safe for your stomach and can be used to get relief from muscle pains and menstrual cramps, arthritis, muscle pain, and knee pain. It is also good for reducing swellings.

16) Valerian Root

[Valeriana officinalis]

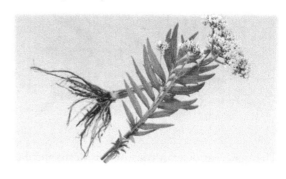

Valerian roots are used to make medicine for sleep disorders. The root is often used with a combination of hops and lemon balms. The valerian root can cause drowsiness and is ideal for those suffering from insomnia. If you are using sleeping pills, then you are advised to treat your insomnia with valerian root.

Women suffering from menstrual cramps and symptoms of menopause can use this herb for treatment. The extracts and oil of the valerian root can be used to flavor different food items and beverages.

17) Arnica

[Arnica montana]

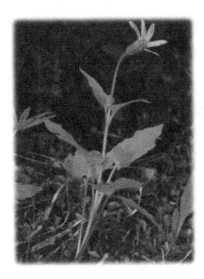

This is an excellent herbal rub that can be used to cure your pain, acute injuries, and pain after surgery, injury, and extreme sports. This herb is useful for its anti-inflammatory properties.

18) Ginseng

[Panax ginseng]

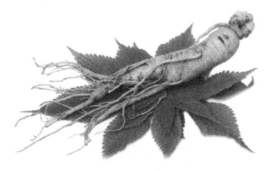

There are various varieties of this herb, and Panax ginseng is the most common variety. It is known as Korean ginseng. It has anti-cancer and anti-inflammatory properties.

19) Licorice Root

[Bupleurum falciparum]

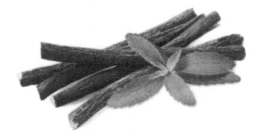

The Licorice roots are used to make medicine, flavor foods, beverages, and tobacco.

If you are experiencing digestive system problems, then you can use it because it is perfect for treating colic, stomach ulcers, and heartburn. It is also beneficial to use for constant gastritis, infections of bacteria, including a cough, bronchitis, and sore throat. It can be used with the combination of Panax ginseng to enhance its benefits.

It is also helpful for the production of essential hormones that enable your body to respond to stress.

20) Aloe Vera

[Aloe barbadensis miller]

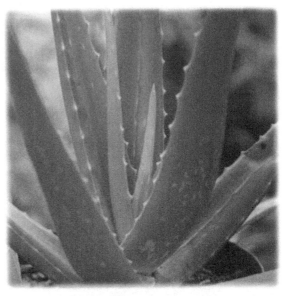

For centuries, people have used aloe vera because the gel of aloe vera is helpful in healing your skin and makes it soft. There are many benefits to the use of aloe Vera, such as it is beneficial to treat constipation and skin disorders. It can fight tumors and colorectal cancers. Aloe Vera is available in the form of supplements and gel. Aloe Vera is famous for its healing properties, and it is specifically used to treat sunburn and relieve pain. You can apply it to your aching joints to get rid of arthritis pain. The key symptoms of arthritis are inflammation and painful joints; you can use aloe vera to treat rheumatoid arthritis.

21) Calendula

[Calendula officinalis]

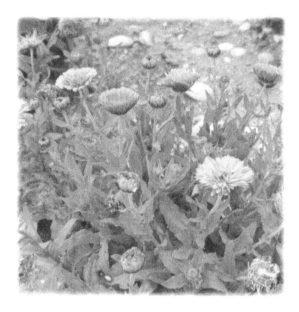

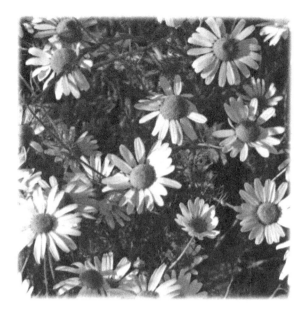

This lovely flower can be used as a vulnerable agent that is a substance to promote healing. The plant is famous for its anti-microbial and anti-inflammatory properties. It is good for topical use to heat abrasions, treat infections and infected mucous membranes. It is easy to buy calendula herbal medicines from food stores and to apply it to your wounds. If you want to treat internal infections, you can make a calendula tea with warm water (1 cup) and one tablespoon of calendula flowers (dried)

Chamomile was a traditional medicine used thousands of years ago to treat anxiety and upset stomach. The herb is used with a combination of other plants to get lots of health benefits. If you are suffering from heartburn, upset stomach, nausea, and queasiness, then you can use chamomile. It also proves helpful for sore mouth and cancer. If you have any skin irritation, chamomile can help you to heal your wounds.

23) Cayenne Pepper

[Capsicum annuum]

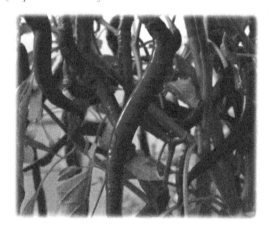

22) Chamomile

[Matricaria chamomilla]

Cayenne pepper is excellent to speed up the blood clotting process at the site of your injury or wound. Thanks to its antibacterial and antifungal properties, it can disinfect your wounds. With the use of cayenne pepper, the injury may stop bleeding in 10 to 12 seconds. You can mix one teaspoon cayenne pepper in 8 oz. water and give it to the afflicted person.

24) Marshmallow Root

[Althaea]

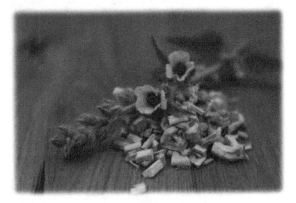

This root is similar to white cylinders and is famous for its sweet taste. The herb is found in the candy segment of the grocery store. The plant has excellent properties to heal wounds wreaked on your body, and it's also great for extracting bacteria and toxins from your injury. It can heal bruises and burns. You can create a poultice with marshmallows and apply it to your wounds for speed healing.

25) Passionflower

[Passiflora incarnate]

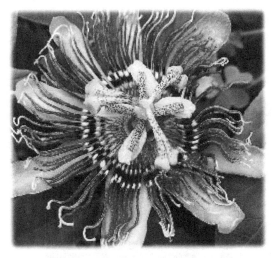

The southeastern United States, as well as Central and South America, are native to the passionflower. It has long been used to aid sleep by alleviating the effects of muscular spasms.

One study found that it can be as effective as benzodiazepine drugs, but the only difference is without the drowsiness. Passionflower may also help you to feel an emotionally balanced and exceptionally beneficial way.

Furthermore, if you suffer from exaggerated emotions, then this is by far one of the most efficient home remedies to deal with anxiety, and it needs to be part of your daily regimen.

26) Green Tea

[Camellia sinensis]

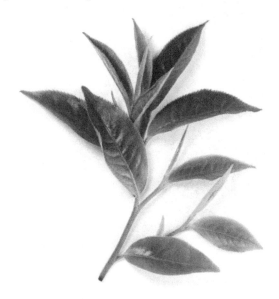

Green tea is obtained from the Camellia Sinensis plant by steaming, pan-frying, and drying plant leaves.

There are lots of health benefits of green tea. By drinking one to two cups of green tea on a regular basis, you will be able to reduce the risk of breast cancer as well as skin, lungs, and colon and bladder cancers. It plays a significant role in dealing with cardiovascular diseases. Green tea has a variety of beneficial components, including EGCG, a kind of plant-based molecule known as catechin. Much of EGCG's popularity stems from its powerful antioxidant capability and ability to alleviate stress and inflammation.

27) Cat's Claw

[Oxindole alkaloids]

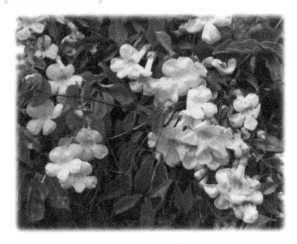

The Cat's Claw is a useful herb to treat stomach problems. It is famous for its exceptional properties to strengthen your body's immune system. It will enable your body to fight different infections. The oxindole alkaloids can enhance the capacity of the immune system to destroy pathogens. You can use this herb to treat painful and swollen joints, and eight weeks are enough to treat different health problems.

28) Astragalus Herbs

[Polysaccharides, saponins]

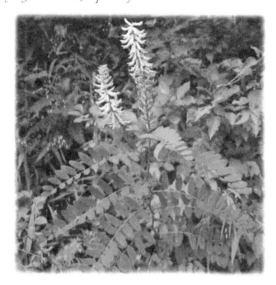

This is a Chinese herb used to stimulate the adrenal gland's immune system and digestion. It is a diuretic herb to help your body to fight against different infections. The herb has polysaccharides, saponins, and flavonoids contents. It can reduce the acidity of your stomach, increase your body's metabolic rate, and encourage the abolition of waste.

The herb can be combined with ginseng to increase the strength and natural defense of the body. The anti-inflammatory properties of the herbs are equally suitable for fever and other allergic reactions.

29) Turmeric

[Curcuma longa]

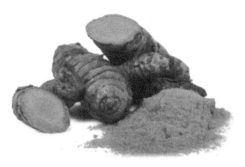

Turmeric contains curcumin that has distinguished antioxidant properties. It has anti-inflammatory, stomach-soothing, and antibacterial benefits. It is good to reduce tenderness by stimulating adrenal glands to amplify the hormone that is useful to reduce inflammation. Turmeric is good for protecting the liver and helps you solve digestive problems.

30) Parsley

[Petroselinum crispum]

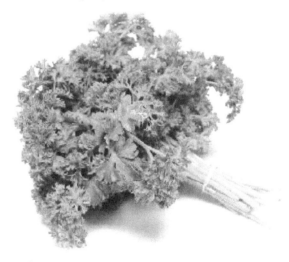

Parsley is mainly grown annually, but it will stay evergreen all winter long in milder climates. Some find parsley just a curly green food garnish, but it lets foods like stews produce a more natural taste. Parsley can help treat indigestions as an added benefit, and it's an excellent source of Vitamins A and C.

31) Mint

[Mentha]

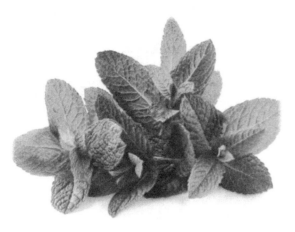

Mint types are numerous. They can be found in cocktails, foods, or simply in your glass of water for the season. It can freshen the air and help relax the stomach.

If you cultivate mint, note that it's an unwanted herb.

32) Dill
[Anethum graveolens]

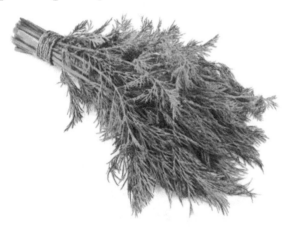

Dill assists in preventing poor breath and has the additional benefits of minimizing swelling and cramps. It's easy to grow dill. It will draw helpful insects like wasps and other aggressive insects to your yard, too. It also saves a trip to Santa Barbara Dentist!

33) Thyme
[Thymus vulgaris]

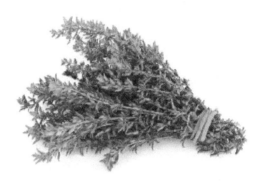

Thyme is a member of the mint family. It is a Mediterranean plant having culinary, medicinal, and decorative use.

Thyme flowers, leaves, and oil have traditionally been used to cure a variety of ailments and concerns such as diarrhea, stomach discomfort, arthritis, and a sore throat.

34) Fennel
[Foeniculum vulgare]

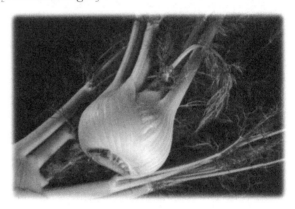

Fennel is found in the Mediterranean region and grows well in dry areas near the coast or on the canal's banks. It's used to treat various digestive issues, including heartburn, intestinal gas, bloating, lack of appetite, and newborn colic. The fennel's strongly aromatized leaves are similar in shape to dill. The bulb is perfect for creating healthy dishes that may be grilled, sautéed, or eaten raw.

35) French Tarragon
[Fines Herbes]

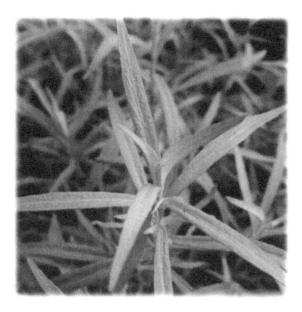

French Tarragon, with its anise taste, is a must-have culinary herb. It will transform an ordinary dish with its flavor into a work of art.

It was found how chewing on tarragon leaves may provide numbing effects, which may assist reduce teeth pain. This might be because tarragon contains eugenol, a natural anesthetic found in clove oil. Eugenol may aid in the battle against inflammation, which explains why it might be an effective pain reliever. Eugenol has antimicrobial effects as well.

36) Catnip
[Nepeta cataria]

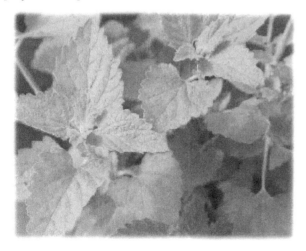

What's more enjoyable than seeing the family cat go somewhat berserk at the catnip smell? Yet catnip is more than merely a stimulant to felines. It contains antioxidants and volatile chemicals with therapeutic properties such as nepetalactone, thymol, and pinene. Catnip may assist in calming the body before going to bed and in encouraging sleep. Its soothing qualities are due to nepetalactone and nepetalactone acid molecules.

A Catnip tea may be used as a diuretic remedy. When you buy catnip outside, mind your cats as they love to crawl in and chew on it.

37) Chives
[Allium schoenoprasum]

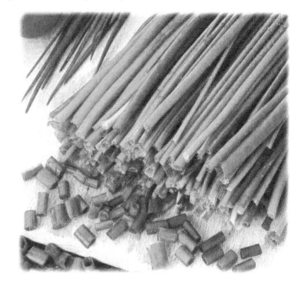

Chives belong to the Alliaceae family and are herbaceous perennial plants. They include elements that are beneficial to sleep and bone health. Some studies have also connected the compounds found in chives and other allium plants to anticancer properties.

Chives are also a healthy source of both beta-carotene and vitamin C.

38) St. John's Wort
[Hypericum perforatum]

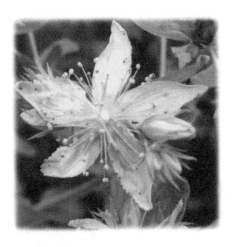

St. John's wort is thought to alleviate depression and anxiety symptoms but should not be considered a cure. It can help relieve muscle discomfort, too. The term "wort" is derived from the Old English word meaning "rose." This rose was called St John's wort as it blooms around 24th June, which is John the Baptist's birthday. It is a common groundcover in gardens, as it is resistant to drought.

It is a well-known herbal remedy for depression but is not used in cooking.

39) Bay Leaves

[Laurus nobilis]

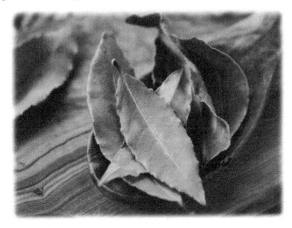

The fragrance of the noble leaves of the bay reminds you of balsam, clove, mint, and some even say, honey! It is best known for its use in heart-rending stews and other long-simmering dishes with a very salty, peppery, almost bitter flavor.

40) Winter Savory

[Satureja montana]

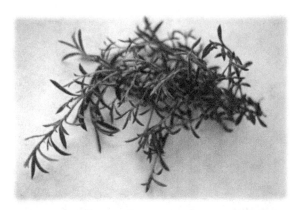

Winter savory is mostly used as a culinary herb, but it also has significant medical advantages, particularly for the digestive tract as a whole. The whole plant, particularly the flowering branches, has moderate antiseptic, fragrant, carminative, digestive, slightly expectorant, and stomachic properties. It is considered to be a sovereign medicine for colic and a cure for flatulence when taken internally, and it is also used to treat gastro-enteritis, cystitis, nausea, and diarrhea.

41) Peppermint

[Mentha piperita]

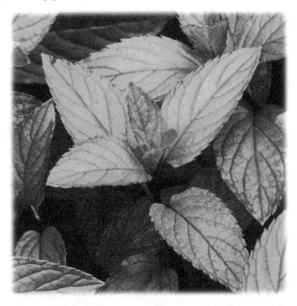

Like other mints, peppermint is famous for digestive help and air freshening. Peppermint enjoys expansive soil and part shade. It spreads quickly like other mints, so try planting it in containers.

Peppermint is also a healthy source of magnesium, potassium, and vitamin B. Peppermint oil may be used as a spice but is also effective as a natural pesticide.

42) Stevia

[Stevia rebaudiana]

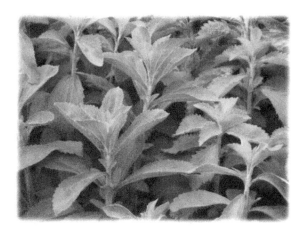

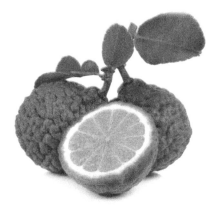

Stevia is an enticing plant in nature and a natural sweetener. The added benefit is that calories don't exist.

Stevia is part of the sunflower family, native to the Western hemisphere subtropical and tropical areas. Though it is a perennial plant, it can only thrive in milder North America. You can add stevia to your summer garden, anyway. Often known as Sweetleaf or sugar leaf, it is grown for its sweet berries. Stevia could be used as a sweetener to replace sugar.

43) Lemongrass

[Cymbopogon]

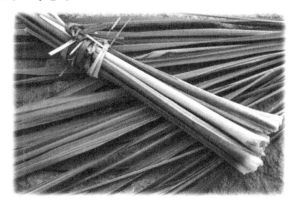

Lemongrass contains antibacterial and antifungal qualities, according to studies. It's been used for centuries as a pain reliever and fever reducer. Citral, a natural plant chemical with anti-inflammatory properties, is found in lemongrass.

Whether commercially prepared or made from fresh lemongrass stalks, Lemongrass tea is the best way to enjoy it.

44) Bergamot

[Bee Balm]

Bergamot has a long tradition of being used by many Native Americans as a healing herb, including the Blackfeet. Blackfeet Indians used this hardy herb in poultices to treat small injuries and bruises. A tea made from the plant could also be used to treat infections of the mouth and throat triggered by gingivitis, as the plant produces large amounts of a naturally occurring antiseptic, thymol, used in many brand name types of mouthwash.

45) Oregano

[Origanum vulgare]

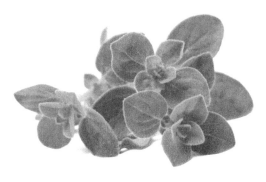

Oregano belongs to the mint family and is native to Eurasia and the Mediterranean warm climates. For thousands of years, people have used it to flavor foods and curative medical issues. Oregano comes in many varieties, and the most prevalent is oregano vulgare, commonly known as Spanish thyme and wild marjoram.

Oregano's anti-inflammatory, antioxidant, and immunity-boosting qualities are attributed to phytonutrients, particularly carvacrol. Some research suggests that the phytochemicals in oregano may aid ease coughs and muscular spasms, as well as combat infections. Oregano also includes a variety of minerals, vitamins, and other useful substances.

46) Comfrey

[Symphytum]

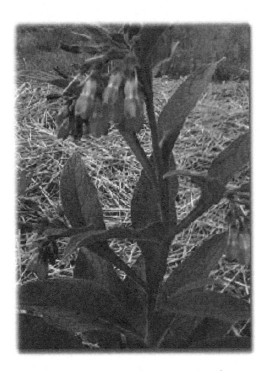

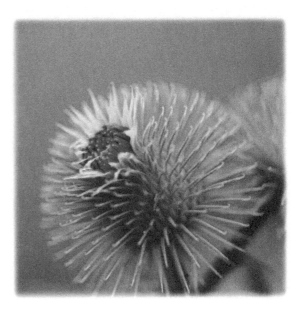

Cooked, mashed comfrey roots used as a topical remedy are good for inflammation, fractures, burns, and sprains. A new study suggests that eating it in abundance is toxic to the liver, don't eat it. Root formulations are dangerous for internal usage owing to differences in the pyrrolizidine alkaloid content because they are considered pyrrolizidine-free. While historically used comfrey root tea, the danger of its pyrrolizidine alkaloids is substantial. Therefore, arrangements for comfrey root and young leaf need not be made in-house.

47) Burdock

[Arctium]

The roots and leaves form an outstanding tonic for the liver and help purify the body and blood. Most people use burdock root to help them get rid of acne symptoms, and that has a really good impact on a variety of skin issues, such as eczema. Render the dried root tincture in alcohol and drink 10–20 drops of tincture a day. You may also consume the fresh leaves and roots upon boiling them in water and discarding the water to eliminate bitterness.

48) Dandelion

[Taraxacum]

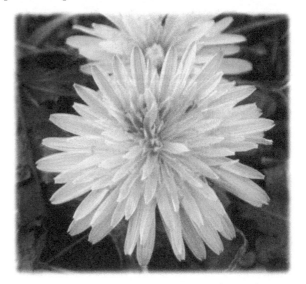

Dandelion has traditionally been used as a diuretic, increasing the volume of urine produced and eliminating fluid from the body. Place one teaspoon of the dried root in one cup of hot water as a general liver/gall bladder tonic and to promote digestion. A root-made tincture can be used three times a day.

One or two teaspoons of dried leaves may be applied as a moderate diuretic or appetite stimulant to one cup of boiling water and consumed as a decoction up to three times a day.

49) Black Walnut
[Juglans nigra]

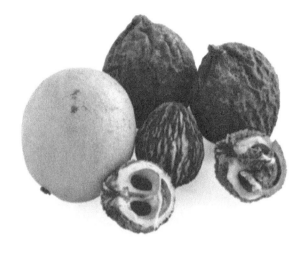

Black walnut is used to cure parasitic worm infections as well as a variety of other ailments such as diphtheria and syphilis. It's also used to treat leukemia.

Some individuals gargle with black walnut, apply it to their scalp as hair color, or apply it to their skin to cure wounds.

Black walnut has significant levels of tannins, which are compounds that help relieve pain and swelling as well as dry up bodily fluids like mucus.

50) Willow
[Salix babylonica]

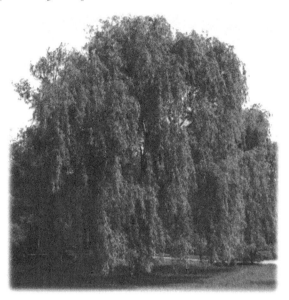

Weeping willow grows in all of North America. Though not local, it thrives in any moist environment, and its droopy twigs and branches can be recognized. Over millennia the leaves and the bark were used as medicine.

The bark of many other willow family types, including the black willow, has been in use since 400 B.C. for inflammation and pain management. Black willow bark, a precursor of aspirin, produces salicin. It was once normal for people to directly chew for pain and fever relief, on the rasped bark.

Willow bark has a similar effect to aspirin and is used to treat pain, such as headaches, muscular or joint discomfort, menstrual cramps, rheumatoid arthritis (RA), osteoarthritis, gout, and ankylosing spondylitis, a spine illness.

CONCLUSION

Native Americans used herbs to treat ailments. They also used them to alleviate many other problems in their lives, such as pain relief, toothaches, and childbirth. The use of herbs in the Native American way of life is an ancient practice that has existed for thousands of years.

Herbs have been used for food, medicine, and religious practices. Native Americans traded with one another to obtain the herbs that they required. They bartered with tribes that lived far away from their location to obtain the herbs they needed.

Herbs were used in teas, tonics, poultices, drinks, and infusions. Women would use the tea method to treat injuries after giving birth for bonding with their child by drinking it themselves. Poultices were used for drawing out infections of infected wounds. Tonics were made of different herbs to be drunk as a liquid that was very bitter tasting for better health benefits

Native Americans used herbs for many different reasons. For one, they used them as food or as beverages for drinking. They also used it as teas as well as poultices. Poultices were used to treat sores and to soothe burns. The Native Americans also used herbs for medicinal purposes.

Herbs have been an important part of Native American culture since the beginning of time. The Native American s learned early on how valuable they were and began using them for a number of different reasons.

Once discovered, herbs were quickly integrated into the Indian way of life. This is not only due to the fact that they were readily available but also because of their numerous uses and benefits within their community. In addition, there was a wide range of herbs that could be found, each with its own unique characteristics, which made them easy to integrate into daily life.

Native American medicine seeks to treat the whole individual and thus employs a holistic approach to healing and treatment. We know that health requires some kind of balance. These days we come across medical problems like some types of cancer, which defy all types of treatments. Yet, when natural remedies are taken, and the environment is taken care of, the water, the air we breathe, and the food we eat, all of these bring some kind of balance in every sphere of life, not just the physical

With this book on your shelf, you will always have the ancient wisdom of Native Americans at your fingertips. Remember to investigate every substance you take and don't delegate responsibility for your healing to anyone but experts.

BOOK 4

HERBALISM ENCYCLOPEDIA VOL. 2

Learn About Native American Herbs and Their Beneficial Properties

Citali Galwen

INTRODUCTION

Native American medicine was once a vital element of life in Northern America. It was essential for the people's health and capacity to fight off illnesses. Then came modern medicine, and people began to dismiss natural cures that had existed and been successful for a long time. Instead of -free and natural treatments provided by the earth, the desire to make huge profits from people's illnesses has now become the primary impetus behind our medical system.

In recent years, people are beginning to investigate if humans can benefit from the lifestyle of people who existed hundreds and even thousands of years ago. Based on research, these people had fewer medical problems than what we have today and could have good health with very few resources.

Did these Native American people know what we do not know now? Do they have the answers to some of the most dangerous health problems that we have today, including cancer, Ebola, and HIV/AIDS?

Despite all of our knowledge and technology, contemporary medicine has significant limits. If it didn't, we wouldn't be paying millions of dollars every year to cure illnesses and diseases that are significantly more common today than in the past.

Native Americans comprehended the interconnection of all life and that a person's well-being depended on the mind, body, and spirit working in harmony. Illness comes from an imbalance in any of the three. These ancient people discovered that certain plants could heal specific imbalances in the human body through their close connection to the natural world.

Through their collective learning, Native Americans catalogued over 500 different plants and their medicinal uses. This knowledge is even more impressive because it was all done through oral tradition, as their knowledge was not written down until modern times.

In this book, I would like to recall 50 of the best herbs that aided Native Americans in their healing practices.

CHAPTER 13:

TIPS FOR USING NATIVE AMERICAN HERBS SAFELY

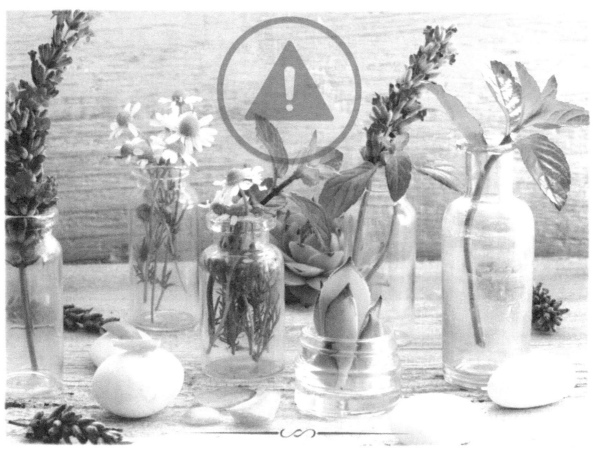

When reading a book on this subject, the first thing you should recognize is that these herbs may be quite harmful if taken wrongly. If they are not used appropriately, they may cause serious health problems, including death.

The manner in which these herbs are consumed is critical, and they should be done in ways that were natural to the people who used them. If you come across any of these ancient recipes, double-check the ingredients to ensure that they are safe. The majority of these plants have been researched for hundreds of years. And the vast majority of them are absolutely safe when used correctly.

Here are a few safety precautions to take while utilizing Native American herbs:

Do Not Use Any Toxic Herb

It may seem obvious to say, but it's never too much to remember.

There are many different types of plants that can be used as medicinal herbs in Native American culture. However, there are several that may be dangerous or deadly if taken incorrectly. If you don't know what it's for, it's better to avoid using it entirely.

Always Start With A Small Amount

If you are new to home remedies and Native American medicinal herbs, you may be tempted to use at least a few of them immediately. However, that is not the best thing to do because it will cause your body to shock and make you sick. Instead, just try out one herb for starters and then work your way up from there when you know your body has adjusted to it.

Take Your Medicine On Time

When practicing Native American herbal medicine, one of the essential things to remember is never to forget your proper doses. If you do, it will not have any of the desired therapeutic benefits. Instead, make sure that you set the alarm or use a watch not to miss it. Then try to repeat this process as often as possible until your condition has completely healed.

If you take these steps into account, many people have found that using Native American herbal remedies can help them overcome their illnesses and they start healing faster than ever before. So, if you have been looking for a natural cure for your ailments, then it may be time to look into this type of herbal medicine a little bit more.

Do Not Combine Too Many Different Herbs At Once

When utilizing any form of the medicinal plant, you should always begin with one and observe how it affects your body before adding other herbs. Not only is this safe, it will also help you to understand better how each herb affects your body and what your body needs the most at that particular time.

If Any Herbs Are Out Of Season, Do Not Use Them

Always use the herbs during the right time of year. Otherwise, they will become poisonous when they aren't in their correct season. Take this into account and only use the herbs that are currently available to you at the time of your request.

When First Starting With Native American Herbal Medicine, Don't Use Too Much Of A Single Plant

If you begin by using too much of a particular plant, you may experience nausea and vomiting. However, if you start with the right amount, it will help aid in the healing process; be aware of how much you are taking and make sure that you stick to a proper schedule.

Do Not Begin Utilizing Some Herbs Until You Have Been Properly Educated

Many herbs may be used for the same reasons but have varied consequences in the body; thus, not all of them will operate the same way for all of us, despite their similar purpose. For example, a few Native American herbs such as the Stinging Nettle can help with conditions such as diabetes or cancer. But if you have no education on these herbs, how do you know if it is the right herb for your particular condition? You may find you are using the wrong herb or might not even work for the intended purpose.

Use Herbal Medications Only If You Understand What The Plant Can Do And Its Function

Many plants serve a variety of functions in different cultures. In some cultures, they are used for healing, but are used for purifying or cleansing in others. If you know what they are used for in Native American culture, you can always use this information to your advantage.

But if you don't know and just pick up a random herb and decide to use it anyway, there could be consequences; you could either do more harm than good, or it could even become poisonous if used improperly.

If You Are Out Of Balance, Do Not Use Any Of The Herbs

To use any medicinal herbs properly, you must first be in a correct state of mind, which means that you must be strict with your diet and exercise regularly. This will ensure that your body is balanced and in the proper state to heal. It is best not to use any type of herb or plant until this has been done.

Do Not Utilize Any Wild Herbs Or Plants Unless You Are Certain They Are Edible And Only Edible

There are many different types of wild plants that can be used for medicinal purposes in Native American culture, but several can be poisonous. You must be positive that you do not use any of these items since they may negatively affect your health and wellbeing. However, if you know what the plant is used for, everything will be okay; just make sure to do your research before using any plant or herb from the wild.

Herbs Should Not Be Used For Any Ailment That Is Not Specified In Native American Culture

For example, if a particular plant was utilized for a specific purpose in Native American culture, you should stay with what works and does not hurt. But if it is used for other purposes that you may not be familiar with or have heard of before, then it could do more harm than good or even become poisonous. Try out the various herbs and see if they work for you.

If You Are Pregnant, Avoid Using Herbs

When pregnant, you should always see your doctor before using any herbs; just because they aren't classed as medication doesn't mean they won't hurt you. Many various herbs, such as parsley and willow branches, may be hazardous to your unborn child; therefore, if you are pregnant, you should see your doctor before trying any new medicinal herbs or supplements.

CHAPTER 14:

NATIVE AMERICAN HERBS

1) Alfalfa

[Medicago sativa]

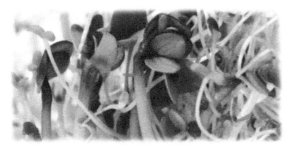

Alfalfa is a digestive cleanser, tonic, and nutritious food and medicine. Both studies and traditional medicine hold that Alfalfa can have healing effects that combat cancer and digestive ailments. Use Alfalfa by eating it as sprouts or leaves raw in meals, or use fresh leaves in a thick infusion every day.

Alfalfa is typically available as an over-the-counter supplement as well.

Alfalfa is a very cleansing digestive detoxifier to the gut. The research observed Alfalfa binding to carcinogens in the colon. European studies suggest regularconsumption of Alfalfa helps lower

cholesterol. Alfalfa leaves are a significant source of Vitamin K, Potassium, Iron, Zinc, and Protein, as well as Vitamins A, B1, B6, C, and E.

Never consume Alfalfa seeds, especially in high amounts daily, as they will lead to developing a blood clotting disorder.

2) Black Haw

[Viburnum prunifolium]

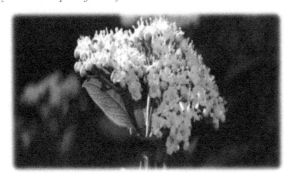

This beautiful bush—with bright red berries and cream-colored flowers—is a cornerstone in United States Southern herbalism. It was once used for all sorts of women's health issues by Native Americans, including childbirth, miscarriage, and labor. Now, it has settled into the comfortable role of allaying uterine cramps that accompany menstruation—but anyone, man or woman, can enjoy its ability to take away intestinal or stomach cramps as well.

A compound in the roots and stems called scopoletin works to soothe spasms in smooth muscles, whether found in the digestive tract or uterus. It also works on the smooth muscle in the trachea, making Black Haw beneficial for asthma symptoms and attacks.

Black Haw should not be used in women who are pregnant, nor in children under 16 or those with Aspirin allergies.

3) Chickweed

[Stellaria media]

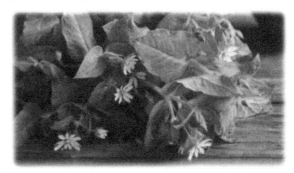

Native Americans used this herb for treating coughs, fevers, and intestinal upset. Chickweed also encourages a healthy digestive system.

4) Black Cohosh

[Actaea racemosa]

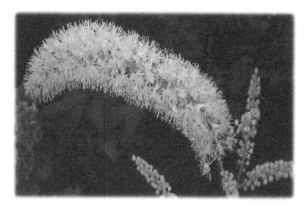

Nature's healing hormonal resource for women.

A native to North America, this stunning plant (once used for snakebites in Native herbalism) has become an important herbal medicine for women today. It contains compounds called "phytoestrogens," which mimic estrogen and fit perfectly in female hormone receptors.

Some herbalists say Black Cohosh is good for women with menstrual problems. It is more precisely relieving for women with low estrogen levels: especially women in menopause. It can provide a natural hormone replacement therapy but check with your physician.

Some menstrual issues are, in fact, due to low estrogen. If you have PCOS (Polycystic Ovarian Syndrome), adult acne issues, and/or irregular menses, consider getting your hormone levels checked and try Black Cohosh. Avoid Black Cohosh if you are pregnant, and make sure you are taking Black Cohosh, not Blue Cohosh, which can be dangerous. Avoid taking it if you have liver disease.

5) Boneset

[Eupatorium perfoliaturn]

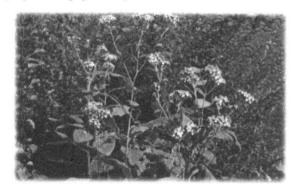

It might be hard not to think this plant has something to do with bones. But actually, its ancient old-time use was for alleviating colds, flu, and fevers so intensely that they literally made your bones hurt! Use the dried leaves of this tall plant in a hot tea or tincture, and take them daily for the duration of minor viral illnesses.

Before modern medicine, Boneset was used to fight dengue fever and cases of malaria that wouldn't respond to quinine bark—making it highly reputable to colds with fevers.

Studies claim that Boneset's effects on colds and flu are due to increased stimulation of white blood cells, which help fight off foreign infection. Do not use the plant fresh, in large amounts, or every day for the long term. It causes diarrhea, nausea, vomiting, and liver damage. It contains pyrrolizidine alkaloids, much like Comfrey, when used fresh or often.

6) Primrose (Evening) Oil

[Oenothera Biennis]

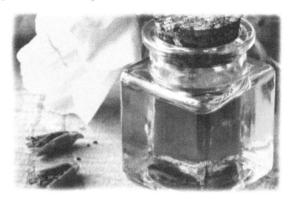

Evening Primrose oil is rich in Gamma-linolenic acid (GLA), which is an omega-6 fatty acid with anti-inflammatory and analgesic (pain-relieving) effects. Women have historically used evening primrose oil to alleviate hot flashes throughout menopause.

7) Evening Primrose

[Oenothera biennis]

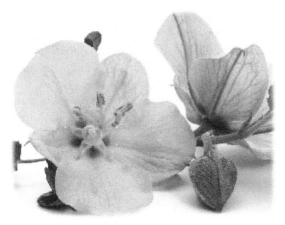

Evening Primrose is a great source for Omega-3 with inflammation soothing.

Because it blooms in the evening, Evening Primrose is given a unique, mysterious name. Its benefits are not so mysterious, though—high amounts of plant mucilage contain Omega-3 fatty acids, making it a target in the herbal world for dealing with inflammatory issues. Evening Primrose is active only in oil form—lookout for oil capsules or topical oils at natural food stores. If you are an advanced herbalist, try making your own sun-infused oil of the seed pods.

Evening Primrose oil (compared to a placebo) helps improve symptoms of inflamed joints in Rheumatoid Arthritis patients due to Omega-3 ability to modulate inflammation.

Like Omega-3 found in anything else, Evening Primrose helps lower cholesterol, blood pressure, and the risk for heart disease.

If experiencing discomforts, discontinue use. Avoid excessive use internally if pregnant.

8) Cinnamon

[Cinnamomum zeylonicum]

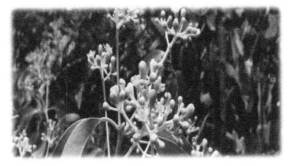

Sweet spice for sweet problems: diabetes and cholesterol.

Ironically, this spice commonly found with sweet foods happens to be excellent at blood sugar control. Cinnamon is the sweet, powdered inner bark residue from mighty evergreen trees native to India and China.

Cinnamon affects insulin receptors and helps create glycogen, a storable sugar. Daily use can perhaps help type 2 diabetics manage their blood sugar levels. Studies from both Japan and Canada revealed that Cinnamon also helps lower blood pressure and bad cholesterol in turn.

Cinnamon essential oils are available but should not be used internally. Supplements of Cinnamon are available, though it can, of course, be used in meals or in a tea or tincture at home. The cinnamon essential oil should not be applied to the skin since it might produce a burning rash.

9) Licorice

[Glycyrrhiza glabra]

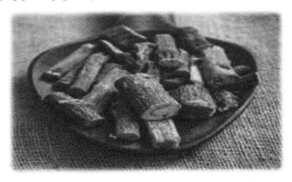

Licorice, also known as Sweetwood, Sweetroot, was widely used by the Blackfoot tribe to treat stomach ulcers. It can also help ease sore throats, heal intestinal ailments and reduce swelling in the body.

10) Eucalyptus

[Eucalyptus globulus]

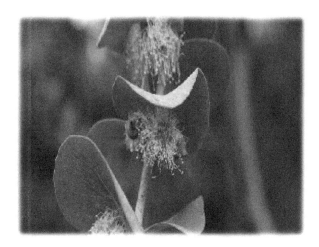

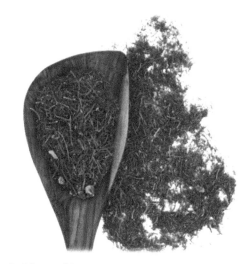

Eucalyptus has snuck its way into many over-the-counter cough medicines—maybe without us realizing we depend on plant healing already!

Oils in the leaves are antibacterial, antiviral, and anti-inflammatory, but the plant is especially best at opening up the lungs and assisting with coughs. Seek out Eucalyptus in essential oils and supplements. Dried leaves are available to make teas, tinctures, salves, and oils for healing as well.

A volatile oil in Eucalyptus, eucalyptol, acts as an "expectorant" and "bronchodilator." These actions help open up air passageways, stimulate productive cough, and produce a thinner mucus that can more easily be expelled.

Eucalyptol is also antibacterial and antiviral, helping kill off illness and infection while also relieving respiratory symptoms. This plant's natural oils are found in many cold-fighting lozenges, syrups, pills, and even chest rubs.

Do not ingest Eucalyptus essential oils for any reason. Diabetics should avoid use, as it might lower blood sugar. Do not use if you take certain medications. Check with your doctor.

Goldenseal is nature's magic, natural antibiotic, and digestive tonic.

Goldenseal's use originated among the Native Americans, who then introduced it to English settlers. Today, it has achieved study and reputation enough to be one of the most wildly popular herbs—though it does hold an endangered status.

Both traditional and

mainstream medicine considers Goldenseal an antibiotic and healer of numerous digestive issues.

Goldenseal's active alkaloid, berberine, has proven efficient at combating stomach or intestinal infections like Giardia, E. Coli, or H. pylori, bacteria that cause peptic ulcers.

Topically, berberine helps fight fungal infections and alleviate psoriasis.

Its powers also enter the arena of the cold-fighting world—Goldenseal's alkaloid also heightens immunity, which can help fight colds (though it cannot kill viruses).

Use the dried root to make a (very bitter) tea, tincture, ointment, or salve. Supplements are available—topical use can help with skin infections, internal for digestive ones.

Do not use if pregnant. Check with your doctor before using Goldenseal if you take prescription medications.

11) Goldenseal
[Hydrastis canadensis]

12) Motherwort
[Leonurus cardiac]

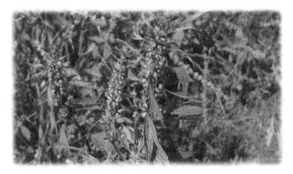

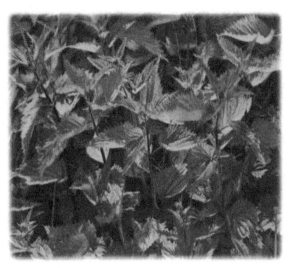

Motherwort is a heart-warming ally for cardiovascular health.

Some may plague Motherwort as a noxious weed with spiny, irritating burrs that attaches to your clothes. Little do they know: a preparation of leaves and flowers could be one of the most astounding natural heart tonics out there! Make and use your own homemade tea or tincture if you desire. Motherwort supplements are not uncommon either and are an option at natural food grocers.

A Chinese study observed Motherwort relaxing cells in the heart muscle. This then modulated blood pressure, strengthened heartbeat, and even showed the ability to regulate certain heart arrhythmias or palpitations.

The same heart effects have the ability to reduce anxiety, tension, and nervousness. People taking clotting medications or with clotting disorders should avoid this.

13) Sumac

[Urtica dioica]

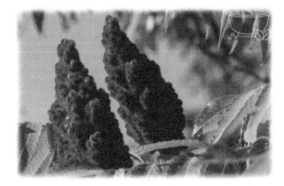

Sumac refers to any flowering plant in the Anacardiaceae family's Rhus, typically consisting of tiny shrubs and sumac trees that yield brilliant red drupes. Sumac has a plethora of advantageous properties. Indeed, sumac may significantly impact blood sugar regulation, heart health, illness prevention, and even pain alleviation.

14) Nettles

[Urtica dioica]

A stinging plant overlooked super food and inflammation healer. Did you know Stinging Nettles are more nutritious than any plants that might grow in your garden? That includes Kale, Spinach, and Lettuce. Think twice the next time you pull on gloves to remove them like a weed.

Keeping those non-flowering, seedless Nettle tops might make for an incredibly nutritious supplement or relief for allergies. Pick with gloves, hang, and dry for 1 hour to remove the sting. Use a tincture or supplement for allergy and urinary issues, or cook up greens from Nettle tops before they flower. Opt for a thick infusion of the leaves for nettles 'nutritional content, excellent for the anemic or undernourished.

Nettles are a significant source of Vitamins A, B6, and C, Antioxidants, Protein, Potassium, Magnesium, Manganese, Iron, and Phosphorus.

Nettles suppress histamine response—great for allergy relief. A noted diuretic can be cleansing for urinary health. Studies even demonstrate an ability to reduce prostate growth in men.

Avoid use if you are pregnant. Avoid long-term use as well with diuretic herbs—they deplete potassium stores and lead to electrolyte imbalance.

15) Oats

[Avena sativa]

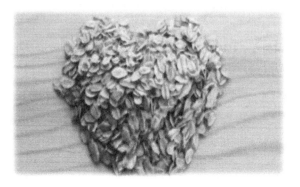

This cereal was used by various tribes to treat skin problems and promote healthy hair. The Cherokee used it in joint support for arthritis and gout. This was especially beneficial during winter and rainy seasons when skin infections were more common.

16) Prunella

[Prunella vulgaris]

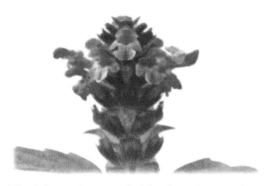

The Menominee used this plant for treating colds, coughs, sores, and diarrhea. It is also considered a diuretic and is used for the treatment of fevers in children. The sap from the whole plant is used to treat boils and ulcers. The crushed leaves are applied to wounds or sores for relief.

17) Lily-Of-The-Valley

[Convallaria majalis]

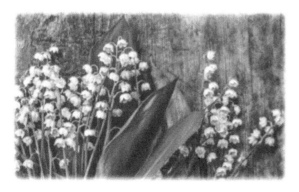

This herb was popular with the Menominee for treating earaches, coughs, and infections. The Menominee also used it as an antispasmodic and tonic.

18) Blueberry

[Vaccinium corymbosum]

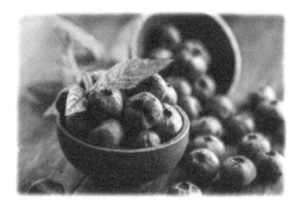

The Cherokee used this herb to relieve a disturbed stomach. For treating diarrhea and calming sore tissues and joints, they used blackberry tea. Blackberry root combined with honey or maple syrup will produce an all-natural cough syrup to cure sore throats. They chewed the leaves to soothe bleeding gums. Often, this plant is ideal for improving the whole immune system.

19) Hawthorn

[Crataegus monogyna]

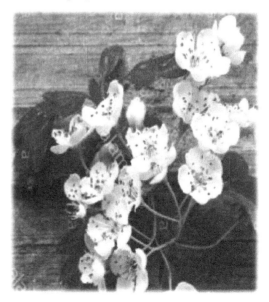

73

This shrub/tree can be found from the mountains of the Mohegan to the soggy shores of Lake Superior. Hawthorn is most widely used to treat heart and blood vessel disorders. It may assist increase the volume of blood pushed out of the heart during contractions, enlarge blood vessels, and enhance nerve signal transmission.

It was also used to make brooms, baskets, and hats. The Mohegans used hawthorn for stunning fish as well as making arrowheads for hunting purposes. They also used it to treat sore muscles and burns and as a tonic for upset stomachs and colds.

20) Black Gum

[Eucalyptus aggregate]

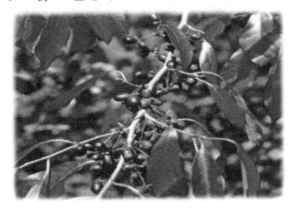

Officially known as Nyssa Sylvatica, from southern Ontario and New England to central Florida and eastern Texas, the tree is native to eastern North America. It is also frequently referred to as Black Tupelo, Pepperidge, or either Gum or Tupelo. Native Americans have used its fruit, bark, and roots as a bath, as well as in decoctions to trigger vomiting, remove worms in children and cure eye problems. Cherokee healers used a gentle tea made from small bits of bark and twigs to ease chest pressure.

21) Black Gum Bark

[Nyssa sylvatica]

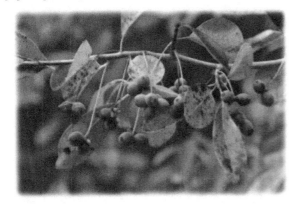

Cherokee used black gum bark for making a mild tea from the twigs for alleviating chest pains

22) Goldenrod (Solidago)

[Solidago canadensis]

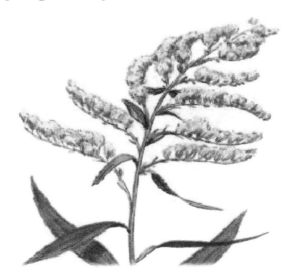

This herb is still an important part of the traditional Cherokee diet and is now known to be excellent for treating skin problems.

23) Hummingbird Blossom

[Buck Brush]

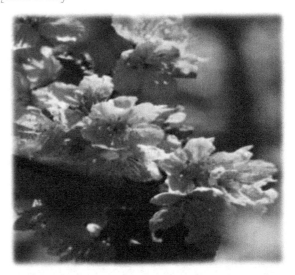

Native Americans used this herb to cure mouth and throat problems, cysts, inflammation, and fibroid tumors. To make the most of it in terms of healing burns, sores, and cuts, it can be turned into a poultice. The roots of this herb stimulate kidney function.

This unique plant was used as a substitute for black tea by the early colonists. The latest findings have shown that hummingbird blossoms effectively treat elevated blood pressure and blockages of the lymph system.

24) Rose

[Rosa]

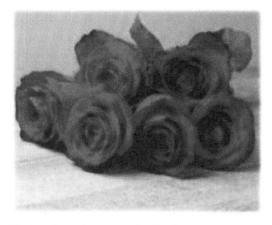

Native Americans used this flower as a preventive measure and a treatment for the moderate common cold. Rose tea is a gentle diuretic for the bladder and kidneys. For a sore throat, they used a petals infusion.

25) Saw Palmetto

[Serenoa repens]

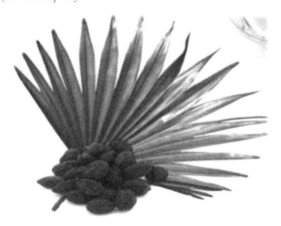

The plant was used for food by Florida's tribes, such as the Seminoles, but healers used it as a natural cure for abdominal pain. It also encourages digestion, lowers inflammation, and promotes appetite.

26) Echinacea

[Echinacea]

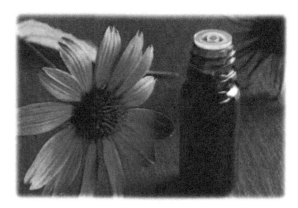

Its popular name is Purple coneflower. Echinacea is one of the most commonly known herbal products among herbalists. It was used widely for centuries by American Indians in North America, and it achieved fame in Europe in the 1900s. While many of its past uses have been linked to topical treatments, one of its key uses, is to support better immune function. It is also one of the most commonly available nutritional supplements and continues to focus on clinical research in natural food stores. With heavy concentrations in Kansas, Arkansas, Oklahoma, and Missouri, nine plants are native to the United States and Canada. These species are perennial, and they are part of the sunflower family.

27) Ginger

[Zingiber officinale]

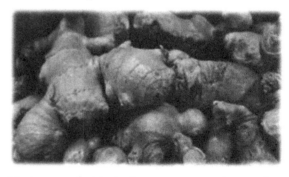

Healers used this herb to cure earaches and ear infections. They also used the rootstock for making a gentle tea to improve the digestive system and alleviate bloating. It also assists in nausea and bronchial infections.

28) Slippery Elm

[Ulmus rubra]

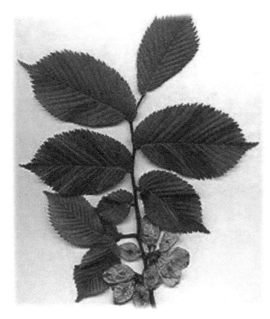

It's one of the most well-known medicinal tree barks. It has a long history of use—North American First Nations people used slippery elm for a range of health problems and gave it to European colonists, who immediately adopted it into their pharmacopeia. According to tradition, first Americans used slippery elm's moistening abilities to relieve thirst by eating the inner bark peeled off twigs. They also provided it as a calming dish, often in porridge for youngsters and the elderly. They also used moist bark on wounds as a bandage. Today, slippery elm is still used in skin care products and topical treatments to provide soothing assistance for skin irritations.

29) Lavender

[Lavandula]

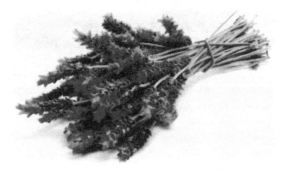

Lavender is often associated with two characteristics: its scent and its color. However, you may be unaware that the lavender flower and the oil extracted from it have a long history in herbal therapy.

Lavender plants are not original to the Americas; Europeans introduced them there, most likely in the 1800s. Although Native Americans did immediately begin using some newly arrived plants as medicine, and folklore about the new plants occasionally arose (dandelions are an example of this), references to "lavender" in Native American folklore and ethnographies are usually referring to desert lavender, a flowering shrub with some physical similarities to lavender but is completely unrelated to lavender. Desert lavender, also known as Lavender bush mint, grows in Arizona, southern California, and northern Mexico and has been utilized as a medicinal herb for a long time by the local Native American tribes.

This herb has traditionally been used to cure healers' insomnia, nausea, depression, headache, and exhaustion. Antiseptic and anti-inflammatory effects are found in the essential oil. Infusions may be used to soothe bug bites, as well as wounds.

30) Honeysuckle

[Lonicera periclymenum]

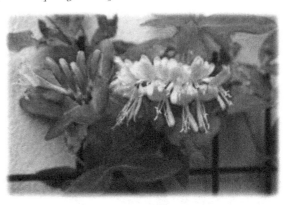

Native Americans utilized this plant to treat and cure asthma, but it has various healing uses, including rheumatoid arthritis, mumps, and hepatitis. It also assists with the upper respiratory tract infections, such as pneumonia.

31) Ashwagandha

[Withania somnifera]

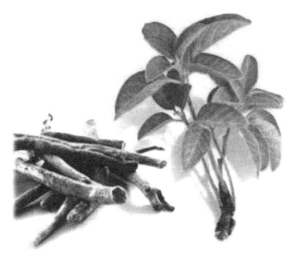

The name ashwagandha is Sanskrit for "horse smell," and it refers to the herb's potential to improve strength—as well as its distinct odor.

It is an adaptogen, which means it may support your body in dealing with mental and physical challenges. Many of the advantages of this plant come from powerful chemicals known as withanolides.

Ashwagandha also contains glycowithanolides, which are antioxidants, as well as alkaloids.

Due to its many rare medicinal applications, this plant was essential for Native American healers. It addresses bone fatigue, stiffness and muscle weakness, missing teeth, loss of memory, and rheumatism. It can also be used as a sedative.

Its leaves and root bark were used as an antibiotic too.

32) Mullein
[Verbascum Thapsus]

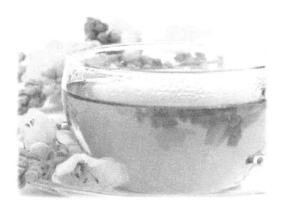

It was a tobacco-like plant that was used mostly to treat respiratory disorders. To relieve swelling in the joints, feet, or arms, the Native Americans made concoctions from the roots. Officially known as Verbascum genus and sometimes known as velvet plants, these flowering plant species are native to Europe and Asia and were first introduced by Europeans to America. A tobacco-like weed has a long tradition of use as a medication for the treatment of asthma and respiratory diseases and is one of the oldest herbs. In the treatment of ear infections, extracts made from the plant flowers are used, and one species, called the Great Mullein, is used as an herbal cure for sore throat, cough, and lung diseases.

33) Barberry
[Berberis vulgaris]

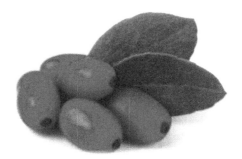

Anthropologists claim that it acts as a spiritual force or a preventative or cure of disease in a ceremonial activity or sacred object, especially by Native Americans. It is the most frequently prescribed treatment in the homeopathic medicine system for kidney pain and kidney stone removal.

34) Eyebright
[Euphrasia officinalis]

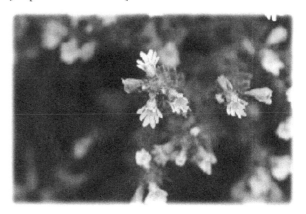

Small white flowers that bloom in late summer or early fall characterize eyebright. When the flowers bloom, the flowers, the leaves, and stems can all be gathered and dried for medicinal preparations. The many uses of eyebright for acute or chronic eye conditions are where the herb gets its name.

The actions of eyebright include anti-catarrhal, astringent, anti-inflammatory, antioxidant, and anti-mucus. Most notably, it is antibacterial, with similar properties to goldenseal, but slightly less potent, which makes it good for use in mucus membranes like the eyes. In addition, infusions help with nasal catarrh, sinusitis, and other congestive states, including irritations to the nose, throat, and esophagus. Add dried eyebright leaves to smoking mixtures as a helpful calming smoke for bronchitis and cough.

The combination of anti-inflammatory and astringent makes it good for many conditions dealing with mucus membranes. A room-temperature infusion of eyebright used as a compress is an effective relief for chronic conditions of the eyes, including redness, stinging, weeping eyes, and oversensitivity to light. Eyebright washes help eyes that are weak or those suffering from eyestrain. It is helpful to aged eyes and is thought to be able to restore vision.

Rare side effects to eyebright can include confusion, nausea, sweating, and pressure in the eye, itchy eyes, and allergic reactions in those who are allergic to ragweed.

35) Reishi

[Ganoderma lucidum]

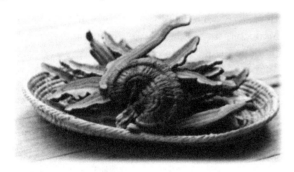

Reishi Mushrooms are highly hydrating, antioxidant-rich adaptogens (substances that help the body adapt to stress and tiredness) and have immune-boosting characteristics that benefit both the inside and outside of the body.

The Chippewa people used this herb for treating coughs, fevers, and diarrhea. It is also considered an anti-inflammatory.

Reishi mushrooms have several skincare advantages as well, ranging from decreasing redness to preventing fine lines and wrinkles.

They may be ingested whole, in extract, or powdered form in terms of health.

36) Black Raspberry

[Rubus occidentalis]

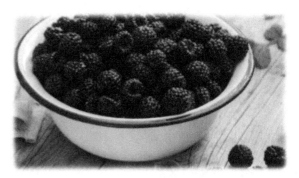

It is also identified as thimbleberry, wild black raspberry, black cap, blackcap raspberry, and scotch cap. It has been found that the shrub's roots, which are boiled into tea or chewed, are cathartic and efficient in curing gonorrhea, cough, and toothache. They were sometimes used for sore eyes, ulcers, boils, and sores as a wash. The root bark was boiled by the Pawnee, Omaha, and Dakota tribes to cure dysentery. In the care of bowel problems, extremely astringent leaves were used. In the treatment of whooping cough, a decoction of the roots, stems, and leaves was used.

37) Hyssop

[Hyssopus officinalis]

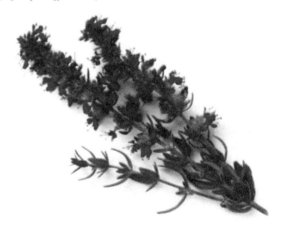

Hyssop was used orally as a drink for intestinal inflammation, bronchitis and respiratory diseases, urinary tract infection, sore throat, coughs, asthma, flatulence and colic, and sedative effects.

Hyssop is used topically in baths to cause sweating and for treating skin irritations and wounds.

38) Fenugreek

[Trigonella foenum-graecum]

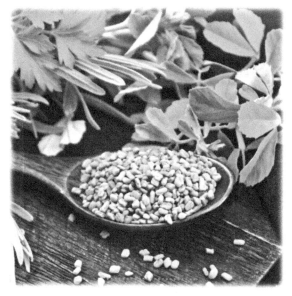

Fenugreek is a legume that has been used as a spice to improve the sensory quality of meals all over the globe. It is well-known for its therapeutic properties, which include anti-diabetic, anticarcinogenic, hypocholesterolemic, antioxidant, and immunological properties.

Besides its medicinal value, Fenugreek is strongly associated with prosperity and wealth. When used in charms and spell bags, it will attract money and prosperity to you. If you take a glass jar and position it in your kitchen (which is thought to be the heart of a home), add a couple of seeds of fenugreek into it every day to increase the flow of money and wealth coming into the home and prevent it from leaving.

39) Prickly Pear Cactus

[Opuntia]

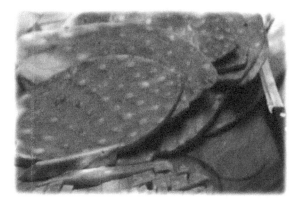

Native Americans developed a poultice as an antiseptic and for healing cuts, burns, and boils from mature pads. Tea was made to cure urinary tract diseases and aid the immune system. The study now suggests that the prickly pear cactus helps lower cholesterol and reduces cardiovascular disease and diet-related diabetes.

40) Frankincense

[Olibanum]

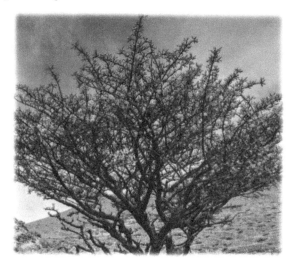

It is an aromatic gum resin derived from trees of the species Boswellia and contains a volatile oil used in incense and fragrances. This resin's essential oil is prized for its ability to beautify and revitalize skin when applied topically and enhance cellular health and immunity and induce a healthy inflammatory response when consumed internally.

When used in incense, it will increase the potency and effectiveness of your spells and rituals. It is perfect for use in magical workings that are meant to increase your determination, self-discipline, and willpower or aid in completing a difficult task. Frankincense will improve your overall level of success, both personally and professionally.

41) Marjoram

[Origanum majorana]

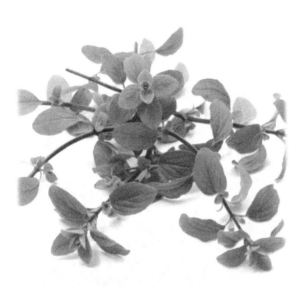

Marjoram, often called sweet marjoram, is a fragrant plant of the mint family. It has been demonstrated to have anti-inflammatory and antibacterial effects. It has been used medicinally to cure several diseases, including digestive difficulties, infections, and painful menstruation. It's most effective when dried, but it may also be utilized fresh. Marjoram is also considered an herb of protection and defense. Hang a sprig of it in your doorway to keep your home safe from intrusion and protect it from malevolent entities. Anoint a ring with oil infused with marjoram and wear it daily to create a personal protection charm. If used in a magical bath for a consecutive week, it will cleanse you of sadness, anguish, and grief.

42) Vervain

[Verbena officinalis]

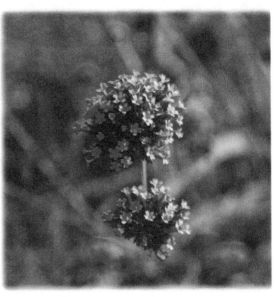

This plant is in the Verbenaceae family and features lobed, serrated leaves and soft, pale-purple blooms. Because of its many benefits, it is utilized as a herbal treatment all over the globe. In reality, it contains over 20beneficial plant chemicals, such as iridoid glycosides, flavonoids, and triterpenoids. These compounds may be responsible for their alleged advantages, including
anticancer actions, nerve cell protection, and anxiety- and convulsion-reducing
characteristics.
It may be taken as tea, tincture, powder, or cream.

43) Myrrh

[Commiphora myrrha]

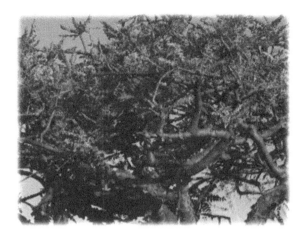

Myrrh is a sap-like material (resin) that emerges from cuts in the bark of Commiphora species trees. Myrrh Essential Oil promotes wound healing by protecting them from infection and reducing tissue inflammation. Its astringent effect prevents wounds from bleeding, reducing excessive blood loss. Myrrh Oil, which has emmenagogue characteristics, regulates menstruation and alleviates its unpleasant consequences, such as hormonal imbalances that cause mood swings.

Myrrh is also known for its magical energies. When added to incense, myrrh is great for consecration, and it's often used during meditation to reach a deeper meditative state and open paths within your mind that are difficult to access. Often myrrh is blended with frankincense to create potent magical blends used in most rituals.

44) Dragon's Blood

[Dracaena cinnabari]

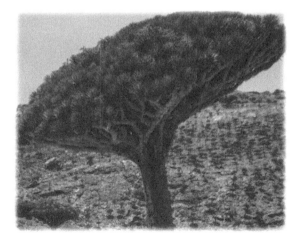

Dragon's blood is a resin derived from a tropical tree species known as dragon trees. It is dark crimson in hue, contributing to the term "dragon's blood."

Dragon's blood has long been used in numerous medicinal traditions across the globe. It has been shown to have anti-inflammatory, antioxidant, anticancer, antibacterial, and wound healing properties.

45) Oregon Grape

[Mohania aquifolium]

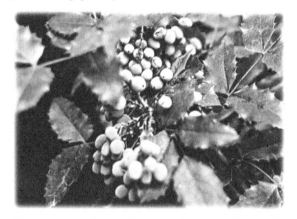

Oregon grape has a similar action to goldenseal and acts as an alternative, antibacterial, anti-inflammatory, antimicrobial, antifungal, cholagogue, laxative, antiemetic, anti-catarrhal, and tonic.

Collect the underground parts of the Oregon grape and the root in the fall. Clean them and cut them into slices before drying.

External preparations of Oregon grape work well to treat chronic and scaly skin conditions, including psoriasis and eczema. Use Oregon grape as a douche for treating vaginitis.

Internally, Oregon grape root helps to calm chronic constipation, nausea, vomiting, and stomach and gallbladder conditions. It can also be effective for indigestion, gastritis, abdominal bloating, irritable bowel syndrome, arthritis, jaundice, and fever.

It works as a blood purifier, tonic, and immune enhancer. It cleanses the liver, gallbladder, and spleen, and clears out microbial diseases.

Oregon grape should not be used while pregnant or breastfeeding. Side effects can include low blood pressure and heart rate, vomiting, lethargy, nosebleed, irritation of the eyes, skin, or kidneys.

46) Elder

[Sambucus nigra]

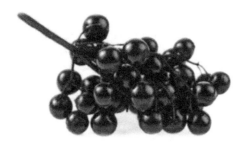

Elder is an esteemed virus-fighter and fever supporter of the herb world.

If you were to combine Echinacea, Boneset, and ginger, you would have an entirely natural herbal medicine to combat any cold or flu that comes your way. Add elder, and all your bases are covered! This vivid, dark purple berry is not only delicious—it also stimulates the immune system and combats viruses. Dried elderberries make a delightful tea or infusion and a tasty tincture. Drink 2–3 cups or take 2–3 droppers a day while sick. Elder supplements are out there, too.

Laboratory studies documented elder extracts acting exactly like antiviral medicine, particularly for combating the flu. The elder might, in fact, help fight any viral or respiratory infection, like colds, flu, or bronchitis.

Elder increases the body's ability to produce inflammatory "cytokines" during fevers, which are responsible for killing infections via the immune system.

Do not eat unripe berries or other parts of the elder plant. All parts, including unripe seeds, are slightly toxic and may produce nausea, vomiting, confusion, dizziness, and fainting. Use cautiously if you have an auto-immune condition.

47) Greek Valerian

[Polemonium caeruleum]

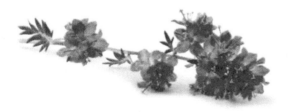

Greek Valerian is a perennial native plant found in lush woodlands, wet terrain, and along shaded river banks across Eastern North America, from New York to Minnesota and south to Kansas and Georgia.

The roots have alterative, astringent, diaphoretic,

expectorant, and pectoral properties and may be used to make an infusion or as an herbal tincture for colds, coughs, laryngitis, bronchitis, and inflammatory disorders, including abscess and skin issues. You can use a plant decoction as a hair rinse.

48) Cattail

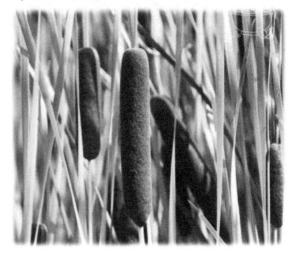

Cattails are marsh plants with a distinctive flowering spike and flat blade-like leaves. They are common plants that grow in huge marshes and on the edges of ponds. Cattail has natural antibacterial characteristics, aids in preventing anemia, offers skincare, aids in cancer prevention, gives a consistent rise in energy, and has cardiac tonic and lipid-lowering effects. Cattail reduces the risk of atherosclerosis, assists in managing diabetes, regulates hypertension, aids in weight gain, improves digestion, and works as an analgesic.

49) Horsemint

[Mentha longifolia]

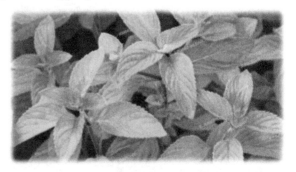

Horsemint, commonly known as Wild Bergamot, is a popular and beneficial medicinal plant.

This herb has been used for a long time by many Native Americans, including the Blackfeet, Ojibwa, Menominee, Winnebago, and others, as a medicinal herb to treat different diseases.

The leaves emit a strong citrus or lemony aroma

when the leaves are brushed or crushed. Horsemint has the most thymol of any mint. It is more than just an antiseptic, mite-killer, and cough syrup component. This herb's tea may be used to treat a range of digestive issues, including PMS cramps, stomach aches, gas, bloating, and indigestion, among others.

Horsemint is also a natural insect repellent, and while it's in season, you may put a handful of leaves on your skin to keep the pests at bay.

It contains the oil citronellol, which is commercially used in commercial insect repellents and creams.

50) Gotu Kola

[Centella asiatica]

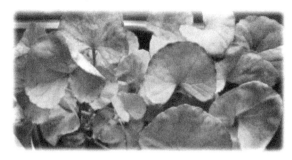

This herb is in the parsley family. Various tribes still use it for preventing baldness and relieving fevers. It is also considered a natural antioxidant.

CONCLUSION

There is a lot of new information to take when you first start looking into herbalism and even more information to absorb once you've decided to start practicing. Luckily, it's easy for anyone to get started with herbalism and the best way to do it is by using the leading practices and methods available which we will see later in this collection. But the first thing is to know all the available herbs and plants well to avoid any mistake when dealing with something related to our well-being

An herbalist needs to know many things in their herbalism journey, and they should know most of them before they even begin.

At this moment, you should be conscious about the number of herbs you can use, and this knowledge will assist you in understanding the following pages better, especially when it's time to show you the best recipes and remedies that Native Americans used for the treatment of their diseases.

BOOK 5

HERBAL APOTHECARY

The Ultimate Ancient Herbal Remedies Guide to Create Your Natural Homemade Apothecary

Citali Galwen

INTRODUCTION

Native Americans were vital in educating us about the critical nature of herbalism. The medicinal and herbal wisdom of the Native Americans has been overlooked by history for far too long. This book aims to bring their medicinal experience and deep knowledge of natural supplements back to life.

The world of Native American herbal medicine is vast and deeply enriching for those who take the time to explore its treasures.

Ultimately, the goal of this book is to provide you with an overview of some of the recipes that are available to you in order to begin to heal yourself and others with herbal remedies in the manner of our Native American ancestors.

Herbal remedies are not only good for your body, but they are great for your mind too. They have been employed throughout history for a variety of ailments, such as pain relief and healing. Today, people use herbal remedies to help with fatigue, insomnia, nausea, among other maladies.

Herbal remedies can help you feel better in many ways. Using herbal remedies and recipes can give you a calming and peaceful feeling as well as improve your overall health and well-being. Since they are very popular today, it is wise to consider using them at least once or twice a week to reap the benefits. The beauty of herbal remedies and recipes is that you can tailor them to suit your individual needs. When taking herbs, you can lower or increase the dosage depending on what you need. You should always consult a doctor before you start using herbs, but you can rely on herbal recipes to deliver the right results.

Herbal remedies are made with natural substances that stimulate the body's natural healing abilities. They, together with herbal recipes, are a great tool for anyone who wants to help themselves feel better. Herbal remedies and recipes are able to do this without the use of any chemicals or medications.

Today, herbal remedies are one of the most popular ways for people to maintain good health. They are useful when you want to maintain or improve your overall health.

Herbal medicines can be taken in a variety of formats, including pills, teas, and powders. Many people choose to drink herbal remedies as teas or add them to water for greater benefits. Herbal remedies are often combined with other natural ingredients like honey or lemon juice to increase their potency even further.

Learning herbalism and plant-based home remedies can be difficult, but I hope—and I'm sure—that this book has been an excellent primer for you to continue your journey, get acquainted with the recipes for different ailments, select which ones work best for you—and to empower healing at home.

CHAPTER 15:

ALLERGIES

Native Americans have been using herbs for healing and spiritual purposes for centuries, and many of these herbs can be found in modern herbal stores. However, because the body's immune system is much more sensitive than it was when Native Americans were using these herbs, people may now be allergic to them. Unfortunately, this often goes unnoticed until the person begins to feel symptoms such as asthma or hay fever.

It's important to always talk with a doctor before taking any new medications or supplements, even if they're natural. And if you experience any negative reactions after taking an herb—whether it's an allergy or something else—stop taking it immediately and consult your physician right away; the negative effects could last much longer than just a few hours.

How To Determine If You Are Allergic To Herbs

Herbs are often used in combination with one another, either with other herbs or with other forms of medication. If you are suffering from an allergy to these herbs, you might also have an allergy to any medications that are used in combination with them since the pharmacology of the two substances is likely similar.

Check the ingredients on all over-the-counter medications or dietary supplements, including vitamins and pain relievers. If you think a product might contain an herb to which you are allergic, it's a good idea to avoid taking it until you have spoken with a physician.

If your allergies are severe or if you suffer from chronic allergies, it's important to be aware of what unrelated medications could possibly cause an allergic reaction for you. In addition, if your allergy symptoms seem unusual for what is normally associated with that particular herb, contact your doctor right away.

Herbs To Watch Out For Side Effects

Some herbs that have been known to cause allergic reactions to include:

Cayenne pepper

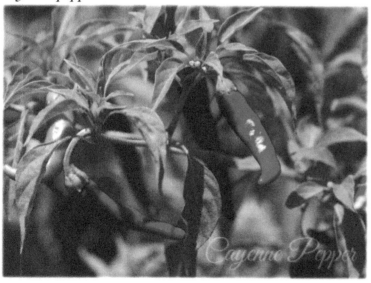

Cayenne pepper has been used by Native Americans for hundreds of years as a natural pain reliever and as a way to stop minor bleeding. It has also been used to treat cold symptoms, heart disease, rheumatism, and arthritis. Cayenne pepper is now widely used as a spice in cooking.

In addition to anaphylaxis, cayenne pepper allergy can cause the throat to swell, as well as itchy skin and hives. In some cases, asthma attacks have also been associated with cayenne pepper allergy.

It is important to note that cayenne pepper sold in stores has been known to contain other substances that may produce an allergic reaction as well.

The chamomile plant

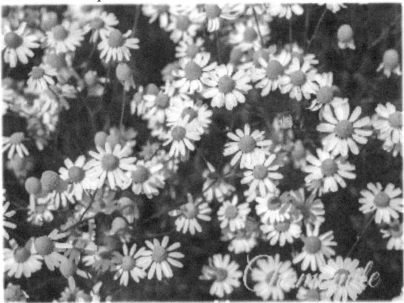

Chamomile is a healing herb used to treat indigestion, ulcers, insomnia, headaches, and heartburn. It can also treat inflammatory problems and can be used to relieve pain.

It's most common for people to be allergic to the flowers of the chamomile plant rather than its leaves. Some of the symptoms of an allergic reaction might include swelling in the mouth or throat that could cause breathing problems, as well as hives or anaphylaxis.

Ginseng

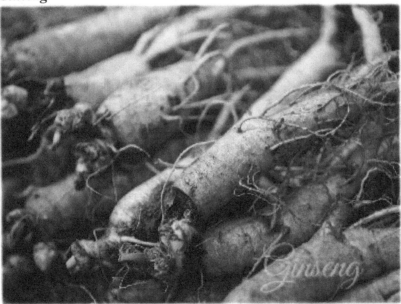

With its ability to boost energy levels and stimulate the immune system, ginseng has been widely used for both medicinal and spiritual purposes. It is also used to treat colds, asthma, heart disease, and many other conditions.

Because of the medicine's popularity, it's important to be aware of side effects such as allergic reactions and different forms of toxicity. Some people are allergic to all parts of the ginseng plant, including the roots or dried leaves. An allergy may develop to various ginseng products that contain only a tiny percentage of the herb itself.

According to Harvard Health Publications, ginseng can cause symptoms similar to those associated with an allergic reaction: swelling in the throat and lips; breathing difficulties; itching; hives or welts on your body; or fainting.

Cinnamon

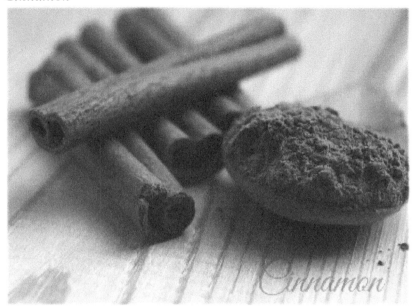

You've probably heard that cinnamon helps sweeten things up, but you might not know that it has also been used for the care of digestive problems. Chronic users of cinnamon may develop an allergy to it, although the condition is uncommon.

Some people who are allergic to cinnamon have only experienced mild side effects such as a rash on their face and neck, while others have had more severe reactions, including breathing problems and difficulty swallowing.

Always Try Small Quantities First

Many people think that they can't try using a small quantity of a particular herb before starting on a large amount. However, because the body often responds positively to small amounts of highly potent herbs like black cohosh and ginseng, it's important to start with very small amounts.

If you have allergies or any other health problems, it's important to always use the smallest quantities possible. Although this may not eliminate all negative effects from trying a new herb or supplement, at least you'll know what the supposed benefits are before taking an entire bottle.

It's also important to consider how long you have been taking a particular herb when you decide whether or not it might be safe for you to continue using the product in question.

You should also be aware that there are many herbs that have multiple uses, and some herbs may not be safe for a person to use regularly. For example, some people have been known to develop a sensitivity to the aloe vera plant. Individuals who regularly use aloe vera on their skin or in their food may experience side effects such as burning, swelling, or itching.

Be Aware Of Herbs' Potential Side Effects

There is no doubt about it: Herbs can help improve your health and make you feel better while they're being used. However, if you try a new herb without first consulting with your doctor, side effects aren't something you should ignore.

Some herbs might be useful for curing an illness, but they could also cause other health issues. For example, people who regularly use the aloe vera plant to treat minor cuts or burns should consider the possible side effects of using this herb.

People who are allergic to aloe vera might not experience any side effects until they start using it regularly. Once their allergies develop, they might develop unpleasant reactions to it. If you notice a rash on your skin after you've been using aloe vera products, it's important to stop using them and contact a doctor right away.

CHAPTER 16:

REMEDIES TO TREAT THE MOST COMMON ILLNESSES AND PAINS

Abscess

Rose and vanilla elixir

It is used to address abscess and for emotional issues, such as depression and loss.

Ingredients:

- 3 to 5 vanilla beans, cut the long way and finely hacked or squeezed 1-16 ounces (470 ml) container approximately loaded up with new flower petals 1 cup (235 ml) excellent, smooth-tasting liquor.
- 1 cup (320 g) unadulterated crude honey

Instructions:

1. Add the vanilla into a container of roses. Consolidate the liquor and honey, blend well, and pour over the roses and vanilla. Spread to the edge of the container and jab with a chopstick to ensure the herbal material is secured. Top the container and store it in a cool, dim spot for 4 days to about a month and a half. Strain and tap into a perfect jug.
2. Take some drops of the mixture straight into your mouth, or add to some hot or cold water or tea whenever you need a touch of motivation, unwinding, or break. It's a phenomenal gut-warming stomach-related guide and is great over vanilla frozen yogurt!

Asthma

Quick-acting asthma tea

This tea helps relieve asthma and can provide quick relief for asthma attacks.

It also has the additional advantage of calming the lungs, which is great for any respiratory problems, such as the flu or cold.

Ingredients:

- 1 teaspoon elecampane root
- 2 teaspoons horehound herb
- 1 teaspoon blue vervain leaves
- 2 cups water

Instructions:

1. Mix them all together in a pot.

2. Boil the mixture for 5 minutes. Because mint has a tendency to concentrate during boiling, it should be done properly.
3. Strain the tea into your cup and drink it during an attack, or use it as a preventive measure against asthma attacks.

Back Pain

Spine's fine tincture

These warming, relaxing, and analgesic herbs relieve the spasms that cause most back pain, whether acute or chronic, muscular or connective and so on. After using this solution topically, if you have infused oil created from fresh goldenrod or ginger, use it as a massage oil. For help sleeping, take 1 to 4 drops of tincture of wild lettuce by mouth—this will also contribute to more pain-relieving action.

Ingredients:

- 1 fluid ounce tincture Solomon's seal
- 1 fluid ounce tincture ginger
- ½ fluid ounce mixture goldenrod
- ½ fluid ounce remedy meadowsweet
- ½ fluid ounce tincture mullein root
- ½ fluid ounce tincture St. John's wort

Instructions:

1. In a small bottle, combine the tinctures. Cap the bottle and label it.
2. Take 1 to 4 drops by mouth 3 to 5 times per day.
3. Additionally, squirt 1 to 4 drops into your palm and massage them into back muscles.

TIP: Increase the mullein root to 1 fluid ounce if the spinal discs are impinged or worn away. It explicitly supports these issues. If you have sciatica or other spreading nerve pain, include St. John's wort. It regenerates damaged nerve tissue.

Sciatic pain tea

This tea helps relieve Sciatic pain.

Ingredients:

- 2 teaspoons crampbark
- 2 teaspoons kava gout root

Instructions:

1. Simmer for 30 minutes.
2. Cool and strain.
3. Take up to one cup per day. This tea can help relieve sciatic pain.

Bedsores

Bedsore topical wash

This wash helps relieve bedsore pain

Ingredients:

- 2 teaspoons marigold flowers
- 1 teaspoon coarse echinacea root
- 1 tablespoon white oak bark

Instructions:

1. Strain.
2. Use as a wash periodically throughout the day.

Bee Sting

Fresh plantain poultice

For 1 treatment.

The modest plantain plant is a green weedy plant that contains aucubin, a powerful antitoxin glucoside. Other components have antibacterial and anti-inflammatory properties, making this basic therapy quite effective. If you can't obtain fresh plantain leaves, you may rehydrate it by soaking a teaspoon of dried, crushed plantain in a tablespoon of water and then use it as a poultice.

Ingredients:

- 1 tablespoon finely chopped fresh plantain leaves

Instructions:

1. Cover the injured area with a cotton towel after applying the chopped leaves.
2. Allow the poultice to be absorbed for 10 to 15 minutes.
3. Repeat as often as needed until the pain stops permanently.

Bites And Stings

Bug bite relief spray

Makes 8 fluid ounces.

This spray helps relieve bug bite pain. If you often pass through clouds of mosquitoes or black flies, or if you live in a chigger-infested region, have this cooling, itch-relieving spray on hand for when you come inside.

Ingredients:

- 4 oz. non-alcoholic apple cider vinegar (or in substitution, witch hazel extract)
- 2 fluid ounces tincture rose
- 1 fluid ounce tincture self-heal
- 1 fluid ounce tincture yarrow

Instructions:

1. Combine all of the ingredients in a bottle/container with a fine-mist sprayer top.
2. Liberally spray wherever you've been bitten.

Bronchitis

Hyssop oxymel

Great to treat colds, flu, and bronchitis.

Ingredients:

- Hyssop, fresh or dried (an herbaceous plant with antiseptic and expectorant properties)
- Honey
- Apple Cider Vinegar (vinegar made from cider that is great for weight loss and heart health)

Instructions:

1. Fill a jar lightly with chopped fresh hyssop. (Only half fill it if you're using dried hyssop).
2. Then, fill the jar with honey just 1/3 of the way, and top it off with the apple cider vinegar.
3. Let it sit for 2-4 weeks in the sealed jar before straining.
4. For a congested cough, you can take 1–2 teaspoons of this remedy every hour. Keep the hyssop oxymel in the fridge for better preservation.

Fire cider

Great to relieve bronchitis pain.

Traditional fire cider recipes are blends of spicy and aromatic stimulating expectorants that will heat you and help you get the gunk out. In this variation, we slip in several immunity boosters and a decent source of vitamin C. If you use prescription blood thinners, do not ingest this.

Ingredients:

- 1 whole chopped head garlic
- 1 (2-inch) piece fresh ginger, chopped

- ¼ cup dried pine needles
- ¼ cup dried sage leaf
- ¼ cup dried thyme leaf
- ¼ cup dried elderberry
- ¼ cup dried rose hips
- 2 tablespoons dried elecampane root
- 2 tablespoons dried angelica root
- 1-quart apple cider vinegar
- Honey or water, for sweetening or diluting

Instructions:

1. Combine the garlic, ginger, and remaining herbs.
2. Fill the pot with vinegar. Place a wax paper sheet under the jar lid before you screw down the ring. (The coating on the bottom of the metal mason jar lids corrodes when exposed to vinegar.)
3. Macerate the herbs in the vinegar for at least two weeks, preferably longer.
4. Finally, strain, bottle, and label the finished fire cider. If the vinegar is too strong for you, add some honey (up to one-fourth of the entire amount) or dilute your dosage with water.
5. Take a shot (about ½ fluid ounce) at the first sign of mucus buildup in the lungs and every couple of hours after that until symptoms resolve.

Sweet soothing tea
This soothing tea helps relieve bronchitis pain.

Ingredients:

- 1 teaspoon marshmallow leaves or flowers
- 1 teaspoon of coltsfoot leaves
- 1 teaspoon mullein leaves and flowers
- ½ cup boiling water, honey

Instructions:

1. Combine the above herbs; steep one teaspoon of the mixture in the boiling water; strain. Sweeten with honey.
2. Take one-half cup, three or four times a day, hot.

Burns And Sunburns

Aloe burn relief
Great for treating the pain of sunburn, mild burns, and psoriasis.

Aloe is a very common ingredient in sunburn ointments. In its natural state, it helps heal and moisturize the skin. It helps with just about any skin issue involving redness and itchiness.

Ingredients:

- 1 piece aloe vera leaf

Instructions:

1. This is probably the easiest remedy you'll come across. If you've never used aloe before, always test it in a small area of your skin first, so you're sure you aren't allergic to it.
2. Simply cut the tip off one of the leaves, making sure to cut at an angle (just not straight across) and leaving at least some of the leaves. With a knife, carefully split the leaf in half, revealing the gel. Rub gel directly on your burn. That's it!

Burn-healing honey
It is the finest burn healing agent: even if you just have basic honey, you'll be okay. It's even better if you infuse it with these medicinal herbs ahead of time.

Ingredients:

- ½ cup fresh calendula flower
- ½ cup fresh rose petals
- 1-pint honey, gently warmed

Instructions:

1. Fill a pint-size mason jar halfway with calendula and rose petals.
2. Fill the pot with warm honey and place it in a warm area to infuse for one month.
3. Gently warm the closed pot until the honey has a liquid consistency. Strain the infused honey into a new pot, pressing the marc against the strainer to express as much honey as you can.
4. After cooking and cleaning the burn area, apply a layer of the infused honey and loosely wrap it with a gauze bandage. At least twice a day, refresh the application.

Sunburn spray
A few spritzes will start to calm the skin and relieve irritation.

Ingredients:

- 1 tablespoon dried peppermint leaf
- 1 tablespoon dried plantain leaf
- 1 tablespoon dried self-heal leaf and flower
- 1 tablespoon dried linden leaf and flower

- 1-quart boiling water
- 4 fluid ounces rose water

Instructions:

1. To make a hot infusion, put the peppermint, plantain, self-heal, and linden in a mason jar.
2. Refrigerate the jar until it is cold.
3. Strain out four fluid ounces of the infusion and transfer to an 8-ounce bottle with a fine-mist sprayer top. Use the remaining input for compresses or a cooling drink. Keep refrigerated for three days.
4. Fill the spray bottle halfway with rose water. Cap and label the bottle.
5. Apply copiously and frequently.
6. When not in use, store the spray in the refrigerator.

Burn poultice

This poultice helps relieve burn pain.

Ingredients:

- 1 tablespoon dried coneflower flower
- 1 tablespoon dried hyssop flowers
- 1 tablespoon dried golden-rod flowers
- 1 tablespoon dried sunflower petals

Instructions:

1. Combine the above ingredients, moisten with boiling water, and place between two cheesecloth layers; let cool and apply to the affected area.
2. When dry, remoisten. Use as often as necessary.

Immunity strengthener

A burn can weaken the body, leaving you vulnerable to illness and infection. Use this tea to strengthen immunity.

Ingredients:

- 30 drops echinacea tincture,
- 20 drops wild indigo root tincture,
- 1 cup warm water

Instructions:

1. Combine the above herbs in warm water.
2. Take up to five times a day.

Canker Sores

Echinacea remedy

Great to treat canker sores.

Ingredients:

- 2 tablespoons sage tincture
- 2 tablespoons echinacea tincture
- 2 tablespoons lemon balm tincture

Instructions:

1. Combine the three tinctures in a dropper bottle. Use one dropper full of the mixture to swish around your mouth 2–3 times daily.

Chapped Lips

Aloe-calendula balm

This balm helps relieve chapped lips' pain.

Makes 2 tablespoons of aloe vera and calendula whichhelps compromised skin to heal, and aloe provides thirsty lips with deep hydration. This rapid method requires readymade calendula oil; however, you may use your own infused calendula oil. This balm may be refrigerated and carefully sealed for up to a year.

Ingredients:

- 1½ tablespoons aloe vera gel
- 1½ teaspoons calendula oil

Instructions:

1. In a medium-sized bowl, merge the aloe vera gel and calendula oil. With a whisk, blend them thoroughly.
2. Fill a jar with a tight-fitting lid with the balm. While it's ideal for keeping your main supply refrigerated to keep it fresh, you may want to have a teaspoon or two on hand in a little squeeze bottle to apply throughout the day.

Cold Sores

Homemade mouthwash

This mixture is a great way to keep your mouth fresh and healthy.

Ingredients:

- 1/2-ounce echinacea tincture
- 1/4-ounce Oregon grape root tincture
- 1/8-ounce plantain tincture (generally used for cooking due to its sweet taste)
- 1/8-ounce propolis tincture

Instructions:

1. Mix all of the tinctures together in a bottle. Add 30–60 drops to 1 mouthful of water. Swish it in your mouth for 20–30 seconds.

Cold sore compress

The ointment in this recipe, made with clove oil, will stop the pain and itching of cold sores very quickly.

Makes 5 cups dried herb mix.

Ingredients:

- 1 cup dried calendula flower
- 1 cup dried plantain leaf
- 1 cup dried chamomile flower, dried self-heal leaf, and flower
- ½ cup dried St. John's wort leaf and flower

Instructions:

1. Mix all the herbs.
2. Store in an airtight container.
3. Lie down and apply a moist cloth to the afflicted region. Place a dry towel on top and place the hot water bottle on top. Get comfortable and wait 10 to 20 minutes for it to take effect.
4. Repeat 2 to 3 times per day.

Cold sore balm

Makes 5 ounces.

This is a homemade salve that is great for soothing cold sores. It also stops the pain and heals it very fast.

Ingredients:

- 1 fluid ounce calendula-infused oil,
- 1 fluid ounce plantain-infused oil,
- ½ fluid ounce self-heal-infused oil,
- ½ fluid ounce chamomile-infused oil,
- ½ fluid ounce St. John's wort-infused oil,
- ½ fluid ounce thyme-infused oil,
- 1-ounce beeswax, plus more as needed

Instructions:

1. Make a salve as usual. If you're going to store it in little jars, make it soft; if you're going to use lip balm tubes, make it slightly harder.

Cold sore mouthwash

This mouthwash helps with the pain and irritation of cold sores.

Ingredients:

- 1 teaspoon echinacea root
- 1 teaspoon yerba mansa root
- 1 tablespoon white oak bark
- 1 cup boiling water

Instructions:

1. Combine the herbs in a glass container.
2. Steep 30 minutes, calm, and strain. Use the solution as a wash to treat cold sores.

Colic

Chamomile infusion

This is great for the treatment of colds, coughs, diarrhea, and general ailments, but I found it very helpful in relieving pain from colic. It is made by boiling chamomile flowers in water.

Ingredients:

- A handful of dried chamomile flowers
- 250ml of boiled water

Instructions:

1. Put the chamomile flowers in a clean mug.
2. Once the boiled water is a little cooler, pour it on the dried flowers.
3. Sieve the infusion, and you have it ready to treat your child's cold.

Herbal gripe water with peppermint, ginger, and fennel

Commercial gripe water often includes high-fructose corn syrup. This homemade version, which includes a little sugar as well as fennel, ginger, and peppermint, relieves pain by relaxing the digestive muscles and releasing trapped gas. When refrigerated, this cure can keep for a week.

Ingredients:

1. 1 teaspoon crushed fennel seeds
2. 1 teaspoon chopped fresh ginger root
3. 1 teaspoon crushed dried peppermint leaves

4. 1 cup boiling water
5. 1 teaspoon cane sugar

Instructions:

1. Combine the herbs and boiling water in a teapot or cup. Allow the mixture to steep for 10 minutes in a covered saucepan or cup.
2. Transfer the gripe water to a sterilized jar with a tight-fitting lid. Add the sugar, then stir well until it dissolves. Allow the gripe water to cool to medium temperature.
3. 1 teaspoon should be placed in a medicine dropper and given to your baby orally. Repeat once or twice a day as needed to relieve colic symptoms.

Constipation

Bowel-hydrating infusion

Makes 2½ cups dried herb mix.

If you have a stomach ache, drink this tea to relieve it temporarily.

Ingredients:

- 1 cup dried linden leaf and flower
- 1 cup dried marshmallow root
- ¼ cup dried cinnamon bark
- ¼ cup dried licorice root

Instructions:

1. Mix all the herbs. Store in an airtight container.
2. Make a cold infusion. Pour in cold water (room temperature will be fine too) and let it steep for 4 to 8 hours before filtering.

Bowel-motivating tincture

Bitters and carminatives stimulate bile flow and intestinal peristalsis, causing the bowels to move.

Ingredients:

- 1½ fluid ounces tincture dandelion root
- 1½ fluid ounces tincture St. John's wort
- ½ fluid ounce mixture angelica root
- ½ fluid ounce medicine ginger

Instructions:

1. In a small bottle, combine the tinctures. Cap the bottle and label it.
2. Take 2 to 4 drops every 20 minutes until relief occurs.

Cough And Cold

Antitussive oxymel

Makes 20 to 60 doses.

An oxymel is essentially a vinegar and honey mixture that combines the astringent and stimulating properties of vinegar with the moistening and calming properties of honey. With the addition of lung-specific herbs, this is a go-to for coughs of all types.

Ingredients:

- 1/3 cup dried pine needles
- 1/3 cup dried sage leaf
- 1/3 cup dried thyme leaf
- ¼ cup dried ginger

- 1-quart of apple cider vinegar
- Honey, as needed to fill the container

Instructions:

1. Fill the jar four-fifths of the way with vinegar, then with honey.
2. Cover the pot and let macerate for four weeks.
3. Strain and bottle the oxymel. Cap the bottle and label it.
4. Take 1 to 3 tablespoons as needed.

Cough syrup

This cough syrup is a great way to relieve a nasty cold or flu.

Ingredients:

- 2 teaspoons coltsfoot leaves
- 1 tablespoon wild plum root
- 2 teaspoons mullein leaves
- 2 cups boiling water
- 1 pound honey

Instructions:

1. Combine the above herbs in boiling water, steep for 30 minutes, and strain in non-metallic containers.
2. Add one pound of honey, heating, and stirring until the honey is dissolved; cool and store in a glass container.

Soothing cough and cold formula

This formula's components may aid in promoting much-needed relief for any respiratory infections.

Ingredients:

- 30 drops echinacea tincture
- 20 drops wild indigo root tincture
- 2 cups white cedar leaf tips tea

Instructions:

1. Combine the above ingredients and take half a cup at a time, hot.
2. Take up to three times a day.

Lakota cough and cold formula

Also known as plantain, dandelion, or yucca root, this is a great herbal remedy for sore or dry throats caused by the common cold.

Ingredients:

- 1 teaspoon goldenseal root
- 1 teaspoon mullein leaves
- 1 teaspoon Osha root
- 1 teaspoon pleurisy root
- 1 teaspoon yerba mansa root
- 2 teaspoons yerba santa leaves
- 2 cups boiling water

Instructions:

1. Combine the above herbs and cover with boiling water; steep for 30 minutes, calm, and strain.
2. As required, take two teaspoons at a time, up to two cups a day.

Lumbee cough and cold formula

This formula is formulated with natural ingredients that help to relieve the discomfort of colds and flu.

Ingredients:

- 3 teaspoons goldenrod leaves,
- 4 teaspoons horehound leaves

- 2 teaspoons white pine inner bark
- 4 cups boiling water

Instructions:

1. Combine the above herbs in cheesecloth; tie closed with a string.
2. Place the bag in the boiling; simmer for 15 minutes; cool; remove the bundle.
3. Take half a cup of the hot mixture at a time, as needed, up to two cups a day.

Quick-acting cough and cold formula

This tea can quickly relieve cold and flu symptoms.

Ingredients:

- 4 teaspoons agrimony leaves
- 2 teaspoons mullein leaves
- 2 teaspoons blue vervain leaves
- 1 teaspoon oxeye daisy
- 3 teaspoons horehound leaves
- 2 teaspoons speedwell
- 2 cups boiling water

Instructions:

- Combine the herbs with water, steep for 30 minutes, calm, and strain.
- Take up to two cups each day.

Expectorating cough and cold tea

This formula contains known expectorant herbs that can help to relieve your cough and sore throat.

Ingredients:

- 2 teaspoons boneset herb
- 2 teaspoons licorice root
- 2 to 3 slices ginger root
- 2 teaspoons wild cherry bark
- 2 cups boiling water

Instructions:

- Combine the herbs with water, steep for 30 minutes, calm, and strain.
- Take up to two cups each day.

Quick-acting mullein cough syrup

This syrup helps relieve cough

Ingredients:

- 1 cup mullein tea
- 1 pound honey

Instructions:

1. Heat until the honey is liquid.
2. Remove from heat, calm, and pour into a glass container. Take a tablespoon at a time, as needed.

Cramps

Muscle rub

These warming herbs promote local circulation while also lowering inflammation and relieving stress. If you're still in a lot of pain when it's time to go to bed after applying the remedies, take 1 to 2 drops of wild lettuce tincture for further comfort.

Ingredients:

- 2 fluid ounces ginger-infused oil
- 2 fluid ounces goldenrod-infused oil
- 2 fluid ounces tinctures ginger
- 2 fluid ounces of meadowsweet
- 80 drops essential oil of peppermint or cinnamon

Instructions:

1. Mix the infused oils, tinctures, and essential oil in a small container/bottle. Cap and label the bottle, and shake vigorously before each use.

2. Drop a tiny bit in your palm. Warm the remedy between your palms before applying it to the hurting joints.
3. Massage the cream into the joints until your hands no longer feel oily. Work the cream into the tissue.
4. Apply the solution 3 to 5 times per day.

Ointment #1
Ingredients:

- 1 tbsp. peppermint oil
- 1 tbsp. meadowsweet oil
- 1 tbsp. ginger oil
- 1 tbsp. ginger tincture
- 1 tbsp. goldenrod leaves oil

Instructions:

1. Mix the oils and tincture in a small, amber glass bottle with a dropper lid. Whenever it is needed, put 5 drops of the mix on your hands, rub it vigorously until you feel the heat, and then massage the cramping muscle.

Ointment #2
Ingredients:

- 1 tbsp. Lizard Tail Root oil
- 1 tbsp. wintergreen oil
- 4 oz. coconut oil

Instructions:

1. Melt the coconut oil in a water bath.
2. Add the herbs, stir and keep on low heat for two hours. Strain and pour in a mason jar, let it cool down, and then close the lid.
3. Apply on the sore part, massaging vigorously.

Cuts And Wounds

Cuts or abrasions are not something you have to underestimate. If not correctly addressed, they can cause unpleasant infections, swellings, and inflammations.

When dealing with a minor wound, the first thing to do is stop the bleeding, and then it is time to wash it properly to remove any sign of dirt and foreign matter and only then proceed with the medication. Of course, serious bleeding and artery damage require emergency care by a medical professional.

Herbs can come in handy to prepare effective washes to disinfect the wound and promote healing.

Wounds wash #1
Ingredients:

- 1 tsp. ashwagandha (root)
- 1 tsp. echinacea (root)
- 1 cup distilled boiling water

Instructions:

1. Boil the roots in water in the indicated proportions for 30 minutes. Let cool and strain. Use to wash the wound.

Wounds wash #2
Ingredients:

- 3 tbsp. calendula (flowers)
- 3 tbsp. echinacea (root)
- 3 tbsp. plantain (leaves)
- 3 tbsp. goldenrod (leaves and flowers)
- 2 tbsp. heal-all (leaves and flowers)
- 1 tbsp. chamomile (flowers)
- 1 tsp. ashwagandha (root)

Instructions:

1. Mix the herbs and store in a mason jar in a shady place. To prepare the wash, boil 4 tsp. of the mix for each cup of water. Let simmer for 30 minutes, cool, strain, and use it to wash the wound.

Diarrhea

Astringent tea
Makes 2¼ cups dried herb mixture (around 14 to 18 quarts of tea).

The tannins in these herbs aid in the re-bonding of loose tissues, allowing fluids to remain where they belong and barriers to maintaining their integrity. Drink a quart of tea throughout the day.

Ingredients:

- 1½ cups dried self-heal leaf and flower
- ½ cup dried meadowsweet flower
- ¼ cup rose petals

Instructions:

1. Mix all the herbs. Store in an airtight container.
2. Tincture variation: make a tincture mix with the same quantities if you wish. Combine 1½ fluid ounces tincture of self-heal, ½ fluid ounce tincture of meadowsweet, and ¼ fluid ounce tincture of rose petal. Take 1 to 6 drops every 20 minutes until relief occurs.

Cinnamon powder capsules
Makes 22 to 24 capsules.

Cinnamon's demulcent property is enhanced when it is extracted into the water as an infusion or decoction. It releases the dry powder, which then absorbs excess water and exerts an astringent effect on the intestinal lining. This quells diarrhea quite nicely. The capsule machine, a handy manual capsule-filling device, helps with this recipe quite a lot.

Ingredients:

- 20 to 24 "00" size empty gelatin capsules
- 2 tablespoons of powdered cinnamon

Instructions:

1. Fill the capsules with cinnamon powder.
2. When you have diarrhea, take 1 to 3 capsules. If you don't feel better after an hour, take another dose.

Eczema

Elderberry extract/tincture

Elderberry extract and tinctures contain a variety of chemicals that may help to relieve itchiness and has a calming effect on irritated skin

Ingredients:

- Dried or fresh elderberries
- Menstruum (vodka or liquor of decision) to cover
- Yield: 1 16 ounces (470 ml)

Instructions:

1. In the case of utilizing dried material, fill a 1-16 ounces (470 ml) container 33% full before including fluid (menstruum is the specific term for the dissolvable or transporter utilized in a concentrate, tincture, or remedy). In the case of using new herbs, fill free to the top.

Fever

Fever-inducing tea

Makes 3 cups of dried herb mix (about 18 to 24 quarts of tea).

I personally use this tea when I have a fever, and after it has gone down, I drink a few cups of this tea to dampen the heat and ease the pain.

Ingredients:

- 1 cup dried tulsi leaf
- ½ cup dried sage leaf
- ½ cup dried thyme leaf
- ½ cup dried yarrow leaf and flower

- ¼ cup dried angelica root
- ¼ cup dried ginger, one garlic clove, sliced, for a real kick (optional)

Instructions:

1. Mix all the herbs. Store in an airtight container.
2. Add the garlic (if using).
3. Reheat before drinking and sip extremely hot for maximum impact.

Fever-breaking tea

Makes 1¾ cups dried herb mix (enough for 14 to 24 pints of tea).

This tea also works for a fever; it has a cooling effect and helps to relieve the symptoms of a headache.

Ingredients:

- ½ cup dried catnip leaf and flower
- ½ cup dried elderflower
- ½ cup dried peppermint leaf
- ¼ cup dried wild lettuce leaf and stalk
- 1 pint boiling water

Instructions:

1. Mix all the herbs. Store in an airtight container.
2. To make a hot infusion, pour 1 to 2 teaspoons of herbs in a pint-size mason jar. Drink this tea slightly more relaxedly than usual.
3. When you have a fever, drink a mugful of this.

GERD

Elderberry pie

Cake for a 9-inch (23 cm) two-outside layer pie

This pie helps relieve GERD pain

This is a heavenly, delicious berry pie for whenever; however, if there's an infection going around, it's only one method to get a portion of elderberry anticipation.

Ingredients:

- 3 cups (450 g) elderberries
- 1/4 teaspoon salt
- 11/8 cups (225 g) sugar
- 33/4 tablespoons (56 ml) lemon juice
- 21/4 tablespoons 18 g) cornstarch
- 2 tablespoons (28 g) unsalted margarine

Instructions:

1. Preheat the grill to 425°f (220°c, or gas mark 7). Line a 9-inch (23 cm) pie dish with one of the outsides.
2. Join the elderberries, salt, sugar, lemon juice, and cornstarch in a pot over medium warmth and cook until thick. Fill the cake-lined pie dish. Spot with margarine. Spread with the top hull. Seal and woodwind. Prick the covering with a fork.
3. Prepare for 10 minutes; at that point, bring down the broiler temperature to 350°f (180°c, or gas mark 4) and heat for 30 additional minutes, or until the covering is brilliant earthy colored and the juices are bubbly and thickened.

Hangover

Quick-acting hangover tea

This tea helps to quickly relieve the effects of dizziness and fatigue due to hangover.

Ingredients:

- 1 teaspoon bayberry root
- 1 teaspoon dried goldenseal root
- 2 cups boiling water
- 1 teaspoon Oregon grape root

Instructions:

1. Combine the herbs in a non-metallic vessel, then cover with boiling water; steep for 30 minutes; strain.
2. Drink several glasses throughout the day.

Spicy hangover tea

This spicy tea helps relieve hangover effects, increasing blood flow

Ingredients:

- 1 teaspoon catnip leaf
- 1 teaspoon peppermint leaves
- 2 cups boiling water
- 1 teaspoon dried chaparral leaves

Instructions:

1. Combine the herbs in a non-metallic vessel, then cover with boiling water; steep for 20 to 30 minutes;
2. Drink half a cup at a time, up to two cups a day.

Headache

Valerian root capsules

Great to treat insomnia, headaches, stomach aches.

Valerian is a powerful medicinal herb with its benefits found in the root. People who don't want to use sleeping pills often turn to valerian root instead. It also eases headaches and stomach aches. It should not be used if you're on anti-anxiety medication.

Ingredients:

- 3000–6000 mg valerian root, dried
- 10 capsules

Instructions:

1. To powder your valerian, use a mortar and pestle or a food processor. Grind until you get a sandy texture. Fill the capsules. If you're using a machine, pour the powdered herb over the machine base into one-half of the capsules. Spread the powder over the capsules to fill them. With the tamper, press the powder down so it's packed into the capsules. Keep spreading with the card and tampering until the capsules are full.
2. Sweep off any extra powder. Go ahead and take the bottom off the stand. Put the top of the capsule machine on the base and press down. The capsules should be packed now. Over a container, press down on the back of the machine's top part to release the capsules. That's it!

Based on research for capsules, we saw that herbalists often recommend shaking a little bit of valerian powder around in the container, so you'll taste a little of the root when you take a capsule. Tasting helps your body recognize what it's consuming, which can help it respond better to the powder.

Warming headache tea

If your headaches strike, you have a pale face, and the pain feels cold, dull, and broad, try this blend. These herbs warm, astringe softly and enhance circulation. (Try this if caffeine normally works as a headache cure for you.) If you experience recurring headaches and discover that this helps, drink a quart or more every day as a preventative measure.

Ingredients:

- 1 cup dried betony leaf and flower
- 1 cup dried tulsi leaf

- ½ cup dried chamomile flower
- ½ cup dried sage leaf
- ¼ cup dried ginger

Instructions:

1. Mix all the herbs. Store in an airtight container. Warm to drink. One cup of this tea should provide some relief.

Peppery headache tea

Rub a few drops of peppermint oil on your temples and forehead, then sip a cup of this peppermint tea to help relieve your headache.

Ingredients:

- 1 teaspoon feverfew leaf
- 1 teaspoon peppermint leaves
- 1 cup boiling water,
- Honey

Instructions:

1. Combine the above herbs in a non-metallic vessel, then cover with boiling water; steep for 30 minutes; strain.
2. Add honey to taste. Take a tablespoon, up to one cup a day.

Heartburn

Cleansing aloe water

This water is used for detoxing, constipation relief, and heartburn relief.

It can help with stomach issues, like constipation.

People also drink aloe water to boost their energy and immunity. If you haven't eaten aloe before, we recommend talking to a professional first.

Ingest only a small amount at a time as aloe can have laxative effects.

Ingredients:

- ½-teaspoon or 1 tablespoon aloe gel
- 1 cup water

Instructions:

1. Scrape out gel from a fresh-cut leaf into a blender or food processor. If you have never ingested aloe before, start with just ½ teaspoon.
2. Blend with water and drink!

3. To make the beverage tastier, you can add other ingredients like 100% fruit juice, cucumber, parsley, or raw honey.

Marshmallow infusion
Makes 1 quart

If you suffer from functional heartburn, the first thing you should do is a marshmallow root infusion. Keep this on hand in case of an assault to help mend the damaged tissue in the esophagus. When you have heartburn, simply drink this carefully, and you'll feel better in no time

Ingredients:

- 2 to 4 tablespoons dried marshmallow root

Instructions:

1. Combine the marshmallow with enough room-temperature water to fill a quart-size mason jar; cover and soak for 4 to 8 hours. Keep refrigerated, where each batch will last 2 to 3 days.

Preventive bitter tincture
Makes 3½ fluid ounces (about 35 to 55 doses).

Take these drops before each meal to restore normal stomach acid levels and decrease the circumstances for heartburn to develop.

Ingredients:

- 1 fluid ounce tincture dandelion root
- ½ fluid ounce tincture catnip
- ½ fluid ounce tincture chamomile
- 1/3 fluid ounce tincture fennel
- 1/3 fluid ounce tincture meadowsweet
- 1/3 fluid ounce tincture self-heal
- ½ fluid ounce tincture St. John's wort.

Instructions:

1. In a small bottle, combine the tinctures. Cap the bottle and label it.
2. Take 1½ to 2 drops 10 minutes before eating.

Hypertension

Softhearted tea
Makes 2 cups of dried herb mix (about 14 to 16 quarts of tea).

Take these drops before each meal to restore normal stomach acid levels and decrease the circumstances for heartburn to develop.

Ingredients:

- 1 cup dried linden leaf and flower
- ½ cup dried marshmallow leaf
- ½ cup dried rose petals

Instructions:

1. Mix all the herbs. Store in an airtight container.

Free-flowing circulation tea

This tea helps in blood circulation

Ingredients:

- 1 teaspoon burdock root
- 1 teaspoon goldenseal root
- 1 teaspoon cayenne
- 2 teaspoons slippery elm bark
- 3 cups boiling water, and two slices of ginger root

Instructions:

1. Combine the overhead herbs in a non-metallic vessel, strain.
2. Two tablespoons at a time, take up to one cup a day.

Arteriosclerosis preventive tea

This tea can help prevent arteriosclerosis or the hardening of the arteries.

Ingredients:

- 2 to 3 ginger slices
- 2 teaspoons ginkgo biloba leaves
- 1 teaspoon ginseng leaves

Instructions:

1. Drink up to half a cup per day.

Immune System

Vitamin C pills

Great for helping to boost the immune system and fight off colds and flu-like symptoms.

Ingredients:

- 1 tablespoon rose hip powder (the fruit of a rose plant, which has a high vitamin C content)
- 1 tablespoon amla (an Indian gooseberry, which has strong antibacterial properties) powder
- 1 tablespoon acerola (a Barbados cherry, which is great for stomach discomfort). powder

- Honey
- Orange peel (optional) (orange is a citrus fruit, and its peel is often used for flavoring) powder

Instructions:

1. Blend the powdered herbs, smoothing out any clumped powder. Pour a few droplets of slightly warmed honey into the powdered mix. Stir, add a few more droplets, and stir again. Mix until the combination holds together without being too sticky or moist.
2. Shape the mix into pea-size balls. Roll these around in the orange powder if you've decided to use it. The mixture should make 45 balls. Store these in an air-tight container to give them an extended shelf life. Take 1-3 daily.

Elderberry gummy bears

Great for an immune system-boosting treat that takes care of your well-being.

Ingredients:

- 50 g elderberries, dried
- 30 g rosehips, dried
- 15 g cinnamon chips
- 7 g licorice root
- 0.5 g pepper, freshly ground (a flowering vine, which is often used for seasoning)
- 3 cups apple cider
- 3 tablespoons gelatin (derived from collagen and used as a gelling agent in food)

Instructions:

- Place all of the ingredients (minus the gelatin) into a medium-size saucepan. Bring the mixture to simmer and continue to simmer for 20 minutes. Strain, squeeze well to extract the juice.
- Measure 2 cups juice (you can add more apple cider to make the mixture fill 2 cups). Put 1/2 cup into the fridge, then after it's chilled, dust the gelatin on top of it. Allow this to sit for one minute.
- Bring the rest of the mixture to a simmer. Combine the hot juice with the cooled gelatin mixture. Stir quickly with a whisk. If you want to sweeten this up more, add sugar or honey.

- Pour this mixture into molds and refrigerate. Eat 1–3 gummies per day, and keep them stored in a sealed container in the fridge.

Indigestion/Dyspepsia

Pre-emptive bitter tincture

Indigestion often refers to insufficient digestion. This solution stimulates all of your digestive fluids, including saliva, stomach acid, bile, and pancreatic enzymes, to ensure thorough and complete digestion.

Ingredients:

- 1 fluid ounce tincture of dandelion root
- 1 fluid ounce tincture of sage
- 1 fluid ounce tincture of catnip
- 1 fluid ounce tincture of chamomile

Instructions:

1. In a small bottle, combine the tinctures. Cap the bottle and label it.
2. Take 1 to 2 drops 10 minutes before eating.

Carminative tincture

This combination warms the core of the body, activating the digestive organs and preventing the intestines from becoming sluggish; if peppermint isn't your thing, use angelica instead.

Ingredients:

- 1½ fluid ounces tincture ginger
- 1 fluid ounce tincture fennel
- 1 fluid ounce tincture peppermint
- ½ fluid ounce tincture licorice

Instructions:

1. In a small bottle, combine the tinctures. Cap the bottle and label it.
2. Take 1 to 2 drops after each meal or whenever your guts feel uncomfortably stuck.

Strong digestive tea

This is an excellent digestive aid, and it can provide fast relief for "flatus" or ringing in the ears, as well as indigestion.

Ingredients:

- 1 teaspoon angelica root
- 1 teaspoon grated ginger root
- 2 teaspoons chamomile flowers
- 2 teaspoons peppermint leaves
- 1 cup boiling water

Instructions:

1. Combine the above ingredients in a vessel.
2. Take one tablespoon of the herb combination and place in boiling water; steep for 30 minutes; cool and strain.
3. Take as needed, up to two cups a day.

Spicy ginger elixir

This is a great digestive aid. It's also great for chest congestion.

Ingredients:

- 1/2 cup (50 g) hacked ginger
- 1 lemon, daintily cut
- 1 (4-inch, or 10 cm) cinnamon stick
- 2-star anise
- 2 cardamom units
- 1/2 cup (160 g) crude nearby honey
- 1 cup (235 ml) 100 proof vodka or liquor
- Yield: 1 cup (235 ml)

Instructions:

1. Add 1/2 tsp. of ginger root to 1 quart of boiling water.
2. Boil for 10 minutes, then allow to cool for approximately 20 minutes.
3. Strain out the ginger with a strainer or mesh cheesecloth, and drink the syrup warm or chilled in water.
4. For stomach ailments, add 2 tbsp. of ground ginger with 1 cup of honey and cinnamon at night before bedtime to help soothe your stomach muscles and ease indigestion or gas pains in the morning.

Insomnia

End-of-the-day elixir

This tea is excellent for relieving stress at the end of the day. It will help to relax any anxiety, stress, or fear and allow you a better sleep

Ingredient:

- 1 fluid ounce tincture chamomile
- 1 fluid ounce tincture betony
- ¾ fluid ounce tincture ashwagandha
- ½ fluid ounce tincture catnip
- ½ fluid ounce tincture linden
- ¼ fluid ounce honey

Instructions:

1. In a small bottle, mix the tinctures and honey in a small bottle. Cap and label it.
2. Take 1 to 2 drops one hour before bedtime.
3. Take another 1 to 2 drops 30 minutes before bedtime.
4. Take the last 1 to 2 drops before going to bed.

Sleep formula

This formula helps with insomnia and other sleep disorders. It's also great for fighting fatigue since lack of sleep causes lethargy.

Ingredients:

- 2 fluid ounces tincture wild lettuce
- 1 fluid ounce tincture betony
- ½ fluid ounce tincture chamomile
- ½ fluid ounce tincture linden

Instructions:

1. Same as per the previous recipe, "End-of-the-day elixir."

Goodnight tincture 1 (strong version)

Ingredients:

- 3 tbsp. betony flowers tincture
- 3 tbsp. valerian root tincture
- 3 tbsp. chamomile flowers tincture
- 3 tbsp. linden leaves tincture

Instructions:

1. Put the tinctures in an amber glass bottle with a dropper lid in the indicated proportions. Label it. Take 3 drops one hour before bedtime. Then 2 more half an hour before bedtime. Finally, 2 drops before going to bed.

Goodnight tincture 2 (soft version)

Ingredients:

- 3 tbsp. valerian root tincture
- 3 tbsp. chamomile flowers tincture
- 3 tbsp. linden leaves tincture

Instructions:

1. Put the tinctures in an amber glass bottle with a dropper lid in the indicated proportions. Label it. Take 3 drops one hour before bedtime. Then 2 more half an hour before bedtime. Finally, 2 drops before going to bed.

Shower for restful sleep

Makes 1 application.

A decent steaming shower implanted with these ingredients alleviates the considerations of the day and their physical appearances.

Ingredients:

- 1/4 cup dried passionflower
- 1/4 cup oat straw
- 1/4 cup (90 g) Epsom salts
- Boiling water

Instructions:

1. Spot the ingredients into a muslin pack or tie into the focal point of a washcloth. Ensure the herbs have enough space to mix without any problem. Spot in a 2-quart (2 L) pitcher (unbending plastic is fine). Boiling water should be poured over the herbs and left to steep for 10 to 15 minutes while you take a shower.
2. Pour the soaks shower tea and bundle into the tub. Absorb a full tub. The magnesium in the Epsom salts makes an extraordinary expansion to the antispasmodic, loosening up the activity of the herbs.

Lupus

Ginger mint liniment

This liniment helps relieve lupus pain.

Ingredients:

- 1/4 cup (25 g) ground new ginger
- 11/4 cups (295 ml) olive oil
- 5 to 10 drops peppermint fundamental oil

Instructions:

1. Warm the ginger and the olive oil together over the least warmth setting for as long as 60 minutes. Expel from the warmth and permit to rest for the time being. Strain the cooled oil through an espresso channel to evacuate all solids.
2. Include the fundamental oil. Fill bottles. Back rub a small quantity on your hand into sore regions tenderly to diminish pain.

Nausea And Vomiting

Rescue tincture

This is great to stop the urge to vomit.

Ingredients:

- 4 tbsp. ginger root tincture
- 2 tbsp. catnip leaves and flowers tincture
- 2 tbsp. chamomile flowers tincture

Instructions:

1. Put the tinctures in an amber glass bottle with a dropper lid in the indicated proportions. Label it.
2. Take 3 drops every half an hour until you do not feel the urge to vomit anymore.

Soothing tea (after vomiting)

Ingredients:

- 1 tsp. catnip dried leaves and flowers
- 1 tsp. chamomile dried flowers
- 1 tsp. powdered ginger root
- 1 tsp. peppermint dried leaves
- 1 cup distilled boiling water

Instructions:

1. Pour boiling water over the herbs mixture. Let rest for thirty minutes—strain and drink throughout the day.

Meadowsweet elixir

Meadowsweet, or Ditassa, is a common herb found in most parts of North America. It is extremely useful for many ailments, including coughs and colds.

It also helps with urinary tract infections, diarrhea, nausea, and vomiting.

Ingredients:

- 100 g meadowsweet flowers (a European flower that is known as 'the stomach corrector')
- 40 ml 50% vodka (a distilled alcoholic drink that consists primarily of water and ethanol)
- 100 ml glycerin (a sugar-alcohol compound often used in elixirs and skincare products)

Instructions:

1. Place the meadowsweet flowers in a jar, and then add the vodka and glycerin. Shake well and let it macerate for 4–6 weeks.
2. Check the mixture often, as sometimes the flowers will soak up the alcohol and glycerin so that the liquid no longer covers the herb. In this case, you either need to use a stone to weigh them down or add more alcohol.
3. After 4–6 weeks, you need to strain the mixture to be ready for use.
4. Drink a shot of this in case of pain.

Rash

Hiker's rash relief

If you have a hiker's rash, this ointment will help soothe the itching and help the rash heal. The best news about it is that it can also be used to cure diaper rash!

Ingredients:

- 1 teaspoon sage leaves (I use "biergarten" for its extremely high proportion of basic oil)
- 1 teaspoon plantain leaves
- ½ teaspoon yarrow flowers and leaves
- 1 teaspoon jewelweed (cut from the get-go in the mid-year when the stems are succulent and delicious)
- 2 tablespoons apple juice vinegar

Instructions:

1. Join the herbs in a container and add apple juice vinegar to cover; permit to soak for a month if conceivable. Strain enough to fill a shower container and use. A small amount on your palm is enough to treat the rash. I leave the rest splashing for as long as could reasonably be expected.

Rash wash

This is a great way to help prevent rashes from appearing, or to help reduce an existing rash.

Ingredients:

- 1 teaspoon comfrey root
- 1 teaspoon white oak leaves or bark
- 1 teaspoon slippery elm bark

Instructions:

1. Mix the herbs with hot water and let it cool. Transfer to a jar or spray bottle.
2. Use as a topical wash, as needed.

Reflux

Salvia fritta

Salvia fritta is a great tea that can help relieve symptoms of the common cold. It's also good for treating symptoms of stomach problems, diarrhea, and even dengue fever.

Ingredients:

- 1 cup (226 g) coconut oil
- 1/4 cup (40 g) flour
- 1/4 cup (30 g) cornstarch

- 1/2 cup (120 ml) soft drinking water
- 16 to 24 flawless sage leaves
- Sea salt

Instructions:

1. Warm the oil in a griddle. While it warms, join the flour, cornstarch, and soft drinking water in a bowl and whisk well.

2. Dig the savvy leaves in the heater. At the point when the oil is acceptable and hot, include 4 or 5 of the leaves in the skillet, and fry until brilliant earthy colored. Remove them from the oil and let them dry on paper towels. Rehash until all the leaves are seared.
3. Spare the oil; you can utilize it for cooking poultry, potatoes, or veggies later.

Sinusitis/Stuffy Nose
Sinus-clearing steam bath
Makes 2 cups dried herb mix (about 6 to 10 steams)

Steaming is a universal remedy throughout cultures for all respiratory system problems, including sinus problems. The combination of heated steam and evaporating volatile oils from herbs makes pathogen survival very difficult and triggers an immune response in the mucous membranes.

Ingredients:

- 1 cup dried pine needles
- ½ cup dried sage leaf
- ½ cup dried thyme leaf
- ½ gallon water
- Five garlic cloves, chopped, per steam (optional)

Instructions:

1. Mix the pine, sage, and thyme. Store in an airtight container.
2. To make and use herbal steam, boil the water in a medium saucepan over high heat.
3. Create a tent through a blanket or towel over the pot and lay it on a heat-resistant surface where you can sit near it.
4. Add ¼ to ½ cup of the herb mixture to the water, along with the garlic (if using)
5. Bring a handkerchief, as your nose will run as your sinuses clear!
6. Repeat 2 to 3 times per day

Sore Muscles
Ginger bath
This bath helps relieve sore muscle pain.

Ingredients:

- 1 cup (100 g) ground or cut ginger
- Yield: 1 application

Instructions:

1. Spot the ginger in a muslin sack and tie safely. Spot the muslin sack in a tub of high temp water and steep for 10 minutes. Or on the other hand, join the sack to the spigot and permit high temp water to go through it. Absorb the hot shower for 20 to 30 minutes.

Sore Throat
Horehound lozenges
These lozenges can be used to soothe a sore throat and promote irritation relief.

Ingredients:

- 1½ cups horehound leaves
- 1½ cups water
- 3 cups sugar
- Three tablespoons corn syrup.

Instructions:

1. Place the horehound leaves in a pan and cover them with water.

Sore throat gargle #1
Ingredients:

- 1 tbsp. sumac root double extraction
- 1 tbsp. Echinacea root double extraction
- 2 tsp. distilled water

Instructions:

1. Combine the extractions and dilute them with water in the indicated proportions. Gargle with it.

Sore throat gargle #2
Ingredients:

- 2 tbsp. dried sage leaves
- 3 tsp. Epsom salts
- ½ pint apple cider vinegar
- ½ pint distilled water

Instructions:

1. In a saucepan, bring the water to a boil and pour the sage into it. Let simmer for half an hour. Let cool, strain, and pour in a mason jar. Add salt and apple cider vinegar. Cover with the lid and shake to make the salt dissolve. Use it for gargling whenever needed. Remember to rinse with clean water afterwards to avoid damage to the teeth due to the apple cider vinegar.

Fire cider

It makes about 1 quart

Traditional fire cider recipes are blends of spicy and aromatic stimulating expectorants that will heat you and assist you in removing the mucus. We slip in several immunity boosters and a rich source of Vitamin C in this version.

Ingredients:

- 1 whole head garlic, chopped
- 1 (2-inch) piece fresh ginger, chopped
- ¼ cup dried pine needles
- ¼ cup dried sage leaf
- ¼ cup dried thyme leaf
- ¼ cup dried elderberry
- ¼ cup dried rose hips
- 2 tablespoons dried elecampane root
- 2 tablespoons dried angelica root
- 1-quart of apple cider vinegar
- For sweetening or diluting, use honey or water (optional)

Instructions:

1. Combine the garlic, ginger, and additional herbs in a jar.
2. Fill the jar with vinegar (when exposed to vinegar, the coating on the bottom of metal mason jar lids corrodes).
3. Allow the herbs to macerate in the vinegar for at least two weeks.
4. Strain the final fire cider, bottle, and label it. If the vinegar is too pungent for you, dilute it with water or add some honey (up to one-fourth of the entire amount).
5. Take a shot (about ½ fluid ounce) at the first sign of mucus buildup in the lungs and every couple of hours thereafter until symptoms resolve.

Ginger emergency formula

It's best to take this formula when you feel your throat swelling.

It will open and relieve the swollen and inflamed glands in your throat.

Ingredients:

- 2 fluids ounces tincture ginger
- 1 fluid ounce tincture catnip

- 1 fluid ounce tincture chamomile
- 1 fluid ounce honey

Instructions:

1. In a small jar or bottle, combine all of the ingredients. Cap and label it.

Sprains And Strains

Soft tissue injury liniment

This liniment is great for treating sprains, strains, and bruises.

It makes about eight fluid ounces.

Ingredients:

- 3 fluid ounces of ginger-infused oil
- 2 fluid ounces of tincture Solomon's seal or Solomon's seal-infused oil
- 1 fluid ounce tincture St. John's wort
- 1 fluid ounce tincture self-heal
- 1 fluid ounce tincture meadowsweet
- 40 drops peppermint essential oil
- 40 drops cinnamon essential oil

Instructions:

1. Mix the infused oils, tinctures, and essential oils in a small bottle or container. Cap and label it. Shake it vigorously before each use.
2. Drop a tiny bit in your palm. Warm the remedy between your palms before applying it to the hurting joints.
3. Massage the oil into your joints until your hands are no longer slick. Work the cream into the tissue.
4. Repeat the application 3–5 times a day.

Stress

Oat straw infusion

This infusion has a cooling and relaxing effect if you feel stressed or anxious and is great for its calming, stress-relieving effect.

Ingredients:

- 2 oz of the oat straw herb (comes from Avena sativa, which has long-lasting energy effects)

- Boiling water

Instructions:

1. Put oat straw into a 1-quart jar, then pour boiling water over the herb. Cap it with an air-tight lid.
2. Allow the mix to rest for 4–6 hours, which will infuse the minerals throughout the solution.
3. Strain it. If you choose to, you can add a little extra to your mixture once it's made; lavender, lemon verbena, rosemary, etc.
4. Oat straw can be used as a base for juices, lemonades, and frozen concentrates. You can use it to create ice cubes or ice pops if you want a variation.

Rescue elixir

This tea can help bring down stress effects and relieve brain fog.

Ingredients:

- 1 fluid ounce tincture tulsi
- 1 fluid ounce tincture betony
- ½ fluid ounce tincture catnip
- ½ fluid ounce tincture chamomile
- ½ fluid ounce tincture elderflower
- ½ fluid ounce tincture rose
- ¼ fluid ounce tincture goldenrod
- ¼ fluid ounce tincture sage
- ½ fluid ounce honey

Instructions:

1. In a small container or bottle, mix the honey and the tinctures. Cap and label it.
2. Take 2 to 4 drops whenever needed.

Calm candy

The herbs in these sweets help ease uneasiness, stress, and overexcitement.

Ingredients:

- 11/2 cups (355 ml) water
- 1/4 cup new passionflower
- 1/4 cup new lemon ointment
- 1/4 cup new chamomile
- Juice and zest of 2 lemons
- Unsalted spread

- 3 cups (600 g) sugar
- 1/2 cup (160 g) corn syrup or honey (if utilizing honey, the sweets will most likely stay clingy)

- Confectioners' sugar or cornstarch for sprinkling
- Yield: 1 pound (454 g)

Instructions:

1. Pour the water, herbs, and lemon squeeze and pizzazz in an enormous pot over medium-low warmth.
2. Stew to lessen the fluid to 1 cup (235 ml). Meanwhile, add margarine to a baking dish.
3. Add the sugar and corn syrup and mix until the sugar disintegrates. Clasp a treats thermometer to the side of the skillet. Increase the warmth, heat to the point of boiling, and bubble to 300°F (150°C), with as meager blending as could reasonably be expected. Expel from the warmth and empty the hot blend into a baking dish. Let cool.
4. While it very well may be taken care of, cut into pieces and sprinkle with confectioners' sugar or cornstarch to shield the pieces from sticking together. On the other hand, pour onto a spread preparing sheet to 1/4-inch (6 mm) thick, and break into pieces when cooled.

Chamomile remedy

The remedy is brilliant for clearing a stuffy nose. Repeat as needed.

Ingredients:

- 2 handfuls chamomile flowers, dried
- 10 chamomile tea bags (a relaxing, rejuvenating herb)
- Boiled water

Instructions:

1. Bring 2 quarts of water to a boil, then remove from the heat, and put in the dried chamomile flowers. Cover the pot and leave for 15 minutes before placing it on a heating pad. Place a towel over your head as you breathe in the steam by leaning over the pot; this will help unblock your sinuses.

CONCLUSION

Medicinal plants are a great way to get the good stuff out of the ground and into your body; they can help with everything from relieving muscle pain to improving brain function. There are many medicinal plants that can be used to treat various skin conditions.

Medicinal plants are an important part of any natural medicine cabinet. They have been used for centuries by humans to help with ailments and diseases. Many medicinal plants have been used by ancient cultures for centuries. Most of these plants contain potent chemicals that can help with a large variety of ailments.

Starting out learning herbalism and plant-based home remedies can be difficult, but I hope, and I'm sure, that this book has been an excellent primer for you to continue your journey.

The world of medicinal herbs offers you and your family a new, natural world of healing. As you progress in your journey, I hope you discover you can reduce your reliance on harsh prescription drugs.

Regardless of the reasons you're interested in herbalism, you'll discover an overall improvement in your life. That's one of the marvelous side-effects of holistic healing. The intention of your specific therapy with that one herb or combination of herbs may not have been to make you feel better emotionally; nonetheless, it happened.

Numerous medicinal plants have been used for ages to heal a variety of diseases, and there's a good chance you don't know them. Maybe you even stopped taking your medication because you found a natural alternative.

For simple ailments, you can always resort to herbal remedies like the ones we have discussed in this book. There is no need to create dependency on prescription drugs. Going herbal is much safer and healthier most of the time. If you may have any doubt, always consult your physician first.

Many physical issues may be resolved by altering our lifestyle and the social relationships we have with people around us. We may alleviate stress and anxiety by caring for people who care about us, allowing us to discover inner peace. Emotional imbalance is a concern just as much as physical disorders and diseases.

To be able to accept holistic treatment and cure, we must first deal with our emotions.

With this book on your shelf, you will always have the ancient wisdom of Native Americans at your fingertips. Remember to investigate every substance you take and don't delegate responsibility for your healing to anyone but experts.

BOOK 6

HERBAL DISPENSATORY VOL. 1

Learn How to Get, Treat and Use the Best Medicinal Herbs

Citali Galwen

INTRODUCTION

Native American herbalism is a practice handed down from generation to generation that is deeply rooted in the culture of Native American communities across North America over centuries. Today, however, this information is often overlooked and misunderstood as Native Americans are often marginalized and oppressed.

One of the main attributes of Native American herbalism is that each individual had their own treatment method that they preferred for treating ailments. They did not follow "one-size-fits-all" regimens for common maladies. In fact, the opposite was true. Indigenous healing traditions all had different methods and remedies for treating particular illnesses and conditions, while some traditions utilized methods that were useful in a broad spectrum of ailments. There was also a vast array of plants utilized across different cultures and communities with unknown purposes or perceived powers.

What Is Dispensatory?

"Dispensatory" is a word that describes a set of beliefs about health and illness, which may be rooted in religious practices or cultural traditions. It is based upon the premise that the entire body has "spiritual" components, such as the air one breathes or the water one drinks. This premise is then used to justify certain plant uses and modes of preparation because plants are seen as having an active spiritual essence. The belief in this spiritual energy and spirit of plants was one of the main concepts behind herbal medicine in Europe when it arrived in North America and other parts of the world. The term "dispensatory" is derived from the Latin word "dispendio," which means to be separated. So, the belief was that plants had an active life force or supernatural energy that they are separated away from as they are grown, cut, and used in herbal medicine. This spiritual force is believed to be exhausted when plants are used for medicinal purposes.

Native American Herbalism Dispensatory

Native American herbalism dispenses a rich diversity of plants with diverse uses. The medicinal and ritual attributes of those plants vary widely, depending on where they are found and the cultural traditions that surround them. The Cherokees, for example, viewed some plants as evil and made efforts to avoid them. Other traditions have a complex classification system that designates certain plants for specific uses and others for different purposes. The Paiute people used pine pitch in sacred ceremonies; the Cree used spruce gum as chewing gum; and the Potawatomi used plum trees' fruit, leaves, bark, and nuts for medicinal purposes.

Native Americans often incorporate herbal remedies into the daily routine of healing ills and treating disease in both their native lands and those of other cultures. A common belief is that all of nature is interconnected with each other, and all parts of the world share an important role in the spiritual realm. The plants are studied for their spiritual value as well, and information about their medicinal uses is handed down through generations as part of that belief system.

A number of Native American communities have different rituals performed for medicinal plants depending on how they will be used, which is another important aspect of herbal medicine in North America. When certain parts of a plant—flowers, roots, leaves, or wood—are used for specific purposes such as healing or ceremonial purposes, there can be special rituals and prayers performed along with the use of those plants to ensure that they are respected.

This book will examine the healing properties of many Native American medicinal plants, their uses, and the history of herbal medicine in North America. Details about plant uses and treatments related to health care and physical ailments will be included.

The Herbalist And His Role

As a child, do you recall your family members offering you a nice warm cup of herb tea? Perhaps you had a grandmother or a loving mother who used herb tea to treat you as a child when you were ill.

If so, do you recall those earlier days as being healthy – days when your classmates were absent from school due to colds and flu, but you were not? You were always present at school and in good health.

If you remained healthy while others became ill, you realized that your mother's or grandmother's 'potions' boosted your immunity in some way. Occasionally, those cups of tea did not taste particularly good, but they did the job.

Perhaps your father was an avid gardener who set aside a special plot for herbs. Each time you passed by that section of the backyard, you were compelled to stop and smell the lovely scents, and it piqued your interest.

Perhaps you've thought to yourself, "I will eventually have my own garden. One day, I'll learn how to cook with these herbs and how to use them to improve my health."

Or perhaps you came from a family or a profession that relied on medical treatments for everything from a cold to cancer, and you witnessed firsthand how medical treatment could be ineffective at times.

You desired something more – something that provided a modicum of assurance regarding healing and recovery – without causing any side effects. You reflected to yourself, "I'm sure there must be something out there that works and can assist Mama and the rest of us in regaining our health. I will eventually locate it."

You reasoned that by learning more about herbs, you could potentially gain control over your own and your family's health.

That is an accurate statement.

The more you know and understand about herbs, the more effective their use will be. Additionally, the more herbs you use, the healthier you will become.

Discovering Herbs Is A Life-Changing Experience

Whatever your reason for being interested in herbs, the good news is that you can learn how to use them medicinally. To do this effectively, you'll want to pursue certification as a Master Herbalist.

A Master Herbalist has studied herbs – their history, how they are used, what they look like, when they can be used, what dosage they require, how they grow, and how to prepare herbal preparations from them.

A Master Herbalist uses herbs to treat a variety of minor ailments that arise at home, such as constipation or diarrhea, determining what to recommend to a friend or family member who is ill, or reviving tired feet.

Becoming A Master Herbalist Enhances Your Quality Of Life

As you can see from this list, a Master Herbalist possesses a wealth of general knowledge regarding how to improve a person's or family's quality of life. Numerous minor issues nag us day after day until we take action.

And frequently, there are few viable options for eradicating them. Eventually, we end up carrying far too many 'problems' throughout our lives. Then we become irritable.

Consider one of your worst days, when your baby refused to sleep and your feet were so tired and painful that you couldn't stand.

What would you do in this situation? Would you know what to do to achieve results and restore everyone's smile?

The issue is that the majority of people experience these "worst days" throughout their lives. Their health problems continue to accumulate as the years pass. Individuals appear as if they've borne the weight of the world – which they have!

Small Signs Develop Into Serious Health Problems

The unfortunate part is that these issues that arise during the darkest days are indicators of future health problems – more serious ones – that will manifest later in life.

PMS may be an early sign of endometriosis, which impairs fertility. Constipation can become chronic and result in colon cancer. Diarrhea may be a symptom of a parasitic infection, which can cause a variety of health problems. That non-sleeping baby will end up disrupting your sleep and making you more prone to accidents. Rodents may not be far behind those ants.

That cousin who is having difficulties with studying may be diagnosed with Attention Deficit Disorder and placed on Ritalin for ten years. Your tired feet could be a sign of plantar fasciitis, heel spurs, or bunions, or other foot problems associated with flat feet. And that case of the flu may develop complications, such as diabetes or rheumatoid arthritis.

We must resolve these minor issues within our own lives. And, in many cases, popping a pill only creates a bigger problem for us later.

One of the reasons I enjoy my work as a Master Herbalist is that I enjoy problem solving. When I do, I am able to maintain my composure regardless of what happens. I'm always prepared. A Master Herbalist is well versed in the use of plants in a wide variety of situations.

Herbalists Are Divided Into Three Types

Herbalists are not all the same. You can train to become one of three types of herbalists:

A Do-It-Yourself Herbalist

This type of herbalist reads about herbs haphazardly and randomly and lacks formal herbal training. Each and every one of us begins as an Armchair Herbalist. While you are an Armchair Herbalist, you are in a state of mind where you are discovering the wonders of herbology, the study of herbs. The wonderful things you read about herbs stick with you and serve as a springboard for further study. What you read frequently provides the impetus to continue – or, if you read negative things about herbs, it provides the impetus to abandon the subject.

However, at this point in your herbal development, you are knowledgeable enough to address a few minor issues that may arise. You will lack the necessary knowledge to deal with difficult cases or scenarios. And during this stage, it is possible to make numerous errors.

An Aspiring Herbalist

When you decide to pursue formal herbology training, you've taken a significant step forward. Herbal knowledge is passed down from individual to individual, culture to culture, teacher to student, and classroom to classroom.

An Herbalist in Training learns thousands of details and stories about how herbs were used in each class. Each class introduces new principles that lay the groundwork for making sound herb selections in a variety of situations.

While an Herbalist in Training does not understand all of herbology's major concepts, he or she does understand some of them and is much more likely to be correct than an Armchair Herbalist. However, a Herbalist in Training improves in accuracy as more classes on herbs and how to use them are taken.

Taking an herbal class provides you with access to a teacher who has been using herbs for several years and is willing to share what they've learned. A teacher is available when you require herbal advice, and it is during these times that you will most likely learn and grow.

The majority of obstacles we encounter in life recur, and the sooner you master their resolution, the sooner you can return to a calm, peaceful life while sipping your next cup of herbal tea!

An Expert Herbalist

A Master Herbalist is an herbalist who is prepared to truly assist one's family, friends, and community. A Master Herbalist may sign their name with the abbreviation "M.H." These credentials are not distributed randomly! A Master Herbalist must complete a comprehensive curriculum that includes classes such as Anatomy and Physiology, Endocrinology, and Chemistry.

However, do not be alarmed. The classes are structured in such a way that you will gradually and steadily increase your knowledge. Each class – and there are many to choose from – has assigned work, and frequently, projects are required. This homework is to ensure that you understand the material completely.

Whoever tells you that these classes are unnecessary is limiting your future effectiveness as an herbalist.

Take the Straight Path, and the Rewards Will Be Numerous

Attendance at classes is insufficient to qualify as a Master Herbalist. You must master information in order to make the greatest impact on those around you.

The Master Herbalist must pass a comprehensive examination covering all of the knowledge acquired over the course of two to three years. Additionally, you must devote considerable time to researching a particular problem and its herbal remedy.

This research is compiled and finalized with your recommendations in a thesis, much like a thesis for a university or college's Master's or Doctorate program. Taking the test and completing a thesis demonstrates that you have mastered the material. That is when you can walk away with the "M.H." credentials.

The path to becoming a Master Herbalist is fraught with peril. Each time you encounter a new situation in life, you will begin to think "herbally" and consider how to overcome the obstacle naturally. Your mind will recall herbal classes and will recall a story or specific and detailed information about herbs that will assist you in resolving the new situation.

You learn to solve problems by conversing with your classmates and instructors. It's also simple to form long-lasting friendships at that time. Herbalists share their knowledge because everyone needs a little assistance every now and then!

Another thing to consider is this: if you were ever seriously ill, who would you want to look after you? "Another Master Herbalist," you would respond as a Master Herbalist. That is because you have witnessed both the wonder and miracles of God's provision for His people through His herbs. You provide a space for hope on days when you're ill, and two, people who share a common belief are preferable to one person who must go it alone.

CHAPTER 17:

GETTING STARTED

Basic Concepts In Native American Herbalism

Native American Herbalism is an herbal system created by indigenous people long before any European system of medicine reached this continent. It is a part of many Native American cultures and continues to be used by the First Nations' peoples today. The roots of this healing tradition are intertwined with the culture, spirituality, religion, and language of these nations.

The primary practitioners were women called "curers" or "medicine women." They would use plants found in their surroundings-the woods, mountains, streams, and lakes—to treat spiritual, physical, and psychological problems in patients as well as in rself. These medicines were also traditionally passed down through families from one generation to the next.

While many sources attribute the origins of Native American Herbal Medicine to the ancient Egyptians, it appears that its beginnings predate this by several thousand years.

In the healthcare system of North America before European settlement, most medicines were made from plants (of which there were approximately two million in North America alone) and animals. Native American herbalism is rooted in traditional societies, as all other aspects of their culture and spirituality. In fact, the use of indigenous herbal medicines is an integral part of Native American spirituality. Many Native Americans view their native plant medicines as gifts from the Creator; treating with them is akin to treating with deities.

Herbal Energetics

Native Americans used herbal energetics for many of their medicinal needs. Herbal energetics is the use or application of herbs to release healing energies or vibrations into a body, disharmonious energy into a body, or to remove disharmonious energy from a body. In other words, it's the practice of using herbs as medicine as well as an alternative medical treatment.

Herbs are used for their healing properties; the different chemical components create unique effects on the body. Many herbs are used for medicinal purposes, but some herbs are also used as an alternative medicine to treat certain ailments, like sickness or pain. Herbal energetics is considered an alternative medicine because it uses herbal preparations to treat specific ailments. For example, it may be used for relieving pain and other symptoms associated with arthritis or gout.

The holistic approach to herbal energetics is a more natural approach compared to the chemicals introduced into the body by western medicine. The differences between western medicine and herbal energetics run deeper than just the differences in methods of treatment. Let's explore how these two approaches offer benefits to the patient and also contrast their shortcomings.

Herbal energetics was commonly used by Native Americans before European colonists came to America.

How Herbs Affect Energy Production

Herbs are classified according to this system of energy production. In Native American herbalism, each herb is characterized in the same way. The herbs are either warming or cooling in nature.

A warming herb increases the body's ability to generate heat and catalyzes metabolism. A cooling herb acts to lower body temperature and tends to slow down metabolism.

In general, most indigenous medicines originating from Western North America were classified as "warming" or "hot." Those from Eastern North America were usually classified as "cooling" or "cold."

There is some variation in this classification. Generally, the colder herbs tend to be more potent in medicinal action than the warmer herbs.

Some herbalists are advocating a return to these original systems of classification.

Many Native Americans now find themselves unable to obtain traditional medicines or plants from their native lands where they originated due to new government policies that prohibit them from possessing such items. They are also at a loss for the proper preparation techniques as taught and passed down by their elders since they have not had the opportunity to learn these skills.

How Herbs Affect The Density Of Tissues

Determining if herbs have a moistening or drying effect is the second level of energy classification.

A drying herb will tend to increase the amount of water that is held in or evaporated from the body's cells. A moistening herb will tend to pull fluids out of tissues or increase the number of fluids in tissues.

Herbs can be classified as neutral or balanced, which means they do not act on water content to create either moisture (drying) or dryness (moistening) but work on other factors in a more free-flowing manner.

We can see how attitudes towards Native American herbalism have changed slightly over time. It was once fairly common to classify Native American herbs as either "cold" or "hot." Now many people have begun to categorize them with a more neutral ability to either restore water or remove it from the body.

Many of these medicines are still available, and many modern pharmacological treatments have a direct relationship to these herbal medicine practices.

How Herbs Affect Muscle Tone, Flow, And Secretion

Classifying herbs as "relaxing" or "constricting" is the third level of energy classification.

A constricting herb will tend to increase the amount of water that is held in blood vessels and other vessels throughout the body. A relaxing herb will tend to decrease muscle tone, flow, and secretion and tends to slow down metabolic processes.

Herbs can be classified as neutral or balanced, which means they do not act on water content to create either rigidity (constricting) or relaxation (relaxing) but work on other factors in a more free-flowing manner.

All in all, the basic theme underlying all these classifications is to take a sample of a plant and look at how it interacts with the body in terms of the three different levels of action.

CHAPTER 18:

START YOUR HOME APOTHECARY

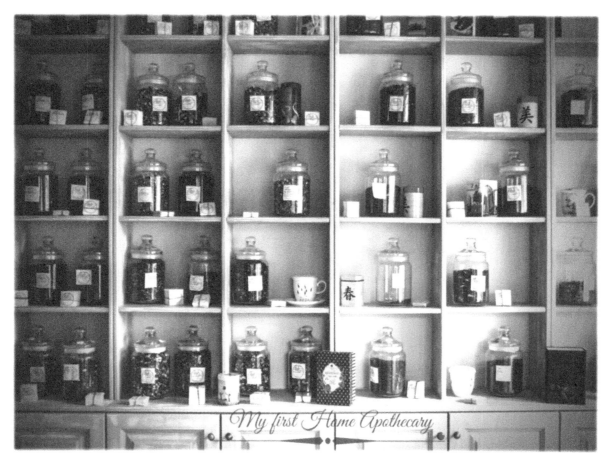

My first Home Apothecary

Start Your Herbalism Journey Where You Live

If you want to have your home apothecary, you need to know how to properly care for herbs. And if you want to learn how, you need to start where the herbs are grown--in your own backyard. You can start a backyard apothecary today with a few basic ingredients.

You will need a closed-door area, out of direct sunlight, that can be sealed off from the rest of your home. A shed or garage is ideal for storage because it's dark and private. If you have a wide-open area in your yard or garden, consider digging a small hole in the ground to store the herbs. You can easily pull it up, cover it with dirt, and plant something else the next growing season.

For your first herbal medicine-making efforts, consider growing easy herbs like comfrey (Symphytum officinale), peppermint (Mentha piperita), chamomile (Matricaria recutita), or calendula (Calendula officinalis). These are hardy annuals that give you a great bang for your buck.

You don't need a lot of fancy equipment to start making medicine. After you learn how to dry and grind herbs, you can buy a set of inexpensive mortar and pestle and start small with these essentials.

What If You Live In The City?

If you live in a city, you may not have a place to grow herbs. But most metropolitan areas have a garden center or a flower shop where you can purchase your herbs. And many groceries and department stores stock them as well.

One thing to remember when purchasing dried herbs is that you are paying for the time, care, and expertise that went into growing them. When purchasing fresh herbs, ask how long they've been on the shelf. If you're buying organic herbs, make sure they haven't been irradiated (a treatment some food and drug stores use to maintain appearance and shelf life).

Apothecary Equipment You Would Need To Start

Mortar and pestle

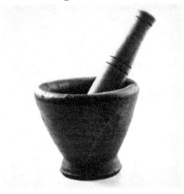

To grind your herbs into a fine powder that is ready to be put into capsules or ointments.

Capsule molder

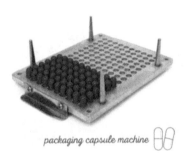

packaging capsule machine

To get the powdered herbs to a size that can easily go into capsules so you can take them with you on the go.

Tea ball infuser

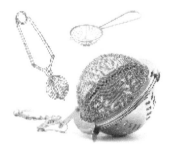

These are great for making herbal teas quickly and easily.

Dropper bottles

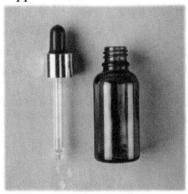

These are used for putting liquids in and dispensing them later on without spilling or anything else going wrong.

Gauze

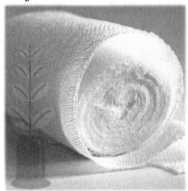

Gauze is used for wrapping around plants or for making herbal poultices.

Pouches and sachets

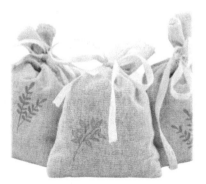

These are used for storing and transporting herbs or powders. They are usually easy to seal tightly so that there is a better chance of them lasting longer than normal.

Dishcloths

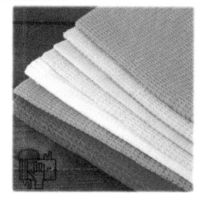

You will need to clean off your mortar and pestle a lot, so having one or two dishcloths ready on your countertop is a good idea.

Measuring spoons, cups, and teaspoons

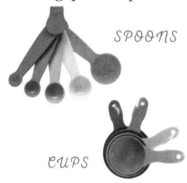

You will need a good set of measuring tools for measuring out the correct amount of herbs in each of your recipes. Always make sure that you have the proper tools when you begin doing this!

Plastic bowls

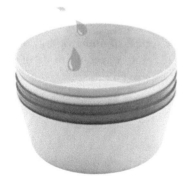

Pretty much any type of plastic bowl that can be washed in hot water is good for this kind of thing.

Bottles with lids

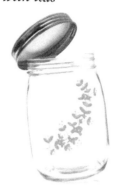

Most liquids are stored in bottles with lids, so if you don't already have enough of them, then you should get yourself a couple of extras for this purpose.

Ziploc bags

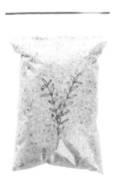

Ziploc bags are good for storing dried ingredients and keeping them fresh. This way, you can use them as many times as possible before making a new batch.

Small tin cans with lids

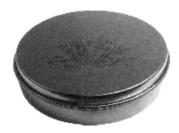

These are useful for storing various things in, especially if they are already sterile when you buy them. They are also useful for storing teas and tinctures in small quantities.

Important Considerations When Building Your Home Apothecary

In ancient times, people paid a great deal of attention to the advice of their herbalists. Whenever someone became sick or fell ill, the first thing that they did was seek the help of their herbalist. Although modern medicines have taken over most of our lives, there are still many who look to herbs for healing purposes rather than using chemical drugs.

This is where the home apothecary becomes very important. It is even more important now that we are aware of what can go into these products and how they affect us on a physical level.

If you live in a place where herbs are not readily available, then it's time to start shopping around for some. This will help you to create your own unique herbal remedies that you can easily take with you wherever you are.

Some people like to have everything in one place for convenience, but others prefer to have their herbs and medicine in several different places for safety reasons.

The next step is to learn how to use the various items that should be a part of your home apothecary. The more you know about your tools and how to use them, the better results you will get from your remedies.

The final step is simply to start gathering your herbs and making your own natural remedies. You should make sure that you do this as safely as possible so that you aren't poisoning yourself, but even if everything is done correctly, there are still things that you need to know about the herbal remedies that can help prevent any dangerous side effects.

One very important thing when it comes to using herbal remedies is not letting them get old. Just like with medications, keeping a stable supply of all of the different herbs in your apothecary will benefit you on a daily basis.

Home Apothecary Downsides

One of the drawbacks to the home apothecary is that you never really know how much dried herbs you will need to create a certain remedy or elixir. Herbalists usually take this into consideration, but regular folk don't often look into it in great detail. This does make it difficult to know which herbs you should grow or get when you are using dried herbs for healing purposes.

When you shop for your herbs and medicine, always try to buy them in bulk. You can do this at most health food stores, but it's best if you can find them lined up along the wall where they have been sitting for years before being purchased by anyone else.

This is because some herbs are very delicate and can lose their potency over a short period of time. It's best to let the professionals store them for you so that you can be sure that they haven't sat on the shelf for years at a time.

The downside to this is that you may end up with more herbs than you need, but it gives you an idea of how much space your apothecary will take up if everything in it is fresh.

Dried herbs are probably better stored in plastic containers rather than glass ones, but that depends on your opinion and the type of herb you have acquired. There are also some herbs that need to be kept as dry as possible. This is usually the case with the more highly-reputed herbs and the ones that take much longer to dry out.

If you like to import herbal remedies from Amazon, then you will want to use a secure shipping option on any packages that contain dried herbs. Generally speaking, gently letting packaged herbs flutter around inside of your mail box for a few weeks is acceptable as long as they are not crushed or sitting in too much moisture.

Tips And Tricks For Beginners

Keep everything super-clean
Even if you think that the only thing you will be using your apothecary for is storing herbs, it's still important to keep everything as clean as possible. This includes the mortar and pestle, any gourds that you may have, and even the various containers in which you keep your herbs.

Get some good storage containers
If you don't have enough storage containers to hold all of your herbal remedies, then it is probably best if you start making smaller batches until you can afford some more storage containers.

Use glass jars for dried herbs
When you start building your home apothecary, it's not a bad idea to use glass jars when storing dried herbs. It may be too early to start using the jars that were used to store jams or pickles, but you can still find some of the canning jars that are used for this purpose at very low prices.

Use liquid containers for oils and extracts

If you are planning on making any herbal oil or extract, then it is best if you use a kit that is currently available on the market. This will include everything that you need to create the oil or extract and is also very convenient. You don't have to purchase a jar of oil and then have to wait for it to become usable; all you have to do is start using it and be sure that everything goes well.

Use the right pestle for your apothecary

Almost every apothecary has a mortar and pestle, but not all of them are created equal. In order to provide the best results, make sure that you get one that is made from stone rather than glass or plastic. This will ensure that your remedies are more effective because they won't be altered by heat from the chemicals in plastic or glass jars.

Study the herbs before you start using them

It's important to know that using some herbs may harm you in various ways. The best way to learn this is to study up on all of your remedies so that you can predict what is about to happen to your body when these herbs are introduced. This will allow you to avoid some of the most dangerous situations and make you feel more comfortable about using natural remedies.

Begin slowly and gradually increase the number of herbs you use.

The home apothecary usually starts with a few dried herbs, but as time goes on, it grows with you and includes more herbal remedies. It can be tempting to use large amounts of herbs all at once, but it's best to start small and increase the amount that you include over time.

Herbal remedies are sacred and often have great power when used correctly. This is why it is important to learn as much as you can about the herbs that you are going to be using before you make the decision to start working with them.

CHAPTER 19:

HOW TO GET HERBS

Buying Herbs

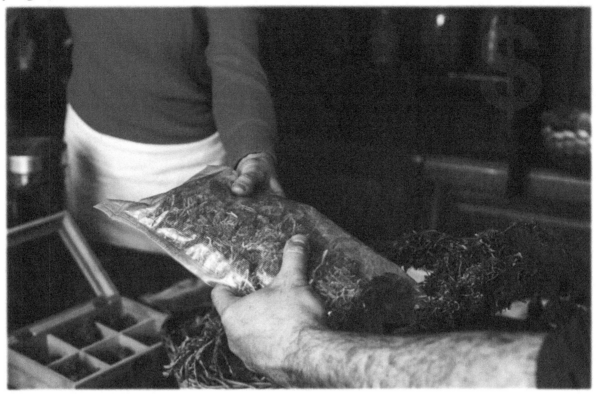

Pros and cons

When you buy herbs, you need to know the pros and cons.

Pros:

- You know in advance what you are going to be using the herbs for, so they are of the finest quality and will work for your purposes.
- You get herbs on sale a lot more than retail stores, and grocery lines would sell them for, therefore making them cheaper than buying new ones.

Cons:

- The convenience of buying from a store is not there; you have to actually go out and find your herbs yourself at an outdoor market or farm, which takes more time and energy than you could ever imagine!
- You should understand how to handle the herbs and look for their proper proportions in other people's formulas.
- You have to know how to make each formula yourself, so you know what is going into it.
- You cannot trust the formulas that come from stores because they are not really tested on anything but paper! What does that mean, you ask? It means they are not used as medicines!

Best place to buy herbs

If you are going to buy herbs from a store, your best bet is to buy from the Indian market or farm. They are of better quality, and you can trust them. If you want the convenience of a store, then go to a natural food store or health food store. They sell herbs for general meditation and cleansing purposes only. Again, if you want the best quality herbs, go to an Indian farm or medicine man's clinic.

In the practice of herbalism, the term "clinic" is used for a place where you can get herbs. The name of the clinic will be written on the front of the window. If you see a nursery or a gardening store, then it is likely that they have two entrances. One will have the word "clinic" written on it and will be open during daytime hours, while another side of their store will have a different name appearing on it, and it will be open only at night.

How to check quality when buying herbs

When buying herbs, check the following:

- Check the color of the herb before you buy it. If it looks dead or green, it is not of good quality.
- Check the strength of an herb's smell before you buy it by actually taking some in your hands and smelling them to see if they smell good or bad.
- Look at the size of each herb (smaller is better). The smaller herbs are stronger, so they are more potent without being harsh on the body.
- Check to see if the herbs are whole or broken. Broken herbs are weak and not good for you.

Tips and tricks for beginners

1. Purchasing from the grocery store: if you want to purchase herbs from the grocery store, make sure you buy at least one of each to see if they are good enough for you. If not, then ask them to let you know when they get more so you can purchase some of the stronger herbs!
2. Purchasing from a nursery: if you want to purchase from a nursery, make sure they have a good variety of herbs. If not, you need to ask them if they would please order more. If you are lucky enough to get some good ones, then take them when you are ready!
3. Purchasing from the farmers market: if you want to purchase from a farmers' market, make sure you know how to tell if they are good herbs. If not, then ask the first person that you see what he/she thinks of them. If they look and smell bad, or the merchant doesn't know what he/she is talking about, then you need to find another market!
4. Purchasing online: if you are going to purchase herbs online, make sure you know you can trust the merchant. Make sure they have at least four stars before buying them! If they don't, then don't buy from them!

Searching Herbs In Nature

Best equipment needed to search herbs in nature:

1. A wilderness survival kit: This is to be prepared for any possible emergencies. If you are not well accustomed to the wilderness, this would also be necessary to have with you so that in case an emergency arises, you will have what you need in order to survive.
2. A hunting knife: This is the only tool needed for preparing these materials.
3. A camera: as a means to document your search for herbs in natural surroundings.
4. A journal: This is your personal collection of all the instances you encounter with herbs in nature.
5. A field guide to native plants of the United States: It is necessary to have this with you if you do not have a background in botany in order to identify the herbs in the process of searching for them.
6. A map: This is for you to be able to search for herbs in the geographical location that you want.
7. A compass: This would be used in order to know the direction where the herbs are.
8. A whistle: This is a means to alert other people on the location of your search and also a means of protection from wild animals or humans while searching for your herbs.

The United States Department of Agriculture has created a wonderful site called the USDA NGR Database (https://data.nal.usda.gov/dataset/germplasm-resources-information-network-grin) for finding native plants in your area! You can even find out which states they are native to and information on how to use them. This is a wonderful reference source! You can also go to the site with just a general location, and it will give you a list of all native plants that grow there!

Pros and cons

When you are searching for herbs in nature, there are a couple of pros and cons to pay attention to.

Pros:

- You get all manner of beautiful and useful herbs for a smaller price than it would cost you at the store or nursery.
- If you are looking for a specific herb, then you can find it more easily since there are all types of combinations of herbs in nature that have components good for a specific purpose.
- You can get some herbs that are scarce in the grocery stores!

Cons:

- Some plants have medicinal effects, and others may not work at all for your condition.
- You have to know what the plants look like and how to identify them.
- If you are not careful, you may get sick from picking the wrong herbs! So, make sure you find the proper ones first, then have them tested to make sure they aren't poisonous.

Tips and tricks when searching for herbs

- Find out what herb you need for what condition ahead of time so that you can search for those herbs in nature! This will save lots of time when searching for your herbs in nature instead of random searching, where it could take months or even years to happen upon your favorite herb (or several years)!
- Ask someone who has experience with herbs to show you how to tell what is good and what is poisonous.
- Make sure you come prepared with a book or a note on your phone, or even a camera to take pictures of the herbs so you can look at them and remember them later if you have to leave in a hurry.
- If it happens that you pick something that doesn't work for you or, God forbid, something that's poisonous, do not despair! Just try another time again!
- If you are going to do any of the following activities, I strongly suggest you wear gloves in order to protect your hands from getting dirt under your fingernails that could cause infections!

How to recognize herbs/plants

There are several ways to recognize different herbs:

- Look at how they grow.
- Look at the color of the leaves and flowers.
- Look at the shape of the leaves and flowers.
- Smell their aroma and feel their taste!
- Look at what they look like in pictures! Many books have detailed drawings of different types of herbs with their descriptions on them, so you can look them up to see exactly what these wonderful little plants look like!

The best moment to search for herbs

Herbs are most abundant when spring is just beginning to bloom. However, you can still find herbs in the fall and winter as well. Just stay out of the rain or snow and don't get them wet while picking them! And don't do anything that will disturb the ground where you are searching. If you do, then expect to have an empty spot where the plants were. So don't dig up the ground or break anything under it!

Growing Herbs In Your Garden

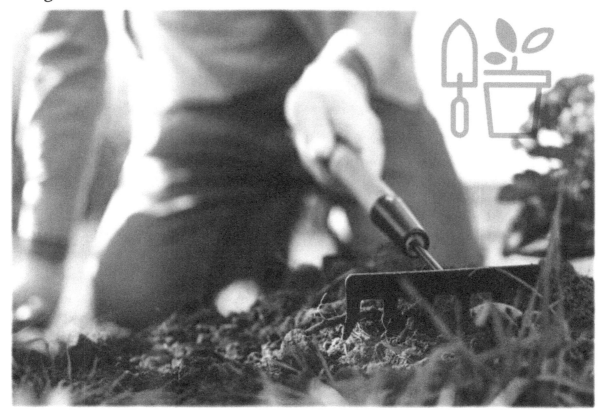

If you wish to cultivate your own herbs, then you have one more decision to make, which is whether or not you will grow them indoors or outdoors. If you have a garden, I would highly recommend growing them there since there is more room and they will get enough light from the sun there. If not, then growing them indoors is fine as well! Just be sure they have enough light, so they aren't weak plants.

Pros and cons

There are pros and cons to growing plants inside. If you want to grow them inside, you will have to do a lot of work on your own:

Pros:

- You can control what they eat and how they are taken care of, so you don't have to worry about the weather or bugs hurting them as much.
- If you have a lot of space, then there is a lot more room for planting many different kinds of herbs outside! So, if you want one herb but not another, then there is no need to buy the seeds for that plant if it is already there! Just avoid stepping on them as well!

Cons:

- If you are in an apartment complex without a yard, then you will either have to purchase a high-quality glow light or spend a lot of money on electricity. Luckily for those of us who want to try to make our own, the sun is always in the sky, and we can easily grow herbs outside!
- You may need more room inside for plants than that which is outside. On the other hand, if there is nothing growing in your garden and the ground is very good, then little to no work may be required from you!
- Do you know flowers from veggies? If so, then you are all set! It will also be much easier for you to have them there than out in the wild! Just make sure the book you are reading is up to date.

Organic vs. Non-organic

If you are growing the herbs in your garden, you must be careful about what kinds of fertilizers and pesticides you use. One way to do this is by buying organic seeds and planting them into the soil that has had no chemicals in it already. If you're going this route, I would suggest looking up a book on organic gardening first! It can be tricky to do!

If you're growing them indoors, then there is a much smaller chance that your plants will grow using these methods. You could try growing them outside on the balcony or on a windowsill where the sun can get to them. However, this is risky. Your plants could die if you aren't careful enough to make sure they can take the cold. Do some research on your specific herbs and how they like to be grown, and then you will know what to do!

Start from your garden: minimum characteristic of the garden

- It must be weed-free
- It must have a sunny position
- It must be well- prepared and fertilized with manure
- It should have an appropriate amount of water and daily irrigation during the entire summer
- The soil should not be very wet or too warm, as it can lead to diseases or even cause plants to die from high humidity in the garden.

The right soil preparation is very important for growing healthy plants, but many people fall short of knowing which herb can grow where they live in their particular climate and under what conditions.

The idea behind establishing a home apothecary is to start from your garden and use it as a tool or a springboard for helping you in case of any medical emergencies. For the summer, usually, the best time to harvest herbs is in July and August because, after that, they stop growing and go into a dormancy stage where they become hard and dry. Most importantly, it is the easiest time to perform the necessary processing of those herbs for making medicine.

In addition, your home apothecary can serve as a great opportunity to educate your friends and family about the wonderful world of natural medicine.

Equipment needed to start growing

You will need the following equipment to start growing your own herbs:

- A shovel that has a long handle so you can easily dig up the ground for planting! This will be important when you are planting many different types of herbs in your garden!
- A digging tool with a sharp end so that you can get to the hard-to-reach places! You will need one if your shovel is too short!
- A watering can and a watering gauge. Make sure you know how much water plants need on a regular basis, so they don't die.
- A nice-looking container for the soil or seeds, whatever it is that you plan to plant inside of. I recommend having at least an inch of dirt above the plant's roots. It helps them as they grow!
- A bag of compost or soil that is made of compost! If possible, get a blend of black soil with some peat moss and some fertilizer in it already. It will help the plant grow better!

Herbs suggested to start growing and why for beginners

As you know by now, I love to tell you guys how to do things that will eventually help you in the long run! This is no different. You can do this at your local library. It shows you all of the different herbs and what they can do. However, that will have to come later. For now, here are some great herbs to start with:

- Rosemary: This herb is great for calming down nerves and helping to lower heart rate. It aids in the relaxation of your blood vessels and reduces stress, which is even better if you are in a hectic and fast-paced way of life.
- Oregano: This herb is great for lowering heart rate and blood pressure! Just put it on fresh cuts or wounds!
- Thyme: You can use it to help fight off the common cold! If you want, you can also use it as a substitute for oregano. It will give your dish more of an Italian flair!

- Mint: Mint is a very common herb that most of us use with our food every day! I love to put it on green tea instead of sugar! It helps aid in digestion!
- Sage: This herb is great for helping calm the nerves and relaxing your muscles. It is also good for helping you to remember things better.
- Parsley: This herb is good as a substitute for high cholesterol foods, like meat!

I would recommend starting with these herbs just because they are easy to grow and can be planted indoors or outside. Having too many of one herb affects the soil quality and makes it harder for other plants to grow, so keep that in mind.

Watering

When you are growing herbs, you want to make sure that you water them the right amount. If they get too much water, they could rot and die. If they don't have enough water, then they could burn out or die from a lack of nutrients. Make sure you water them enough but don't overwater them. Here are the different amounts that you will want to make sure they get enough:

- If you are using a pot that is about 2 inches deep, then it needs about 1/2 an inch of water every week.
- If you are using a pot that is about 6 inches deep, then it needs about 2–3 inches of water every two weeks.
- If you are using a larger pot or a window box, then it needs to be watered much more frequently! About 5–6 inches of water every week!

Growing herbs indoors—suggestions

If you are growing your herbs indoors, then there will be a few things that you will need. I would suggest using pots that are about 2 inches deep for all of your herbs. That way, they can hold the perfect amount of water. Here is a list of things you will need to start off with:

- A glow light if you can afford it! This can help your plants grow bigger and faster, depending on how bright it is. If this is not an option for you, then I would recommend buying some good indoor lights and hanging them up around 6 inches from the plant.
- A pot that has holes at the bottom in order for your water to drain out. This makes it easy for the water to drain out and prevents it from pooling!
- A good, well-draining soil that has compost blended into it! I would suggest buying some soil from a nursery or store if you can't make your own!
- A huge container that can store all of your plants. Smaller pots dry out faster when they are put together in one container and don't give enough room for them to breathe, so they burn out quickly.

Wild Crafting

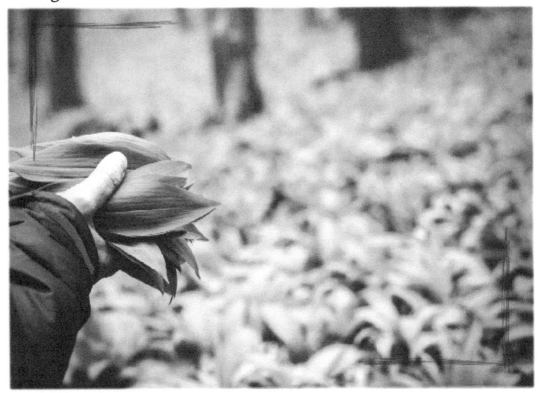

The last way to get your herbs is by wild crafting them. This is a great way to make money if you have the skill set. The only thing is, it will take you longer than just growing them yourself.

Pros and cons

Pros:

There are many reasons why a person would have to source herbs directly from their natural environment. I personally love it. I love being able to identify and harvest plants in the wild, and I feel so much more in harmony with our mother earth.

Also, wild herbs, in addition to being free, tend to have a stronger medicine than cultivated herbs.

Cons:

Clearly, it is not something everyone can do. It requires experience and a good knowledge of plants so as not to damage the environment or harvest something that is harmful to our health

Also, not everyone has a forest behind their house where they can look for herbs and plants. Especially those who live in big cities might find this activity very impractical

Equipment needed

- A good pair of gloves, a hat, long pants, and long sleeves. You never know what you will run into out there! Always be careful!
- A notebook to write down the name of the plant and where it is located. I like to take pictures too.
- A knife or two if you are going for firewood or nuts and berries.
- A basket if you are going for berries or nuts or plants that have thorns on them (such as blackberries). Trust me when I say that you don't want to go back home with your hands full with a basket full of sharp thorns!
- An entrenching tool if you are going for any type of roots.
- A portable stove if you are going for any edible plants.
- A couple of bags to put in your pockets! You never know what you will find, and it will be nice to have some extra bags to put in your pockets so you can carry everything home with you!

Things to check in order to control the quality when wild crafting

- When you make new trails, leave some dead ones behind. If you don't, the plants that are left behind will be more susceptible to die because they have nothing absorbing the water. Not good! Make new trails, so there is no dead plant left behind!
- Check where your plants are growing and if they are getting enough water and sunlight! Make sure you check for weeds around your plants so you can remove them to make room for your herbs and flowers!
- Don't harvest too much of one kind of plant from one spot in order to prevent a "die-off" in that area. Too much of one herb can be bad for the soil since it can kill the other herbs. Just pick up the good herbs and leave some behind so it doesn't become the dead zones of the ground!
- For example, don't pick all of the berries from one bush because then it will become a bunch of dead bushes where everyone knows not to go.
- Leave a trail of little branches or plants all around your camp or area so that other people don't harvest near your spot. This way, you won't hurt any other plants in your area!
- Always check back and see how things are growing. If they are getting more sun, take them further out. If they are getting less, bring them in. This way you can make sure it's the best quality!

The right way to harvest wild plants/herbs

- Let your plants grow for about 2–3 weeks after they have been planted.
- After they have finished growing and the weather is nice outside, harvest all of the herbs you would like to keep in the first week and just pick off all the rest of it! You can leave them if you want, but most people choose to be as humane as possible, so they don't hurt anything else in their area.
- Pick up all of your herbs and place them into a large cloth bag! You can even put hot rocks into one for some extra warmth too!
- Put the bag of herbs in your pocket or have an extra bag on hand just in case you want to pick up one more!

Tips and tricks for beginners

1. Be prepared for wild crafting: Write down the name of your plant, where it is located, and if you can remember any clues to growing or harvesting it.
2. Decide Where to Go: Be aware of your surroundings. Does the area have lots of deer that eat plants? Or bears, or other large predators? Think about it before you attempt to plant!
3. Walk Slowly to Notice Herbs and Plants: Forget that you are on a schedule and stop to smell the flowers. Walk slowly, and check your surroundings as you go.
4. Look in Uncommon Places: Don't walk right through the garden of a neighbor, for example. Simply turn around and go back. You'll probably find some great stuff you didn't notice there before—herbs, berries, or plants that aren't usually in the area.
5. Don't Go Looking for a Specific Plant: Instead, allow yourself to be open to the possibilities, and you'll do even better. If you are looking for rosemary, for example, then the chances are good that you won't have much luck in the deserts of Arizona.
6. Don't Overlook Common Plants: by this, I mean that you shouldn't dismiss plants that are very common as weeds or undesirables. In the landscape industry, these so-called "undesirables" include non-native plants such as garlic mustard (the most invasive in the U.S.) and vinca (similar to periwinkle, a common ground cover in landscapes). Both are edible and medicinal, and both are sold by herbal supply companies!

CHAPTER 20:

AN OVERVIEW OF HERBAL PREPARATIONS, EXTRACTIONS, AND TOPICAL USES

Personal herbal medicine would be an herbal medicine, most likely a combination that you could count on to make you feel better if you ever experienced a fever again. You would become so confident in that remedy over time that you would promote it to others, people you care about. This herbal remedy does not have to be prepared by you. Instead, it could be a pre-made treatment that you've always thought worked every time you tried it.

To begin, you'll need a reason to make herbal medicine; you'll want to use it as a remedy. You will have a result after going through all of the complicated stuff, which may be explained as the mixing process. This outcome may disappoint you in the end, but it only means you'll have to attempt again to locate a fresh and better drug.

The feeling you'll get straight away after successfully using a drug you produced yourself will be priceless.

The next thing you know, you'll be trying to develop newer remedies because you're so confident in your previous success, and you'll be continuously recommending your treatment to those you believe need it.

The majority of herbs are simple to plant in your kitchen garden. It eventually comes to the point where you must be entirely dedicated to it. If you are, you will be willing to plant little quantities of each of these herbs in small pots. You'll also be responsible for these herbs, which means you'll need to water them and take care of their fertilizers. This obligation will eventually grow into a love for those plants.

If you find it difficult to go through all of the steps necessary to make herbal ingredients yourself, you may always head to the nearest superstore. You'll find all of the herbs you're looking for, as well as those you've never heard of.

Macerations

This is the simplest way to prepare herbs. All you have to do is soak your fresh or dried herbs overnight in cool water. Strain the herb in the morning to separate the liquid. This method is typically used for herbs that are particularly tender or fresh, or herbs that contain delicate compounds that can be destroyed by heat or damaged by high-strength alcohol. It's the simplest to adapt macerations to modern western medical practices. Macerations can be made into pills or capsules, or the powder from the ground herbs can be mixed into smoothies, juices, or water.

Fomentation

Compression is a term used to describe the process of fomentation. Fomentations are made up of herbal infusions or decoctions that are applied topically. You can make both hot and cold fomentations, depending on whatever herb you're working with. Both hot and cold fomentations have their own set of benefits.

Hot fomentations are used to relax tight and constricted muscles and to stimulate vasodilation, which improves blood flow throughout the skin. This is especially beneficial when you have painful muscles and legs, and it can also aid with interior congestion.

Cold fomentation can cause blood vessels in the skin to constrict. This aids in the treatment of severe burns, terrible bruising, and other skin inflammations. Fomentations are excellent natural skin remedies that are commonly used to treat eczema, psoriasis, and skin rashes.

Fomentation is made by doubling the power of a decoction or infusion by four times. The mixture is then dipped in a natural fiber like cotton, silk, or wool. The surplus liquid is wrung out of the fabric after it has been soaked in the mixture, and the wet cloth is placed over the damaged region. You can also cover the fomentation with a dry towel or cloth to keep it warm, and wrap it in plastic cling film to keep the liquid from spilling all over the place.

Infusion Techniques For The Domestic Herbalist

Infusions are often liquids, similar to teas, made from medicinal plants that dissolve quickly in water or release their active compounds slowly in oil. An infusion is made to extract an herb's most delicate and therapeutic capabilities. They are frequently made from the plant's softer parts, such as the leaves and blossoms. This varies per herb; for example, the root is employed instead of the leaves or petals in herbs like goldenseal and valerian.

Making an infusion is a relatively simple procedure. Simply pour boiling water over a specified herb and leave it to steep for 15-20 minutes, or until the mixture cools down. After that, sift the mixture to separate the herb from the liquid, bottle it, and keep it for later use. Some infusions should be kept refrigerated, while others should be kept in cold, dark settings. If desired, you can also add honey for added benefit and to enhance the flavor. Honey and lemon are also popular additions. One ounce of herb to one pint of liquid is the most frequent ratio for making herbal infusions.

Boiling water is used to slowly extract the herb's therapeutic qualities from its many sections. Vitamins, carbohydrates, enzymes, and certain volatile oils, as well as tannins, saponins, bitter compounds, glycosides, and other proteins, are slowly released by the water. Boiling water also aids in the release of polysaccharides, pectins, and certain alkaloids from the herb.

Infusions are frequently mistaken for teas. You can make both hot and cold infusions, each with its own set of features and advantages.

Washcloths

Washcloths are an excellent way to get a bath in bed. They can be used on a seriously ill patient who would not be able to tolerate an active bath. Medicine can be easily applied to the skin in this manner, allowing it to diffuse to a deeper part of the body. When specific effects of heating are required, washcloths can be made hot by employing hot infusions of medicine, or they can be made cold by utilizing cold infusions. It all relies on personal preference as well as sickness symptoms. Cold washcloths with unique benefits of ice and anti-inflammatory drugs might be a wise solution for acute injuries, such as brushing and combat sports bouts, to prevent swelling and bruising while also limiting bleeding from fresh wounds. The cold washcloth has anesthetic effects, making it a natural pain reliever.

Warm washcloths can increase blood flow through having vasodilatory properties, as well as provide a relaxing response to the body.

Teas

Herbal teas are just hot infusions of herbs. Herbal tea is enjoyable to drink, and including it into your diet is a healthy choice. The majority of herbal teas offer a calming or refreshing effect. Depending on the herb's qualities, they can make you feel relaxed or energized. Herbal teas, on the other hand, are not as strong as other herbal medicines.

Homemade medicinal teas are simple to create. You can either keep loose tea leaves or make tea bags with dosages that suit your needs. You may then soak them for 10 minutes in boiling water anytime you wish to eat them. You may also make a medicinal tea with regular tea from the supermarket if you triple the amount of tea you use. You can obtain close to the therapeutic efficacy of an infusion by triple the typical amount. Certain herbal teas can be consumed as many times as desired throughout the day without causing harm. Make sure, however, that the teas' characteristics do not create any exaggerated symptoms. Excessive consumption of laxative herbal teas, for example, is not a good idea.

If you're making herbal tea with dried herbs, weigh out the majority and place them in a non-metallic container. It's a good idea to have a kitchen scale on hand to figure out how much herb to put in your tea. As previously stated, one ounce is the suggested dosage. Herbal teas are usually consumed at room temperature. If you wish to induce sweating or if you have a cold or cough, drinking really hot tea will help. It is also useful to lose weight by drinking hot green tea. You can drink the tea anytime you want; the recommended dose is one to four cups, although this varies totally on the herb you're using.

Here are some advantages and disadvantages of drinking infusions:

Pros: Infusions are the simplest to make of all the herbal treatments. Only herbs and water are required. Infusions are often enjoyable to drink, and they have few side effects because of their mildness. Herbs have an easier time releasing their therapeutic compounds into water than other chemicals, such as alcohol, which is used to make tinctures. If you use raspberry leaves, for example, they will release more medication in hot water than in alcohol. Conducting research is the best approach to determine which herbs will work best in your infusion. Your research will reveal which herbs will benefit you the most and enhance the flavor of your infusion the most.

Cons: Even though infusions are very easy to produce, not everyone enjoys the flavor of several herbs combined. This is especially true if you're utilizing herbs that are astringent or bitter. You may feel nauseous before drinking the teas made from these herbs; adults, let alone children, may have difficulty swallowing them. There is, however, a very simple method around this.

If you add anything to enhance the flavor of these infusions, it will not affect their potency or effectiveness. To eliminate the bitter taste and make the tea more drinkable, add honey, agave, maple syrup, brown sugar, or lemon to your infusions. Not all herbal teas, however, share the same issue. Some herbal teas are truly tasty and enjoyable to drink.

Decoction

Infusions are comparable to decoctions. Herbs are softly cooked to unleash their therapeutic qualities in this approach. Decoctions, unlike infusions, can incorporate an herb's stems, bark, roots, and rhizomes. Infusions are typically created with the herb's leafy, delicate sections, whereas decoctions are made with the herb's tougher components.

The herbs are simmered with water as it comes to a boil in a non-metallic container. If you're making a decoction with roots, the boiling time might be one and a half to two hours.

One ounce of dried herb (hard parts) or two ounces of fresh herb parts to one pint of water is required to make a decoction. You'll need to chop the herb as finely as possible and combine it with the water in a small pot. Instead of an aluminum pot, a decoction should be made in a stainless steel, glass, or enamel pot.

To prepare the decoction, simply cook the herbs in the water until it boils. When it comes to a boil, turn the heat down as low as possible and reduce it to a low simmer for at least 20 minutes. The liquid must next be strained, which can be done with a cheesecloth. To get the greatest results, wrap the cheesecloth around a colander and squeeze out as much liquid as possible. Fill the cup with the liquid and consume it while it's still warm.

Decoctions employ the same amount of herbs as infusions, therefore there aren't many differences. To keep your decoction, make sure it's in a container with a tight-fitting lid. A mason jar would be the perfect container to utilize once again. Simmering takes about 20 minutes on average, but it might take longer depending on the herb.

You can drink the decoction immediately once it cools, or you can steep it overnight, drain it, and drink it the next morning. Make sure you don't keep your decoction for too long; it's preferable to drink it as soon as it's cool enough.

When comparing a decoction to an infusion, decoctions take longer to extract since they require constant hot and boiling water on the stove. Because decoctions are formed from the thicker, more resinous parts of a plant, they are the greatest way to extract the herb's medicinal powers. Infusions are regarded softer than decoctions since they are made with the more delicate portions.

Because herbs have different qualities, some function better as infusions and others as decoctions. It all depends on the nutrients you want to get out of the herb. Some herbs may be better suited to cold or nighttime infusions, as hot water can actually destroy some of the herbs' medicinal effects. You may learn which plants are ideal for hot or cold infusions and which herbs are great for decoctions by doing some research online.

You can use your infusions and decoctions as a base for a variety of herbal treatments once they're ready. They can be used for a variety of things, including douches, enemas, herbal baths, fomentations, and steam inhalations. Water-based herbal preparations, rather than alcohol-based tinctures, are commonly recommended for extracting mucilaginous plants. Some herbs, such as hemp and myrrh, are more soluble in alcohol and are utilized in tinctures instead.

Here are some advantages and disadvantages of creating decoctions:

Pros: One of the most effective ways to extract medicine from dried roots or other tough, woody portions of the herb is to make a decoction. Because these components of the herb are harder and won't release all of their medicinal compounds by just soaking in boiling water, a decoction is required for this process. Decoctions are more potent than teas, and among all herbal preparations, they are among the most potent. Because they are easily absorbed by our bodies, they act more swiftly and effectively than other herbal medicines.

Cons: Decoctions are extremely powerful. Because they've been simmered, they're incredibly concentrated, with a really robust and intense flavor. People with delicate digestive systems or finicky eaters with sensitive palates may have difficulty drinking this.

Compresses

Compresses are warm medicinal pastes that are formed from many potent herbs. Compression is a very traditional technique, which is also caller "Marham" in Arabic, and it is the most used technique in Indian ayurvedic as well. Warm herbs in the form of compresses can stay longer than washcloths on the skin and can be a great source of constant delivery of herbal medicine. The feeling of warmth itself is soothing, and it also helps in reducing muscle spasms when applied. It also helps in vasodilation in specific areas to speed up recovery. Some herbs are delightful in fragrance and thus can provide the body with an unusual odor. Any natural fiber, a cloth with pores or a muslin bag, can be used to form compresses from medicinal herbs. In traditional herbal medicine, compresses were formed by putting them in direct sunlight to get the effects of warmth. In modern days, ovens can be used to achieve the temperature and thus applied to the skin in comfortable ways. Microwaving should be avoided when other natural sources are available because of the health hazards of artificial heating. Different and multiple layers are also used over a single compress to achieve maximum absorption as well as the mixing of herbs. It also protects from overheating and bruising.

Juicing

Juicing a fresh plant is sometimes the greatest way to extract nutrients from it. Specific plants, such as freshly picked nettles or wheat grass, are particularly healthy when juiced. For greatest nutritious benefit, utilize different juicers to blend herbs with different vegetables, such as carrots and celery. To increase flavor, combine herbs with fruit juices in a blender. When mixing fruit juice with herbs, however, you must be cautious because oxidation can develop quickly. If you don't want this to happen, filter the liquid before drinking it. You may also squeeze the herbs to extract the juice if you have a food processor.

Tincture

An herbal tincture is a concentrated liquid version of an herb. It's usually taken a few drops at a time while being placed under the tongue.

It's a good strategy, but it necessitates some planning and rest time. If you're considering using tincture to heal yourself, think long-term. You won't be able to utilize it for several weeks. However, tinctures are beneficial, so the work is worthwhile.

Tinctures exemplify the saying "little is more." You get more herbal phytonutrients from a few drops of tincture than you would from a cup of tea. You also get them sooner. The material is assimilated more quickly by your body.

Yes, the tincture takes longer to make, but it also has a much longer shelf life than fresh or dried plants. A tincture's efficacy can be retained for up to five years - occasionally even longer.

A tincture can be prepared from almost any portion of the plant that would be used in another preparation. The leaves (dried or fresh), bark, roots, and berries are all included.

Collect the plant pieces you'll be using. They should be washed and coarsely chopped. If you have a mortar and pestle, now is the time to put it to good use. In a canning jar, put four ounces of the herb. Add a pint of 80 proof vodka or any other grain alcohol to this. This type of alcohol extracts the most therapeutic qualities. If you like, you can make your tincture with apple cider vinegar, but it won't last as long.

Allow the magic to happen by sealing the jar and placing it in a cold, dark spot. Shake the jar every day for the first week to ensure that the healing properties are evenly dispersed. Shake it once a week from the second to the sixth week.

Allow this to remain for at least six weeks before straining the mixture. You can use a wine press if you have one, but it isn't required. A piece of cheesecloth will suffice. Simply move the cloth every now and then to ensure that all of the liquid is drained.

You can also strain the tincture with a potato ricer (I told you it would come in handy). Empty the contents of the jar into the ricer's basket, and it will take care of the rest. Fill an airtight dark-colored glass container halfway with the tincture.

A word of caution: remember to identify it. Not only the name of the herbal tincture, but also the components of the plants you utilized and whether they were dried or fresh should be included. Put the date you first made it as well. It's also a good idea to identify it with the appropriate usage.

Essential Oils

Essential oils are substances extracted from plants. The volatile, oily portions of aromatic plants, trees, and grasses are used to make essential oils. Various oils are derived from microscopic glands found in the leaves, roots, flowers, resins, and wood of these plants.

Essential oils can be extracted using one of four ways. Steam distillation, solvent extraction, effleurage, and expression can all be used to extract them.

The oil is produced from the herb via steam distillation, which involves processing it with heated steam. The herb is then selectively condensed with water before being separated. When you use expression to extract essential oil, the oil is extracted either through centrifugation or by applying pressure on the herb.

Solvent extraction involves dissolving the oil in a volatile solvent, which evaporates to leave a heavy, naturally waxy product known as concrete. The liquid that remains after the mixture has been removed from the concrete is known as an absolute. The absolute is the most concentrated form of the smell, making it an extremely powerful essential oil.

Effleurage is the most time-consuming method of obtaining essential oil. The oils must first be dissolved in animal fat before being separated with alcohol. Essential oils are utilized in cosmetics and aromatherapy, and they offer a variety of therapeutic and restorative characteristics. Essential oils are never used internally.

Salves And Ointments

After you've mastered creating oils, preparing ointments and salves becomes quite simple. Herbal salves are created by combining infused herbal oil with beeswax, as well as other forms of topical butters, such as cocoa butter or shea butter, for their skin-nourishing properties. The preferred base is beeswax; beeswax is thick, thus salves have a thicker viscosity than ointments and creams. Because the salve has a thicker consistency, it can stay on the skin for longer. This allows them to penetrate deeper into the muscles and tissues, allowing them to operate more effectively.

Making salves is as simple as decocting herbs in oils and filtering them out. Simply add beeswax to the oil after the herbs have been filtered and set aside to cool. Salves can be used as restorative ointments for the skin as well as a lip balm for dry, chapped lips.

If kept in firmly sealed containers in a cold, dark environment, salves can last for several months. If there is any mold or evidence of rotting, throw it out right away.

Salves and ointments are comparable. You receive a solid mixture of wax or fat after you remove the simmering herbs from the liquid, which contains the therapeutic elements of the herbs. If you want a thinner ointment with a jelly-like consistency, you can use petroleum jelly or paraffin wax.

Syrups

Syrups are typically created by heating an herbal berry jam or making a powerful herbal decoction from an herb's blossoms, bark, needles, or leaves, then adding glycerin, honey, or sugar to the mix. For centuries, people have used herbal syrups and cordials to treat sore throats, colds, coughs, and other mucus-related respiratory problems. A syrup is a means to make bitter and pungent herbs more appealing to children and finicky eaters, making the cure more accessible to them.

Syrups are used when honey alone isn't enough, and they're a fantastic alternative for vegans who don't eat honey. To improve the flavor of syrups, you can use unrefined cane sugar or peppermint. These are some of the best-tasting herbal treatments, but due to their sweetness, they should be used sparingly.

Poultice

They are suitable for both hot and cold use. Heat stimulates circulation in the affected area, allowing an abscess to be drawn out or removed. The cold variety is excellent for decreasing inflammation and relieving discomfort.

There's a simple way to apply the plant if you need a quick poultice. Place the chopped herbs in a clean white cotton sock and tie the top. Soak the sock in boiling water in a sink or dish. Then you're ready to put it into practice.

In some cases, the paste can be applied directly to the wound without the use of a cloth between the poultice and the skin. Then, to keep it in place, wrap it in anything from gauze to muslin to plastic wrap.

Dried Powders

Another way to get a plant's medicinal benefits is to use dried powder herbs. It's sometimes required by a tea formula or recipe. Some people prefer putting powdered herbs into capsules and taking them that way. If you're interested in trying this, you may buy empty capsules online.

You might also use the herbs you've made this way in your body powder or toothpaste.

One disadvantage of this approach is that it quickly loses its effectiveness. This means you should use them right away rather than letting them sit around.

It's simple to make powdered herbs, and you've probably already figured out how to do it. Before putting the herbs in a spice grinder, make sure they're completely dry. Only a small amount at a time, around a tablespoon or so, should be ground at a time. You'll be sure to grind everything tiny enough this way. A mortar and pestle is used by some herbalists, although a grinder is speedier and produces a lovely powdery product.

After that, you can put them to whatever use you like.

I noted that they don't keep well, but you can extend their shelf life by storing them in airtight containers and keeping them chilled. Avoid storing them in direct sunlight or in a humid environment.

Capsules And Powders

This is also a simple method for making an herbal cure. Many herbs are available in powder form, which you can purchase. You can also use a tiny coffee grinder or a small processor to powder whatever herbs you wish. The job can be done with a capsule blender or chopper.

If you choose to grind your herbs, be sure to do so properly and sift any large pieces out of the mixture before using.

Powders are quite concentrated, so you don't need to take a lot of them, especially if you're taking them orally. To make it easier to ingest, you can put the powder in a capsule.

You can take the loose herbal powder in a variety of ways, depending on what you want it to do for you and whatever route of administration is most convenient for you. For example, if you're taking herbal powder to help with bodily imbalances, you can combine it with a medium like apple sauce to make it simpler to consume than just water. Some herbs irritate the throat or intestine in some people, so consuming powders directly may not be the best option for them.

Powdered herbs can also be encapsulated to make them easier to consume. To produce capsules, you can use a capsule machine. If you're a vegan or vegetarian, you can choose between gelatin-based capsules and plant-based capsules. Capsules take longer to work than powders, but they are a better way to get the complete plant into your system.

Most capsules can be taken with water or a warm herbal tea. If you use cayenne in your capsules, avoid taking them with a hot beverage since they can burn the back of your throat.

Pastilles, or rolled herbal pills, are another classic way of herbal preparation. Herbal pills are prepared by combining powdered herbs with dates or honey and forming little pill shapes out of the mixture. The pills can then be dehydrated or refrigerated and taken as needed.

Suppositories, Pills, And Lozenges

Pills, lozenges, and suppositories are all manufactured in the same manner. You'll need to powder your herbs first, then combine them with a liquid until a stiff dough forms. The mixture can then be shaped as needed.

Pinch off a small amount of dough from the dough ball to produce a pill or a lozenge after you have your dough. The size of a lozenge is slightly larger than that of a pill. Flatten the dough by rolling it into a small ball and pressing it between your fingers. Carob powder or more slippery elm can then be applied. Then, either place your tablets or lozenges in a low-heat oven or leave them out in the sun for a day. They'll last a long time once they've dried out.

Suppositories are a convenient technique to get herbs directly into the vaginal or rectum. They are usually taken as pills. They may appear messy after they dissolve and whatever is left behind spills out, but they are still more convenient to use than enemas or douches.

When it comes to vaginal infections, many individuals prefer suppositories to douches because the pressure from the douche infusion can actually push the virus farther up the cervix. Suppositories are also a better way to get more resinous herbs into your system, which don't extract as well as they should in water-based therapies.

Mix the powdered herbs with melted cocoa butter to form a suppository. This is a simple and effective method of delivering herbs directly into the vagina or the rectum. Nasal passageways are treated with certain suppositories.

Ice Cubes

Ice cubes are a great way to get herbal extracts into your system, and they're easy to use. Teas and decoctions can also be used to make it. After boiling and rapidly chilling, liquid herbal medicine can be frozen, a process known as thawing. It also has pain-relieving properties that are unique to cold therapy. Ice cubes can simply be transformed into homemade sweet popsicles by inserting sticks into them. This method of administration is extremely popular among children. To avoid problems, the ice bags and trays should be labeled appropriately.

CHAPTER 21:

SAFETY TIPS AND ABUSE OF HERBS

Because of their potency, Native American herbs are some of the most amazing ways to take care of our health. Here, we'll go over some safety precautions as well as how people abuse plants.

Herbal medicine has traditionally been used by Native Americans to treat themselves and their family members. Many herbs, such as peppermint for an upset stomach or cedar for a hurting chest, can be used for a variety of purposes. Tobacco is a sort of herb that has been used for a variety of reasons in Native American culture; it can be smoked, chewed, or just smelled while held in your hand. Tobacco can also be provided as a kind of worship to the Earth Mother (or any other god).

Native Americans were typically poor and lacked the financial means to purchase high-quality or even effective medicines in the past, but that didn't mean they didn't know what herbs may be utilized for therapeutic purposes. On Native American reservations, several herbs grow wild and are utilized for a variety of purposes, including cleansing and purification.

Native American civilization has a lengthy history, and it's probable that they knew about the medicinal benefits of plants long before Europeans did. When European immigrants arrived in America in search of new territory for new crops (and more land for themselves), they brought with them some knowledge of medicinal plants. Eventhen, most of this was just passed down from generation to generation as legend.

Safety Tips

When utilizing Native American herbs, keep the following safety recommendations in mind:

If you're expecting a child, avoid using herbs.

You should always see a doctor before taking any herbs while pregnant; just because they aren't categorized as medicine doesn't mean they won't injure or harm you. Many herbs, such as parsley and willow branches, can harm your unborn child; therefore, if you're pregnant, consult your doctor before attempting any new medical plants or supplements.

Use herbal medicines only if you understand what they can do and how they fit into Native American culture.

Many plants are used for a variety of purposes in various civilizations. In certain cultures, they are used for healing, while in others, they are used for purification or cleansing. You can always use this information to your advantage if you know what they are used for in Native American culture.

However, if you don't know and pick up a random plant and decide to use it anyway, there could be consequences; you could cause more harm than good, or the herb could even become poisonous if used incorrectly.

Do not begin utilizing some herbs without first receiving sufficient training.

Many herbs can be used for the same goals but produce distinct consequences in the body, thus even though their purpose is similar, not all of them will operate the same way for everyone. A few Native American herbs, such as the stinging nettle, can aid with diabetes and cancer, for example. But how can you know if the herb you're using is the proper one for your illness if you haven't studied it? You can discover that you're using the incorrect herb, or that it doesn't even perform for the stated purpose.

Use only a few different herbs at a time.

When utilizing any form of medicinal plant, start with one and see how it affects your body before adding more. This is not only safe, but it will also help you better understand how each herb affects your body and what your body requires at any given time.

If a condition isn't mentioned in Native American culture, don't use herbs for it.

If a given herb was utilized for a specific function in Native American culture, for example, you should just use what works and doesn't harm you. However, if it is used for purposes you are unfamiliar with or have never heard of, it may cause more harm than good or even become poisonous. Experiment with different herbs to determine if they work for you.

If you're using wild herbs or plants, make sure they're edible and only edible.

There are numerous types of wild plants that can be used therapeutically in Native American culture, but some of them are dangerous. You must be certain that you are not using any of these items, as they may harm your health and well-being. Everything will be fine if you know what the plant is used for; just make sure to do your research before using any wild plant or herb.

When using Native American herbal medicine for the first time, don't use too much of any herb.

If you use too much of a certain herb at first, it can lead to issues like nausea and vomiting. However, if you start with the proper dosage, it will aid in the healing process; just be conscious of how much you're taking and stick to a strict schedule.

If you are out of balance, don't use any of the herbs.

To properly employ medicinal herbs, you must first be in a healthy frame of mind, which involves sticking to a strict diet and exercising regularly. This will ensure that your body is balanced and in the right state to recover, therefore don't use any herbs or plants until you've done this.

Start with a modest amount and work your way up.

If you're new to home remedies and Native American medicinal herbs, you might be tempted to use at least a couple of them straight away. However, doing so is not the ideal option because it will shock your body and make you sick. Instead, start with one herb and work your way up from there once you've established that your body has adjusted to it.

Poisonous or toxic herbs should not be used.

In Native American culture, there are many different types of plants that can be used as medical herbs. However, if handled incorrectly, several of them can be dangerous or even deadly. If you don't know what it's for, it's best to stay away from it entirely.

If any herbs are out of season, don't use them.

In Native American culture, there are many different types of plants that can be used for therapeutic purposes, but some must be utilized at specific times of the year. Otherwise, if they aren't in the right season, they will become poisonous. Consider this and just use the tools that are currently available to you at the time of your request.

Remember to take your medications on time.

When practicing Native American herbal medicine, one of the most important things to remember is to never forget your doses. If you do, none of the healing results you're hoping for will occur. Instead, make sure you set an alarm or wear a watch so you don't forget. Then, as often as feasible, repeat this treatment until your problem is entirely healed.

Many people have discovered that employing Native American herbal remedies will help them overcome their illnesses and heal faster if they follow these guidelines. So, if you've been looking for a natural remedy for your disease, it could be time to investigate this form of herbal medicine further.

Native American herbs abuse

The use of herbs for personal gain or "self-treatment" is sadly very common among those who do not know any better. Thankfully, most of these people are readily apprehended because many customs and regulations are derived from indigenous communities across the country. If you're interested in Native American herbal treatments but want to learn more about them, it's time to pick up a book or two on the subject. You'll be surprised at how much knowledge there is and how much of it is freely available if you explore around. When reading a book on this subject, the first thing to keep in mind is that these herbs can be quite hazardous if used inappropriately or poorly. If they are not used appropriately, they can cause serious health problems, including death. The method you eat these herbs is crucial, and it should be done in a way that was natural to the people who used them in the first place.

If you come across some of these old recipes, double-check the ingredients to be sure they are safe. The bulk of these herbs have been studied for centuries, and the vast majority of them are entirely safe when used correctly.

The first thing you should do before beginning any form of research project is to take a look around your home. You'll want to look for pages from magazines or medical publications' volumes. Many things relevant to this topic can be simply found in an old book or magazine saved somewhere in your home. It's probably smart to save any old periodicals or medical publications you come across for future reference. You'll be able to swiftly refer to them in the future when you attempt to complete new jobs.

When looking for information about Native American herbal remedies, be cautious of what you find because there are so many different "facts" out there that it can be difficult to distinguish what is accurate and what is not. So, the next time you're seeking information about these kinds of herbs, be sure to complete your homework first because it will help you get better grades and keep your body safe when using any type of herb from this culture.

However, if you have been severely harmed or have been diagnosed with an illness that modern science has not been able to cure, it may be time to attempt these therapies as well. After all, they've aided others in the past, so why not trust them?

CONCLUSION

Herbal therapy has been reintroduced in the guise of alternative medicine in a variety of methods. Aromatherapy, acupuncture, herbal treatment, and other forms of alternative medicine are examples of this. Herbal treatment uses herbal medicines in the form of supplements, tea ingredients, oils, and powdered ingredients to cure common ailments and other health concerns. Native American herbs are sold by certain professional herbalists to cure disorders such as arthritis, skin problems, asthma, fractured bones, hormonal issues, and a variety of other ailments. However, in order for the herbs to be effective, they must be taken in the correct dosage and combined according to instructions. They should also be bought from reputable, quality-assured sources.

The goal of this book is to introduce you to some of the traditional medicinal plants. Herbs that have been used for millennia and are frequently passed down from generation to generation.

Herbs are used by a large number of Americans, and a growing number of doctors are recommending them to their patients. Researchers have discovered in labs what Native Americans discovered thousands of years ago: that the universe of plants contains a fantastic regular medication shop. Many of the drugs we use today contain components that are nearly identical to those found in nature.

A large percentage of our treatments are unavoidably produced versions of herbal extracts that Native Americans used to great success. Plant-based treatments are known as herbal remedies. These drugs have a lengthy history of being used to treat a variety of ailments. This is because the plants employed in traditional herbal therapy have been shown to have healing properties. Herbal medicines have less adverse effects than pills or antibiotics manufactured in laboratories and sold under a brand name, which is why some patients prefer them to regular therapies. Herbal medicines are still popular today since they are a cheaper alternative to the expensive pharmaceuticals that doctors often prescribe.

Native Americans are well-known for their knowledge of medical plants. It is thought that plants and herbs were originally used for healing after observing animals consume such plants when they were sick. To prevent these plants from over-harvesting, the medicine men used to select every third plant they found. Native Americans viewed life from a spiritual perspective. Finally, to be healthy, a person must have a sense of purpose and must follow a fair, harmonic, and balanced life path.

BOOK 7

HERBAL DISPENSATORY VOL.2

Best Preparation Methods for Your Natural Remedies

Citali Galwen

INTRODUCTION

Herbal medicine can be used to treat a variety of diseases and disorders. Because it does not include doctors or medications, it is the most cost-effective method of medicine. Herbal medicines come in a variety of forms and are used to treat a variety of medical disorders, particularly those that affect the body's internal organs like the neurological system, digestion, heart, lungs, and immune system.

When it comes to herbs and plants as cures, they tend to concentrate on the local growths of plants and herbs. When using Native American herbal and plant treatments, it's important to choose the right plants for the job. To treat a fractured bone, you would search for the type of bone that has been broken and treat it accordingly. To avoid something adverse from happening or inflicting greater pain than usual, you'd have to consider what kind of harm was sustained. Some herbs are used to treat specific injuries, while others are used to treat a wide range of ailments.

Alternative medicine has reintroduced herbal medicine in a variety of methods. Aromatherapy, acupuncture, herbal treatment, and other forms of alternative medicine are examples of this. Herbal treatment uses herbal medicines in the form of supplements, tea ingredients, oils, and powdered ingredients to cure common ailments and other health concerns. Native American herbs are sold by certain professional herbalists to cure disorders such as arthritis, skin problems, asthma, fractured bones, hormonal issues, and a variety of other ailments. However, in order for the herbs to be effective, they must be taken in the correct dosage and combined according to the instructions. They should also be bought from reputable, quality-assured sources.

CHAPTER 22:

PREPARATIONS USING FRESH HERBS

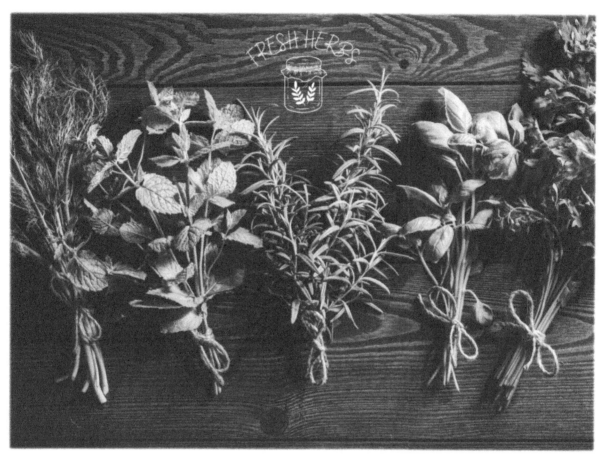

When you are planning to use fresh herbs or plants medicinally, you need to be aware of the nature of these substances. The herbs and plants that you will utilize need to be harvested in a way that is consistent with their energetics, which is different for each plant or herb.

A few herbs are not harvested at all because they are too difficult to process. These include burdock roots, red clover tops, and horsetail (not the hemlocks!).

One thing to consider when harvesting fresh herbs is how much yield you want in relation to your container size. If you plan on using fresh ingredients in liquid form and don't want them sitting on the counter, then a small amount is better. If you want to make a larger container with herbs or plants, then you should plan on having a greater amount of ingredients.

The next thing to consider is the energetics or flavor of the fresh plant or herb. For example, if you are using fresh mugwort leaves in an infusion, it will taste very different if you harvest it before the flowers bloom. The energetics for this plant are largely based on its lightness and clarity, and that comes from its flowers. Harvesting mugwort before its flowers have blossomed will result in a somewhat astringent taste.

Equipment Needed

The following is a list of equipment that you need:

- Container to hold the plant or herb.
- A knife or scissors for harvesting.

- A strainer for the container. This allows you to pour off the liquid while leaving the solid parts in your container while filtering out any debris that might be inside of it, such as dirt, small twigs, and leaves.
- A bowl or cup to hold your herbs and a spoon if necessary to scoop them out with while transferring them into your strainer container or storage container.
- A drying rack that can be used to dry or not.
- A cutting board for harvesting.
- A clean cloth to place over your container and dry the herbs while they are still moist, such as a dish towel or handkerchief.
- A jar that can be easily cleaned with dish soap and water. If you plan on using fresh herbs in liquid form, then you will need to transfer them into a glass container that will fit into your refrigerator after they are harvested and dried.

Harvesting: Step By Step Guide

Harvesting at the right time

Most herbs and plants need to be harvested at the right time in order to have the best overall outcome. Some will tolerate more than others depending on their light needs, but for most, their maximum growth and potency are when they are receiving the right amount of light.

Although it is recommended that you harvest your plant or herb before its flowers blossom, this does not mean that you cannot harvest from it after it has bloomed. Once it has bloomed, you can rest assured that it will continue to send its energy into the air around itself as a form of sexual pollen or seeds for each flower. If you harvest early enough in the season, the energy from the plant will continue. If it is only just beginning to bloom, you might have trouble with its energy leaving you through its leaves and flowers.

Therefore, consider harvesting your fresh herbs and plants at different times in order to harvest from them at their peak of potency before they begin to pass their energy on to the next generation, or if that is not a concern, then be sure that your container has no stagnant air or water or grime (dirt) in it.

Harvesting the right part of an herb

When harvesting an herb, you need to consider where the main part of the herb is, and this is what will determine how you process it. To do this, make sure that all of the leaves are removed from a plant or herb before harvesting any parts of it. The stems, woody underside, and flowers can be left on the plant or gathered after your plant or the herb has bloomed. Try not to tear off too many leaves because this can cause damage to the growth, and leaves will eventually dry out and die off anyway.

The main part of a plant or herb is often the middle or any lower part, such as a root, tuber, stem, leafy underside (no flowers), and sometimes bark. Harvest from the middle downward to get the most for your effort.

It is also important that you know if your plant or herb is harvested in certain ways, then you will change its energetic potential. Harvesting an herb at certain times will affect its energetics, and this can cause them to be more potent at certain times than others.

Best way to bundle & label plants after harvesting

You can bundle the stems together with string, thread, yarn, or rubber bands to keep them together and label your bundles with a pen, so you know what each bundle contains.

Harvesting the fresh herbs and plants is a good time to take a moment and thank the plant or herb for sharing its energetic potential with you. You can also give them a blessing or ask their permission before harvesting them, which will go a long way to making your herbs more potent when it comes time to use them.

To make sure that you have the most for your effort, harvest in accordance with the energetics of each plant or herb. Plan on drying half of everything that you harvest, as many herbs need to be dried out quickly before their energetic potential drops significantly.

Drying: Step By Step Guide

Best time and practice to dry herbs

Herbs and plants need to be dried out to get the maximum energetic potential from them during the time they are being harvested. This is because their freshness and energy are being held in their outermost layers of leaf, stem, or root (the outside part of live things). If you wait until they have dried more than halfway before removing them from the ground, then it might take a very long time for their energetic potential to dry out completely.

Hanging herbs upside down are the simplest way to dry them. The gravity will pull all of the moisture out of them. This process is called drying. The best time for this is early morning at first light, just as the sun comes up brightening the day with its productive energy.

Methods to dry herbs

1. Air Drying: This is done by spreading your herbs on a screen, bed sheet, or paper towels and letting them sit in a breezy spot for about two weeks. You can also dry them with the aid of an electric fan.
2. Microwave Drying: Prepping herbs for microwave drying is much like prepping vegetables for the oven: you want to remove any dirt and cut off leaves that are too large, so they don't burn during microwaving. Then, place your herb sprigs in a paper towel-lined bowl and cover it with another paper towel, so the steam from the microwave doesn't escape from all sides of the bowl. Cook on high heat for 4 minutes or until most of their water has been dried up.
3. Oven Drying: Doing this can take anywhere from 5–20 hours, so you'll have to keep checking to see if the process is done. You also want to make sure that your oven is not too hot as you don't want your herbs to burn. Once done, you can store the dried herbs in air-tight containers.
4. The Sun and Air: This method is ideal for those living in regions with warm climates and who do not own a microwave or electric fan. This method will take about two weeks and requires your herbs to be spread across a screen and placed outside in an area that receives direct sunlight throughout the day.

You can also dry fresh herbs by placing them in large sponges or between clean rags placed on a sturdy surface.

To dry fresh herbs without losing any of the leafy green colors, you can place them between two clean sheets of paper towels or a piece of cloth, and you can also use glass containers with air space for your drying method. If you choose to use glass containers, then be sure that they have no cracks or chips in the glass itself to prevent your dried herbs from absorbing harmful radiation.

CHAPTER 23:

PREPARATION USING DRIED HERBS

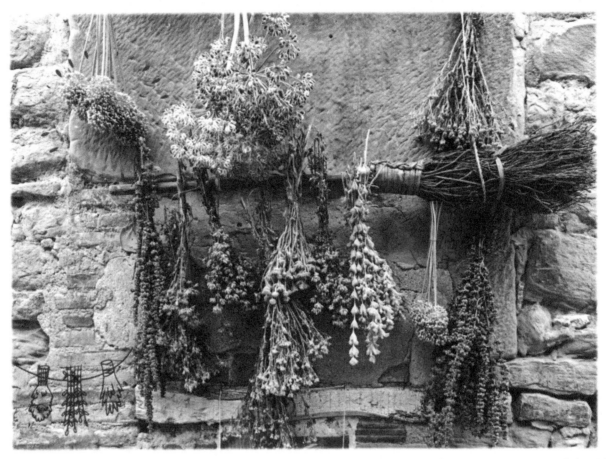

All herbs should be dried in direct sunlight, in a dehydrator, or in the oven at 180°F for 4–10 hours until dry. The oven must be turned off when herbs are fully dried.

The best way to store dried herbs is sealed in airtight jars. If you prefer to put them away in sealed packets, you can use aluminum foil or plastic wrap over the top of the packet.

Make sure that your jar lids are airtight before sealing them shut so that nothing can react with the herbs and cause chemical changes during storage which will alter their natural properties.

Remove any stems from freshly picked herbs. Any stems that remain on the plant will become bitter and will not store well.

A great deal of the healing power of herbs is lost when they are used as cooking ingredients. When using herbs as spices, it is best to use them fresh, as most of their medicinal properties are lost within a few days after drying. However, there are some exceptions, such as spearmint and thyme.

Equipment Needed

Here is the equipment needed when you use dried herbs:

- A mortar and pestle (or electric grinder)
- A large bowl or casserole dish to hold the herbs
- A spoon to help mix the herbs with the liquid

- Funnel to help pour your tincture into a bottle or container.

Bulk Herbs

Using bulk herbs is an excellent way to save money because you can buy them in bulk and make your own herbal medicine for the entire year. Herbs, however, are a living thing, and each batch of herbs has a life span. If you purchase your herbs from the same dealer each time, then you'll get herbs with similar properties and potency. You can also purchase bulk herbs at a discount if you buy them in larger quantities, say by the pound or half-pound.

Quality Control Issues When Buying Dried Herbs

When buying dried herbs, a common complaint is that the quality can vary greatly from one batch to another because different herb suppliers may use different methods. Although this may be the case, you can still purchase herbs and mix them with alcohol and make a tincture that will work for any diseases that your family may be developing or dealing with.

To buy bulk herbs, you might have to visit herb shops in your area on occasion because each herbalist will use their own method of drying the plant material so that it doesn't lose its properties when you dry it out. In order to prepare the herb for use, you'll need to grind it with a mortar and pestle.

Unfortunately, herbalists don't label their herbs with what diseases they are good for. Because of this reason, you'll have to do some research into each plant material so that you will know how they can be used.

Capsules

The first step is to grind the herbs and then fill empty capsules with them. You can buy empty gelatin capsules at most health food stores because they usually carry a variety of sizes that you'll need when you create your herbal medicine.

Many herbs are too bitter or strongly tasting to take raw. For these herbs, it can be more pleasant to take them in capsule form.

Step-by-step instructions:

1. In a mortar and pestle or in a blender, crush the chosen herb into approximately the consistency of a coarse meal. Store in a glass jar.
2. Add a small amount of powdered vegetable glycerin. This adds to the body of the capsule so that it will dissolve more easily when swallowed, or it can be used along with an enema for cleansing.
3. Fill the capsules 2/3 full with this paste. After this is done, add the remaining mixture to fill them completely (an extra 1/3).
4. Store in a cool place until ready to use.

Tablets

You can also create tablets for acute problems such as an upset stomach. To do this, you'll mix an herb with gelatin and then shape the mixture into a tablet. You can crush the tablet into a powder before swallowing it, or you can mix it with water and drink it like tea.

Tablets are simpler to use than capsules, but they are less stable over time. You can get a longer duration from the more stable capsules.

Step-by-step *instructions:*

1. Make an Infusion. Using the method described in Making Infusions, combine dried or fresh herbs with filtered water to produce your mixture.
2. For each tablet, combine the correct quantity of herb powder with powdered vegetable glycerin.
3. Fold in a kitchen towel for several minutes until all the grains are completely embedded in the substance.
4. Add approximately 1/2 teaspoon of any flavoring oil or butter to help facilitate swallowing. This may be necessary if you are having problems with tablets sticking to your tongue or throat after taking them.
5. Using a spoon, scoop one-fourth of the mixture into rounded flat cherry-sized balls. These consist of about 1/8–1/4 teaspoon each.

6. When done, wash your hands and dry them. To minimize the possibility of transmission, use your bare hands instead of a spoon to scoop up the mixture.

If you are unsure how these will affect you, first begin with 1/8th teaspoon doses for 24 hours, diluting if necessary with water on the second day. If it affects you adversely, increase to 1/4 teaspoon or less for 24 hours, then dilute again, if necessary, on the third morning.

Nut Butter Balls

You can make nut butter balls, which can be used to help heal coughs such as whooping coughs or to ease sore throats. You'll need to grind the nuts first, and then you'll mix them with organic honey or date syrup. The next step is to mix with dried herbs and then form the mixture into small balls before putting them into their containers.

Some people prefer the taste of nut butter, too. With the addition of a little powdered vegetable glycerin, it is possible to make nut butter-like balls yourself.

Step-by-step *instructions:*

1. Combine the herb powder with powdered vegetable glycerin, just as you would for tablets-infused oil or butter. These are much tastier than plain nuts and have many times the potency of tablets eaten alone.
2. Use 4–8 servings per batch for more potent medicine.
3. Roll these into balls about 1/2" across and place them on a cookie sheet covered with waxed paper or tin foil to protect them from exposure to air or moisture.
4. Refrigerate until you are ready to eat them or store them in a cool place for a longer time.

If you have trouble swallowing the nut butter balls, grate a little over-ripe banana on top of each one, and they will dissolve in your mouth without too much effort.

In conclusion, it's important to have a good herbal medicine cabinet because it contains natural medicines that will help your family when they are dealing with certain issues.

CHAPTER 24:

INTRODUCING EXTRACTION

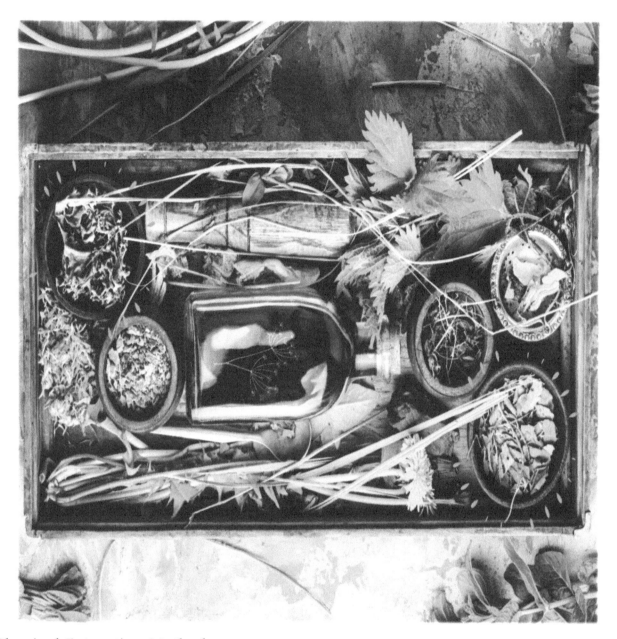

Classical Extraction Methods

Native Americans used extraction techniques passed down to them through generations. Many times, the Native American's tools were simple, and in some cases, there were no tools used at all.

Hot water extraction

Water was warmed in a pot with hot rocks. The material the Native Americans were trying to extract would be dropped in the water, and the mixture would be kept hot for several hours. The mixture was then strained out and cooled.

Cold water extraction

In cold water extraction, the native people used boiling water to infuse herbs. They later took the liquid, separated it from the solid, and infused it again with fresh herbs until they got what they needed for their medicines or food.

Boiling/steaming
Boiling was a common method of extracting oils, waxes, resins, or other chemicals by use of heat and moisture over an extended period of time.

Maceration
Maceration was a process where plant material was steeped in hot water for a lengthy period of time, and the liquid was used as needed.

Alcoholic extractions
Plants were soaked in alcohol to extract oils, resins, and liquids that may have been useful for food, medicines, or cosmetics. These extracts were prepared with Herbal tinctures and infused alcohols like vodka.

Glossary Of Terms

Solvent
A liquid dissolves a solid material and releases the solute, making it possible to separate the solute from the solvent.

Solvent extraction
Using a solvent to dissolve plant material and separating it from the solvent at a later time is extracted through solvent extraction.

Essence
The essential oils of plants are often extracted in various ways to attain their individual effects, as well as creating combinations with other plant materials and herbs for specific needs.

Oil
The waxes or fats from plants are extracted using heat and pressure in an oil extractor (expeller).

Garbling
A process that takes place when liquid is mixed with another liquid, usually water or alcohol. The result is a viscous substance.

Percolation
Percolating simply means mixing two liquids together and allowing the liquids to mix and separate at various points throughout the mixture.

Decanting
Decanting is the process of removing excess liquid in order to make it possible to pour the liquid that is desired.

Sterilization
Sterilization is the process of heat treating material for long periods of time and under high temperatures specific to certain materials in order to kill all microorganisms.

Distillation
Distillation is used when distilling alcohol, which requires heat, pressure, and a substance that will evaporate or change states at a certain temperature, which separates an element from another by reducing it to its purest form and returning it back to its original state. The end product is known as an extract or essence.

Precipitation
Precipitation is the separation of a solid from a liquid. This can be achieved through filtration, sedimentation, and even reverse osmosis.

Equipment Needed

Jars
A jar is a glass container with a narrow rim that is used to collect small plant fragments and liquids.

Rubber spatula
Rubber spatulas are used in the extraction process when dealing with large amounts of plant material. They are made with durable rubber, so they can withstand high temperatures.

Mortar and pestle

A mortar and pestle are tools made of stone or wood that have been smoothed out on one side to create an uneven surface meant for crushing or grinding herbs and roots. The other side usually has some type of handle or groove for easy grip or use.

Coffee grinders

A coffee grinder is a tool used in the preparation of many different types of plant materials. It is used to grind herbs, leaves, and other plant matter into a fine powder for use.

Vitamix

Vitamix is an appliance used to grind a variety of materials, especially for those who are looking to make herbal tinctures. The blender itself is very powerful and can be found on the market for around $600–$1000, depending on what model you choose.

Strainers

Strainers are used to separate plant material from its liquid in order to make sure none of the liquid gets carried into another compartment with unwanted materials mixed in it.

Mixing bowls

Mixing bowls are very useful when dealing with herbs, as well as for mixing other plant materials. They are used to mix all the different ingredients and to keep everything at an even temperature throughout the entire process.

Herb press

Herb presses can be used in herb or flower pressing sessions and do not require a lot of water or oil of any kind in order to operate properly.

Scale

A scale can be used to weigh down tinctures, teas, or other substances that need specific amounts of weight simply by using a scale's base unit weight that is calibrated in grams, ounces, or pounds.

Digital thermometer

A digital thermometer can be used to measure the specific temperature of the plants, herbs, and other substances that need to be exercised at specific temperature ranges and measurements for specific time periods for different types of tinctures.

Measuring cups

Measuring cups can help you get exact amounts of the liquid that you are interested in extracting from a plant or herb by using an accurate measuring cup or measuring spoon. This can be especially helpful when dealing with essences and tinctures that require different amounts of ingredients depending on how potent they need to be in order to make them work properly.

CHAPTER 25:

PREPARATIONS FOR MAKING EXTRACTIONS

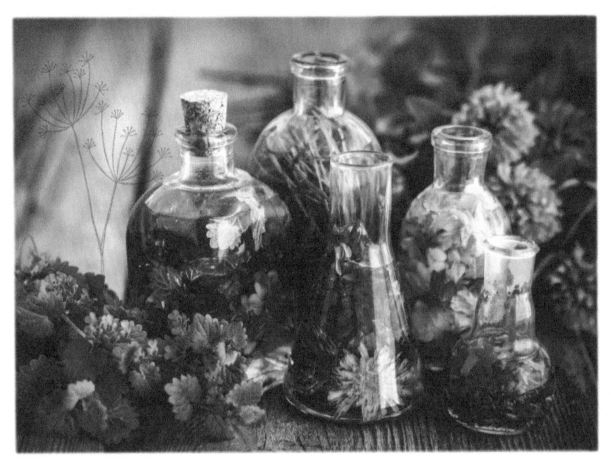

Water-Based Extractions

This is the most common method and is probably the easiest to use. For this type of extraction, it's best to prepare your herbs in the whole form or loosely ground so they will be easier to work with. Following these simple steps will help reduce the chances of killing off some of the plant's beneficial substances. Additionally, it may be helpful to choose high-proof alcohol that is suited for your intended use, such as Everclear (190 proof) or Everard (210 proof).

Infusions

Unless your herb is a leafy type, you will want to chop it up. If it is a leafy type, then you may simply tear or break off a piece to use in the infusion.

1. With a small saucepan, fill with water and turn on medium heat.
2. Add your herbs to the water and let boil.
3. Simmer for 10–15 minutes according to your recipe or until water has absorbed all of the essential oils from the plant material.
4. Turn off the heat and set aside to cool before straining out herbs with a cheesecloth or fine mesh strainer.

Decoctions

1. Chop your herbs into small pieces to help release the active components within.
2. Place herbs in a pot and cover with water, then bring to a boil while reducing the heat as needed (you may need to add more water during this process).
3. Let it simmer until very little liquid remains, about 15–20 minutes; upon this point, do not allow it to evaporate off completely else you run the risk of burning off some of the plant's beneficial substances.

4. Strain through cheesecloth or muslin cloth into another container, squeezing any remaining liquids out of your herbs.
5. Decanting: Pour the mixture from your cloth or cheesecloth back into the pot, then fill a container with alcohol and pour it over the herbs.
6. Cap and label, letting it sit for 2–3 weeks in a dark place at a warm temperature such as 65°-85°. Shake it daily, if possible, to extract all of the beneficial substances out of the herbs.

Alcohol Extractions

There are two distinct ways of making alcohol extracts. The first is by using a double boiler in which the herb sits directly on top of the boiling alcohol. This method works best when the herb is finely ground to release as many of its beneficial components as possible. Alcohol burns off at a higher rate than water, so it'll need to be reduced somewhat after you have added your ground herbs into the pot.

The alcohol types that you can use for this purpose are wine, vodka, beer, and brandy. Some strains of the plant will work with less alcohol than others. The key with these extracts is to make sure it isn't too hot, and you don't let the herb sit too long at a high temperature as this can actually damage your extract.

Tinctures
For this process, it is best to use Everclear (190 proof), Everard (210 proof), or any higher-proof alcohol you can find.

1. Place your herbs in a pot with alcohol and place the pot on the stove on medium-high heat. Add enough alcohol to just cover the herbs; occasionally stir until all of the material has been dissolved. Adding hot water can help build pressure and release more of the active components from your herbs, while cold water will slow down this process.
2. If necessary, reduce heat to low and let it simmer for about 40–60 minutes; ensure that the alcohol does not burn off during this process.
3. Strain through cheesecloth or muslin cloth into another container, squeezing any remaining liquids out of your herbs.
4. To make a tincture, add 1 part alcohol to 1 part water in a jar and shake for 30 seconds before placing the lid on tight and keeping it in the dark, room-temperature area for at least 2 months before utilizing; shake well before each use to extract all of the beneficial substances out of the herbs.

Dried herbs tinctures (macerations)
This process is similar to making tinctures, but instead of using alcohol-primarily, the herb is soaked in an herbal liquid for 1–2 months. The goal in this process is to release as many of the active components as possible while preserving their original beneficial properties.

1. Place your herbs in a jar and fill it with a concentrated herbal liquid such as alcohol or vinegar; cover with the lid and shake well before each use to extract all of the beneficial substances out of the herbs.
2. Allow it to sit for 30 days, shaking daily if possible. After 30 days, strain through cheesecloth or muslin cloth into another container, squeezing any remaining liquids out of your herbs.
3. to make a tincture, add 1 part alcohol to 1 part liquid in a jar and shake well before each use to extract all of the beneficial substances out of the herbs.

Fresh plant tinctures (macerations)
1. Grind your fresh herb
2. Fill a jar just less than halfway with your ground herb.
3. Fill the empty space in the bottle with a high-proof alcohol (Everclear should be used if you are just starting out.) but keep an eye out for this as it evaporates faster than water.
4. Shake the bottle to blend the components well for around 10 minutes, then close with a lid and let it sit in a warm place for at least 4 weeks. Shake regularly every few days to help release active ingredients from plant material, etc.

5. After 4 weeks, strain through cheesecloth or muslin into another clean bottle, then add 1/4 cup of glycerin (optional) and re-cap tightly.
6. Label and date your new herbal extract and store it in a dark place (kitchen cabinet) for future use.

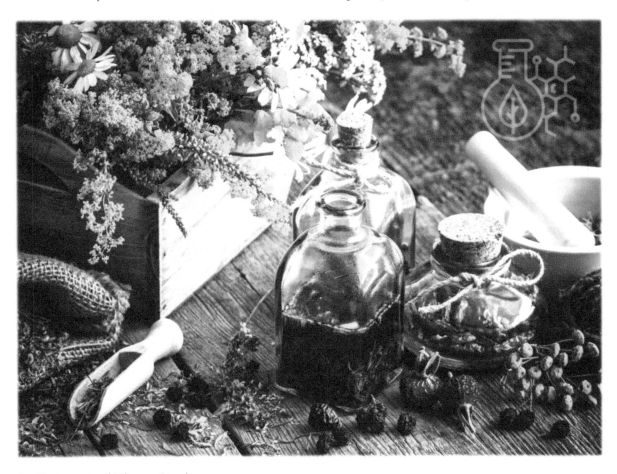

Glycerin Extracts (Glycerites)

Glycerin is an emollient; it acts to soften skin, making it more supple by helping the skin retain moisture. Glycerin also increases smoothness in formulations for the treatment of rough, dry, or cracked skin.

How glycerites are made
1. In a jar, cover your herbs with vegetable glycerin; close with the lid and shake well before each use to extract all of the beneficial substances out of the herbs.
2. Allow it to sit for 2–4 weeks, shaking daily if possible; after this time has passed, strain the mixture through cheesecloth or muslin cloth into another container, squeezing any remaining liquid out of your herbs.
3. Cap and label, letting it sit for 2–3 weeks in a dark place at room temperature before using; shake well before each use to extract all of the beneficial substances out of the herbs.

Seales simmer

This method of extracting a medical tincture follows the same principles and methods as above but with great modifications. For instance, in this method, the herbs are placed into a simmering pot on low heat instead of the oven, filtered through a muslin cloth or cheesecloth before placing into an amber jar.

1. Place your herbs in a container with water and calcium water (1 teaspoon of calcium carbonate for every quart); place the pot on the stove on low heat to begin the heating process.
2. Continue to heat the water throughout the duration of your mixture while stirring every few minutes; then turn off the heat and allow to cool before placing the herbs in a freezer.
3. Place herbs in the freezer for 3–5 days, stirring daily to ensure that all of the beneficial substances are extracted from your herbs.

4. After 3–5 days, remove your herbs from the freezer and place them through muslin cloth or cheesecloth into another container, squeezing any remaining liquids out of your herbs.
5. Cap and label, letting it sit for 2–3 weeks in a dark place at room temperature before using; shake well before each use to extract all of the beneficial substances out of the herbs.

Extracting In Vinegar

1. Place your herbs in a pot with vinegar; place on stove on medium-low heat to begin heating process.
2. Continue to heat the vinegar throughout the duration of your mixture while stirring every few minutes; then turn off the heat and allow to cool before placing the herbs in a freezer.
3. Place herbs in the freezer for 3–5 days, stirring daily to ensure that all of the beneficial substances are extracted from your herbs.
4. After 3–5 days, remove your herbs from the freezer and place them through muslin cloth or cheesecloth into another container, squeezing any remaining liquids out of your herbs.
5. Cap and label, letting it sit for 2–3 weeks in a dark place at room temperature before using; shake well before each use to extract all of the beneficial substances out of the herbs.

CHAPTER 26:

TOPICAL PREPARATIONS

What Is A Topical Preparation?

Topical preparations are made from plant material that is prepared in a way so that it can work topically on the body. For example, a topically applied preparation could be made by macerating herbs in a carrier oil and then applying the oil to the skin (a topical ointment) or by grinding herbs into powder and then applying that powder to the skin (a topical scrub) or by boiling plants whole, seeds, bark, leaves, etc. of their appropriate genus in water and then applying the solution to dry areas of skin for local application (for example foot soak). This preparation would typically be applied before bedtime or during hot weather for foot care.

Oil-Based Herbal Preparation

Making an herb oil preparation is fairly easy and only takes a few minutes to a few hours of your time and small equipment.

Equipment

- Mason jar with lid, grinder (mortar and pestle, coffee grinder, hammer, or stone)
- Stainless steel or glass pot/pan (if using stovetop)
- Spoon, cheesecloth, or other strainer bags (like a coffee filter)
- Funnel
- Glass bottle to store finished product in

Ingredients:

- Fresh herbs that can be ground finely or have leaves that can be chopped easily. A good ratio is 2–6 tablespoons of herb to 1 cup of carrier oil.

Process:

1. Grind the herbs in a mortar or coffee grinder if possible. If not, use a hammer or stone in a glass bowl to crush the herbs until fine and then transfer the herbs to a small pot/pan.
2. One of my favorite methods is to put everything but the oil in a mason jar and then put that jar on top of the stove burner on low heat and leave it simmering for about an hour until it starts to change color and smell.
3. At this point, you can remove the lid and pour off about half of the liquid into a strainer bag (1/2 cup at a time) to remove debris and let it drain. When you have strained out all the liquid, pour it into your blender with the rest of your oil. Blend everything at low speed until it is fully mixed and then strain again through a cheesecloth or other strainer bag to remove all of the ground herb bits and pieces.
4. Now you have your herbal-infused oil! Pour it into storage bottles and label appropriately.

Extracting Herbs In Oil Or Fat

A different way to prepare a topical herbal preparation is to soak the herbs in oil or fat. This method can be very simple or very complex, depending on what you want out of your preparation. If you are making a salve, then the process should be fairly quick and simple. If you are making an infused oil for internal use, then it should take considerably longer. For a salve, simply combine equal parts herb and oil (or fat) and heat until the herbs become saturated.

Local Applications

The most commonly used topical applications are salves and ointments. Salves are greasier and typically made with beeswax, lanolin, or other plant waxes as a base. Ointments are typically oilier and can be made in a variety of ways but typically include some sort of vegetable oil or animal fat (like lard). Another easy way to make an herbal ointment is to mix melted shea butter or cocoa butter with an infused oil.

Herbal salves and ointments have been used historically for both internal and external applications such as scrapes, cuts, burns, dry/cracked skin, bleeding wounds, bug bites/stings, etc.

CHAPTER 27:

ADVANCED EXTRACTION METHODS

Percolation Extracts

This technique of extracting the volatile oils from plants is typically used to make "latakia," a type of tobacco.

This extract is made by placing the plant parts in a pot and allowing them to simmer for 12 hours or more.

An additional solvent such as hexane or alcohol may be added, which might cause some impurities that remain after distillation to separate as a layer on top of the liquid. This layer can then optionally be removed and discarded before boiling with more salt, water, and/or herbs.

Next, heat some cold water in the pot, so it is around 100–120°C (212–248°F) until both sides are frothing.

The froth is removed with a ladle, and more water is added, then the pot is heated to around 180°C (356°F).

Put in some more cold water to make it froth again, remove the froth, add even more cold water, and heat the pot until a layer of oil appears on top.

Put in 100 grams of salt for every 30 milliliters of liquid (1 Fl oz) and boil this for another hour or so.

Remove it from heat and leave it undisturbed to settle for at least 12 hours.

At this point, the oil will begin to separate from the water and herb matter.

Remove the layer of oil and discard it.

Repeat this process two more times, each time removing some of the water in between boiling stages for a few hours or days for each extraction.

After that, you have three layers: the bottom layer of oil, a bottom layer of salt and herbs, and then most of the remaining liquid above that with the least amount of plant matter included (this is also where you can add alcohol or additional solvent if needed).

You currently have four compositions:
1. Total resinous oil with a much higher proportion of resin than leaf or stem water (but contains no alkaloids). The amount of resin in this layer is based on the initial plant material and the amount left after you discard the top layer.
2. Water with an alkaloid content was neutralized by adding salt to make it more soluble. If a lot of water is left behind, it can be used as a wash for poppets, but not for smoking.
3. Herb-washed water with an alkaloid content that is low enough so it can be used as a wash for poppets and incense sticks, but not for smoking.
4. A third liquid above the herb-washed water that is composed of alcohol, salt, and the plant matter (stems tend to leave more of this behind than leaves). This is also where the oil will separate from the water, and it should be discarded.

Note that even though this method is called "percolation," it does not equal "percolation distillation." Percolation extracts as much of the essential oils as possible without burning them off. This method is used to turn plant material into a fluid that can be used for things like incense. It transforms a solid or semi-solid material into a fluid that can easily permeate paper or fabric.

Equipment needed
1. Percolation Cone—You can use a parchment cone, like a coffee filter, but made out of parchment paper. It should have at least three layers (five is better) and a hole towards the top for the oil to pass through.
2. Jar—this can be any glass jar or container that you can fit the percolation cone into, and it will hold water (a Pyrex bowl works well). It should have some holes drilled in the bottom for it to drain with gravity into a larger jar where you will store it.

3. Filter—this is usually made by stretching cheesecloth over something like a funnel or empty bottle cap, so its contents can easily pass through without leaving unwanted plant matter behind. It can also be made by cutting off the bottom part of the percolation cone and just using that.
4. Weight—anything that will keep the filter or cheesecloth in place over the lid of the large jar will work. You can use anything from a book to a brick, etc.
5. Lid—this is to prevent evaporation because it is very slow-going and difficult to evaporate small amounts of oil at high temperatures as you would need for this method.
6. Heat source—a hot plate or burner with a flame is usually used for this, but you could use an alcohol lamp or even sunlight if need be (though that would take much longer).

Preparing the plant material
1. Wash the plant parts, and then dry them using a fan.
2. Grind the plant material using a grinder or food processor to make it as fine as possible. You will not need anything that is very fine, but you don't want it to be coarse either.
3. Pour enough cold water into a small pan to cover all of your plant material (about 1 liter) and fill up the pan with cold water until it covers all of your dry plant matter by at least 1 centimeter (1/2 inch).
4. Put the lid on top of the jar and let sit for 24 hours or so (longer if necessary). Make sure that no condensation forms in the jar.
5. After it has sat for a while (about 12 hours), you will notice that the water has turned a brown or dark color, and the plant material will be floating at the top.
6. Strain out all of the plant material using a cheesecloth, and then discard it.
7. Pour this liquid into the percolation cone until it is about 2/3 full (you want to leave a bit of room for expansion). Then put your weight on top of it so that it won't fall over when heated.
8. Heat the percolation cone in a small pot or on a hot plate or stovetop burner, and when it begins to steam, remove it from the heat. Let it sit undisturbed until most of the water has evaporated, at which point you should see a layer of oil has formed on top (you will notice that this is lighter colored because it has extracted more of the resinous oils than either water or herb residue).
9. Carefully remove the cone from your material and place it upside down in your jar, then pour out any remaining liquid.

Fluid Extracts

Now you have a substance that is composed of essential oils and an alcohol solvent extract. It is very similar to the oil of oregano you can get in health food stores, except this has a higher concentration of the essential oils and would not be good for swallowing.

It can be used to:

1. Make pillows or poppets where you will place a little bit of this inside, then wrap in cheesecloth or something similar and add a bit of resin to make incense that can be used in a brazier or incense burner.
2. Make smoking mixtures where you add it to kerosene or a solvent like ether, and make an oil that can be smoked (this is a highly effective method but is potentially dangerous if not done properly).
3. Make smudge sticks by soaking sage leaves, cedar bark, mullein leaves, etc., in this substance for a few days. Then you dry the herb by heating it in a frying pan with a little bit of vegetable oil, and then compress it into a stick-like incense.
4. Add this to a mixture that can be burned on charcoal disks to increase the potency of your incense.
5. Make anointing oils by adding this to olive or vegetable oil and using it to anoint candles or poppets that will be used in rituals.
6. Mix this with alcohol and water to create an herbal tincture (this is another highly effective method but is potentially dangerous if not done properly).

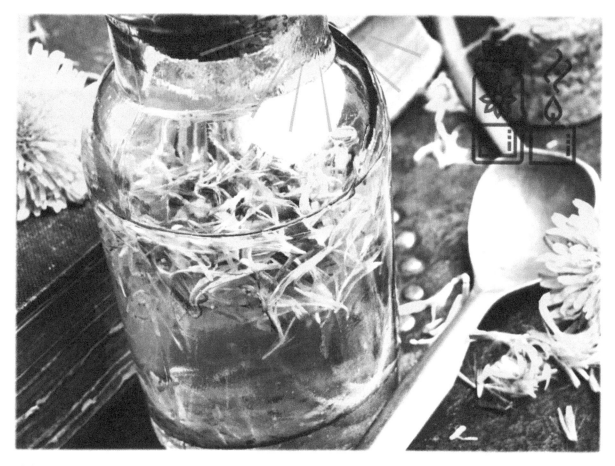

Soxhlet Extracts

This method is the most difficult, but it also produces a more potent product. It uses heat and pressure to extract the essential oils, but because it's not a precise process, some of the compounds that you don't want to extract (like tannins and plant matter) are usually extracted as well.

Most people prefer to use a distillation setup for this method because it is safer and more effective. However, if you don't have access to one of those setups, you can easily make your own using common household items.

Equipment needed
1. Large pot or pan that has a lid (the lid should fit well so that pressure can build up inside).
2. Pan for boiling your plant material in.
3. The jar will fit inside the pot and hold enough water to cover your plant material when you put it in (these usually come with lids as well).
4. Two large bowls, one to sit on top of the jar (with a hole drilled through it) and one that will sit on top of the pot, with a hole drilled through it as well (about the same diameter as a pencil).
5. Clamp or vice grips so you can hold the jar snugly in place or wire to secure it so it won't float up when you put water around it.

CHAPTER 28:

HOW TO STORE HERBS AND KEEP THEM SAFE

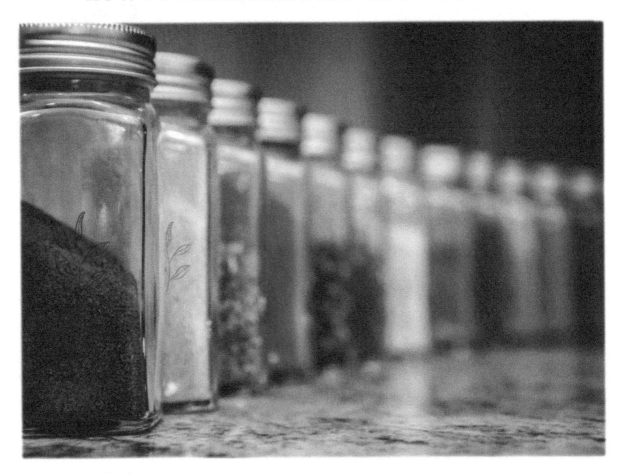

Different Methods Of Storage

Drying

The easiest, cheapest, and safest method of storage is drying. It requires little preparation except for cleanliness.

Freezing

Freezing is very convenient because you can freeze your herbs in small, medium, or large batches. Just open the freezer and dump your herbs on a tray or in a container to freeze, and within minutes, they are freezable. This method requires little preparation as well, but you should take into account that it takes at least 24 hours to thaw before eating them, so this method might not be appropriate for when you need them quickly.

Canning

Canning is one of the best methods of storage. The jars are air-tight and will keep your herbs for years to come. This method requires much preparation, so you need to read the directions carefully.

Herbal butter

Making herbal butter is a very easy and healthful way of storing herbs. You can use this method instead of a freezer or canning jar. It keeps the herbs fresh for about 2 weeks; just make sure that you label it with the date it was made, so you know how long it has been in your medicine bag!

Herbal tea

Making herbal tea is also a great way to store herbs for a long time. To make herbal tea, just place your herbs in the pot, cover them with boiling water, and steep for about 15 minutes. When you are done, you can serve it with honey or add some lemon or orange juice to make it healthy.

Dry herbs

Starting with dried herbs might sound like an expensive way of storing herbs, but this is not the case when you look at how much money you can save in the end! You just have to figure out the amount of herbs you need per dosage so that the amount left will be enough on your trip. Then you can hang your herbs in a cool, dry place, and this will last for years. Herbs can be re-hydrated in boiling water or the amount of water needed reduced by blanching the herbs first.

Best Equipment Needed To Store Herbs

Plastic containers

One of the best containers to store herbs in is plastic because they are durable, and you can see the contents easily without opening the container. You will need at least 1-ounce, wide-mouth jars with lids to hold one day's worth of herbs for one person. This way, you can keep your herbs as fresh as possible and make cleaning easier.

Mason jars

Another good way to store your herbs is in mason jars with canning lids. They are ideal for freezing or drying herbs because they seal tightly so that no air or other people contaminate them! They are multipurpose and great for storage even when dry goods are not needed!

Air tight lids

If you are using canning jars, you will need a jar with an air-tight lid. This way, no bacteria or mold will get inside of them!

Mason jars are also excellent for storing herbs because they are designed for dry goods and keep them fresh for years. In addition, these jars may be used for canning!

If you are using plastic containers, then you need to make sure that your containers have a low sweating point.

Tips And Tricks For Perfect Storage

1. Keep your herbs in a clean, cool, dry place that is out of the way of children and pets.
2. If you are storing your herbs in plastic containers, keep them away from water and humidity! The containers will melt if they come into contact with water!
3. Store your jars away from sunlight so that your herbs stay fresh! Sunlight will fade the herbs, and the colors usually turn brown or yellow instead of green!
4. You can store herbs for a long time if you keep them in air-tight containers. But make sure you close the jar tightly when storing them!
5. If you want to preserve herbs for an extended period of time, and if the jars are glass, then they will need to be kept in an air-tight container to prevent mold from growing on them. The jars should also have a rubber seal (like for canned foods) so that they don't collapse when they heat up!
6. Herbs should not be stored in metal containers because this can create an electric charge which could shock people or animals!

CHAPTER 29:

SPECIAL#: DAILY HERBS

Many people are unaware of, and certainly do not consider, the importance of Native American herbs. Native American medicine, on the other hand, may not be as well-known as other medical options such as Chinese medicine. Still, these herbs are recognized to be beneficial, especially for persons who utilize them on a daily basis. Of course, Native American healing and medicine was about more than just herbs, even if herbs were a big part of it.

Shilajit

The resin of this herb is well-known for being high in vitamins and minerals, which are necessary for a long and healthy life. Shilajit is a common ingredient in Ayurvedic treatments. It's an effective and dependable supplement that can improve your general health and fitness over time. Shilajit may protect against free radicals and cellular collapse since it is high in fulvic acid, a powerful anti-inflammatory and antioxidant. As a result, regular shilajit use may contribute to a slower aging process, increased longevity, and overall improved fitness.

Shilajit is available as a powder or a liquid. Apply vitamins as directed on a regular basis. If you acquire the Shilajit supplement in liquid form, dissolve a pea-sized or a grain-sized piece in liquid and drink 1-3 times per day (depending on directions).

Even better, you can take shilajit powder with pure milk twice a day. Shilajit is taken in doses of 0.3 to 0.5 g per day. Please consult with your doctor before using shilajit as a treatment.

Bogbean

Bogbean is a herb with leaves that are commonly used in herbal therapy.

12 cup distilled water + 1 gram dried bogbean leaves. Bring the water to a boil, then steep the tea for 7–10 minutes before filtering out the solids. You can drink this tea three times a day if your herbalist recommends it.

1 1/3 cup distilled water + 2 grams dried bogbean herb. Before removing the teabags and steeping them for 10 minutes, bring the distilled water to a boil. Once a day, preferably in the morning, drink the tea.

Because a specific dosage varies from person to person, you should always contact with an herbal medicine specialist before using any herbal cure.

To relieve arthritic symptoms such as joint stiffness and pain, take 2 mL liquid bogbean extract twice daily.

Chestnut Horse

Horse chestnut seed extracts efficiently treat varicose veins, and the gels contain anti-inflammatory effects (it's important to remember that inflammation can induce swelling and fluid retention).

A compound containing horse chestnut extract has been discovered to improve sperm quality. Aescin, the main active ingredient in horse chestnut infusion, has been proven to provide numerous health benefits in humans. Its bark, seed, flower, and leaves are all utilized to produce medicines. If eaten uncooked, horse chestnut contains significant quantities of esculin, a toxin that can be fatal.

Horse chestnuts can be available in lotions, liquid drops, essential oil, pills, and tablets at stores and online.

Aescin is commonly found in horse chestnut infusions (10–20%). The dose of aescin utilized in most studies is 0.1–0.15 milligrams per day. As a result, the possible hazardous effects of higher doses remain unknown. As a result, it's best to stick to the recommended dose schedule.

Every day, this equates to around 2–3 pills or capsules. Liquid supplements do not have a regulated reference. Supplement bottles frequently have additional dose instructions.

Infusions and creams containing two percent aescin can be used three to four times per day when applied topically.

Note: When using horse chestnut seed extract topically, the proper dosage appears to be 0.100–0.15 g aescin per day in supplement form and three to four daily cream or infusion applications.

Catnip

Catnip is well-known for its catnip-like effects. Did you know that this herb can also be used by humans? Catnip has a wide range of medical uses.

Catnip has a sedative or weary effect, which has helped many people with sleeplessness.

Pour seven to nine drops of catnip tincture into 12 cups distilled water and consume half an hour before bedtime.

Catnip, to the surprise of many, is also effective in alleviating the symptoms of a common cold.

2 teaspoons dried catnip flowers dissolved in 6 12 ounces pure water. Bring the mixture to a boil, then remove it from the heat and let it aside for 10 minutes. Remove the flowers from the water and set aside. This infusion should be taken twice a day.

1 12 cup distilled water + 12 teaspoon dried and crushed catnip. Remove from heat after roughly five minutes of boiling. Allow the tea to steep for a few minutes. For one to two weeks, strain and drink once a day.

Plantain

Are you aware that plantain leaves are extremely effective in the treatment of sunburn and acne? Chemical components found in the leaves aid in the healing of injuries. Calorie-wise, boiled plantains are similar to potatoes in terms of nutrition, but they have more specific minerals and vitamins. They're high in vitamins A, B-6, and C, as well as minerals such as potassium and magnesium. Plantains are also high in fiber. Fiber is important because it helps to maintain gut health. Fiber softens your stools and increases their overall weight and volume.

Are you aware that huge stools are considerably easier to pass and, as a result, reduce constipation? Plantains contain a significant amount of vitamin C, which is recommended for regular consumption. This vitamin is an antioxidant that may help support the immune system. It may protect your body from free radical damage linked to heart disease, aging, and even some types of cancer as an antioxidant.

Plantains contain a lot of potassium, which is important for maintaining the cell and body fluids that control your heart rate and blood pressure. Plantains' fiber helps to decrease cholesterol, which maintains your heart functioning at its best.

It can be used by children for immediate relief! A leaf can be eaten into a mash and the full juicy lump applied to a bee sting is well known. Simply instruct the child to chew the leaf and apply it to the bee sting! This drug will provide immediate pain relief. If the child refuses to eat the leaf, smash it between two pebbles and tell him or her to add a little spit if necessary.

The plantain leaf may be easily damaged, applied to a wound, and bandaged. The astringent properties of the leaf's juices will have removed any pollutants from the terrible injury the next day.

Plantain can also be used in skin-calming therapies, especifically ingredients for newborn rash. If you have a baby with a diaper rash, try breaking up some leaves and putting them in the diaper, precisely where the problem is.

Plantain tea can be taken internally to treat diarrhea. The tea is also good for yeast infections, and because it's an expectorant, it can help with a cough. Finally, plantain's humble appearance conceals a plethora of beneficial cures.

Camellia

Camellia, or green tea as it is more widely known, is a medicinal herb.

From time to time, we all require a focus boost. Perhaps you're preparing for a big presentation at work or a long night of studying. There's nothing wrong with using medicinal herbs to cultivate a more focused mindset for whatever reason.

1 teaspoon dried camellia leaves or 1 prepared camellia teabag in 8 ounces pure water. Allow ten to twelve minutes for it to steep before drinking.

Camellia extract may aid weight loss in some persons. You might be able to get a lot of mileage out of this herbal cure for weight loss after speaking with your herbalist to see whether it's good for you.

To lose weight, drink 400 mL of camellia/green tea extract twice a day for three weeks.

According to several research, drinking tea brewed from camellia leaves can help lower cholesterol levels in some people.

1 teaspoon dried camellia leaves, 8 12 ounces distilled water, 1 teaspoon dried camellia leaves, 1 teaspoon dried camellia leaves, 1 teaspoon dried camellia leaves, 1 teaspoon dried camellia leaves, 1 teaspoon dried camellia. Allow for an eight-minute steeping period. 2 cups of this should be consumed on a regular basis. Take 1 cup after breakfast or your first meal of the day, and another cup after dinner for optimal benefits.

Cardamom

Cardamom is utilized medicinally in various civilizations due to its capacity to treat a variety of ailments.

Cardamom is a great way to enhance your metabolism and lose weight in a healthy way. This cure may be able to assist you in regaining control of your metabolism.

To enhance metabolism, take 230 mg organic cardamom powder with food twice a day for two weeks. If you've never tried cardamom before, talk to your herbalist about finding the right dose for you.

Halitosis is a disorder characterized by persistently foul breath. If you've been diagnosed with halitosis, this herbal cure can help you get rid of it and breathe more freely.

Heat one cup of distilled water with 12 teaspoon organic cardamom powder for ten minutes or until boiling. Remove from the heat and set aside to cool somewhat before sipping. Take this once a day, preferably after a meal for optimal results.

You may be able to manage your high blood pressure without the use of pharmaceutical drugs if you work with a herbal medicine specialist. You can attempt this cure if your herbalist approves.

To manage high blood pressure, use one cardamom capsule twice a day for up to three months.

CHAPTER 30:

SPECIAL #2: LONG LIFE HERBS

As a Botanical Medicine expert, I've always been interested in living a healthy lifestyle. As I grew older, though, I decided to do everything possible to live to be a centenarian. I set out on a journey to study the work of the world's top aging experts, and I came across some fascinating research on how to live longer, healthier, and younger lives.

To live longer, one of the most pleasurable and simple tools I learnt was to utilize more herbs and spices. I learned that by including the following herbs in your everyday meals, you can add more seasons to your life.

5 Herbs For A Long And Healthy Life

Ginseng
Ginseng is a slow-growing perennial plant of the Araliaceae family belonging to the Panax genus. Ginnsuu is another name for the plant in some locations.

Ginseng is a plant that is thought to have heart-protective qualities. It helps to deliver blood to the heart when oxygen levels are low by increasing blood flow when used in cooking.

Ginseng's enhanced blood flow also helps to reduce blood platelet stickiness, which lowers your risk of blood clots.

Cloves
In all systems of traditional herbalism, cloves have a digestive system-supporting effect. Because of their warming and digestion-supporting properties, they've also been used to maintain a healthy immunological and respiratory system.

In the kitchen, the spice "cloves" is a lesser-known herb. In research labs, however, this spice is prized for having the highest ORAC (Oxygen Radical Absorbance Capacity) score of any spice.

Meaning?

The most antioxidants are found in cloves. Cloves also eliminate parasites, fungi, and bacteria in the intestine.

Oregano
Oregano is a plant with purple flowers and olive-green leaves. Mint, thyme, marjoram, basil, sage, and lavender are all connected to it. Fresh and dried leaves are frequently used in cooking. On occasion, it's also utilized as a medication.

Oregano oil and fresh oregano herb are excellent complements to any cuisine. It offers four times the antioxidant activity of blueberries per ounce!

The antioxidant content of a single tablespoon of fresh oregano is comparable to that of a medium-sized apple.

Beta-caryophyllin, found in oregano oil, helps to reduce inflammation.

Ginger
Ginger is a shrub with leafy stems and yellowish green blossoms. The ginger spice comes from the roots of the plant. Ginger is native to the warmer regions of Asia, such as China, Japan, and India, but it is also grown in South America and Africa. It is currently grown for medicinal and culinary reasons in the Middle East.

Geraniol is a cancer-fighting chemical that can be found in the ginger plant.

Ginger is also an anti-inflammatory, so it's beneficial for your heart and prevents blood clots.

This herb is supposed to aid in the strengthening of the immune system as well as the prevention of atherosclerosis.

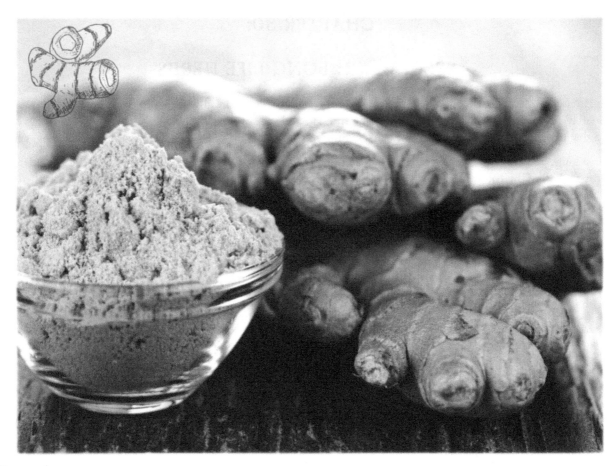

Turmeric

Turmeric is a spice made from a natural plant that is used in a variety of recipes. It's a long-established Indian plant. Turmeric's active ingredient, curcumin, is also known as turmeric. When used as a culinary spice, turmeric powder is yellow.

Adding turmeric extract to your meals reduces your risk of heart attack by 56 percent, according to research published in the American Journal of Cardiology.

Turmeric also improves cardiovascular health as much as aerobic activity, according to a 2012 study published in the Nutrition Research journal.

It contains "curcumin," a bizarre but actual "primary polyphenol."

Turmeric/curcumin has also been linked to brain protection, reduced inflammation, and cancer treatment.

CONCLUSION

Native American herbalism was a practice of healing and prevention through the use of plants by indigenous people in North America. The practice is relatively small compared to modern medicine. Per capita spending on native American herbalism was probably less than one-tenth of one percent. However, this is not due to a lack of efficacy, as many of the original herbal remedies are still in use today. In addition, the idea that Native American herbalism is archaic and ineffective because few Native Americans now harvest medicinal plants is false. There are currently approximately 2,000 tribes in the United States. Many of them have active programs for harvesting medicinal plants and herbs today.

Native American herbalists used plant preparations for both physical and spiritual ailments. Plant medicines were used both to make the body well (as a primary treatment) as well as to support physical healing from other treatments such as surgery or other medical interventions (as a secondary treatment). Plant-based treatments were used widely among Native American tribes before the arrival of European settlers in North America.

I hope that this book will be helpful to those who are interested in learning more about herbalism and the role that plants and herbs have played in treating disease.

BOOK 8

HERBAL REMEDIES
FOR CHILDREN

A Selection of Natural Herbs and Remedies to Treat
the Most Common Diseases of Your Children

Citali Galwen

INTRODUCTION

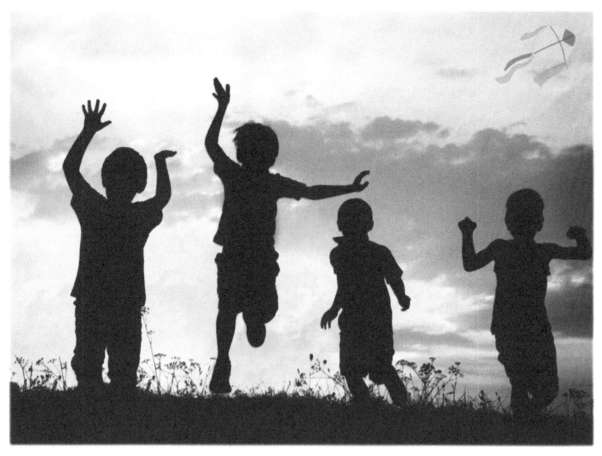

You should ensure that your child is given plenty of rest and sleep. It will make a huge difference in their overall health, growth, and development if they get sufficient rest each day. Getting enough sleep also helps improve one's immune system since it allows the body to be fully restored with energy and protects against illness.

One of the best things you can do for your child's safety is to keep them away from germs and bacteria. Ensure that you wash their hands frequently and always teach them not to touch their mouth with their hands. If they have colds, it would be a good idea to make sure that they are taking medicine or going to the doctor.

You should also make sure that they play outside with friends as opposed to playing video games indoors. This will help them socialize and interact with other people who will keep their immune systems healthy. You should also consider taking your children to a health spa when it is cold because this can help improve their energy levels.

You should make sure that you get your children vaccinated. When it comes to young children, this is very important since they are still very susceptible to many diseases. Some of the diseases they could contract include rashes, measles, chickenpox, meningitis, and type 1 diabetes. The first three of these diseases can cause quite a lot of harm, especially for small children so it is important to protect against them by giving them proper vaccinations.

The first vaccination that should be given is a triple vaccine, which protects against three diseases. The second vaccine is a combination vaccine, and the third one is the meningitis C injection. In most cases, this is enough to help protect your child from these diseases.

It would also be best if you give your children plenty of exercise regularly. That will prevent them from becoming overweight, and it will also make their immune system stronger.

CHAPTER 31:
15 PLANTS PERFECT FOR YOUR CHILDREN'S HEALTH

1) Elderberry

[Sambucus nigra]

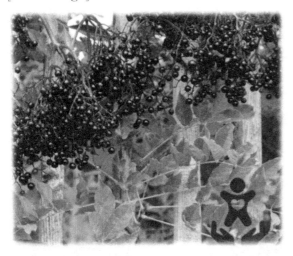

The elderberry is useful when added to the skin while treating wounds. Elderflower is used orally in many nations, including Germany, to combat respiratory illnesses such as colds and flu. Some evidence suggests that chemicals in elderflowers and elderberries may help reduce inflammation of mucous membranes, such as the sinuses, and help alleviate nasal congestion. Elder may have propensities to be anti-inflammatory, antiviral, and anticancer. Dosage is simple. Eat jam or wine made from elderberries only. But be mindful that the raw berries are slightly poisonous. They could have medication reactions with diuretics (water pills), diabetic medications, antibiotics, laxatives, theophylline (Theodor), or immune suppressant medicines.

5) Newborn Dill

[Anethum graveolens]

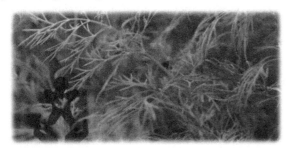

This herb is used by healers to treat earaches and ear infections. Healers also found a gentle tea for the rootstock to stimulate the digestive system and reduce bloating, and it also aids in bronchial diseases and exhaustion..
This herb oil is good for colic, flatulence, and indigestion.

2) Garlic

[Allium sativum]

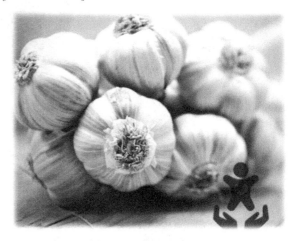

For cholesterol levels and control of blood pressure, garlic is used. It has antimicrobial effects. Reports from minor, short-term, and badly defined trials suggest that slight decreases may be induced by total and LDL cholesterol. The German research results on garlic's cholesterol-lowering influence have been distorted, however, with a positive result, the FDA says. The possible role of garlic in cancer prevention is currently being studied by researchers. The FDA considers garlic to be safe. It should not be mixed with warfarin since large amounts of garlic can induce clotting. Big doses must not be administered until oral surgery or surgery for the same reason.

3) Ginger (The Root)

[Zingiber officinale]

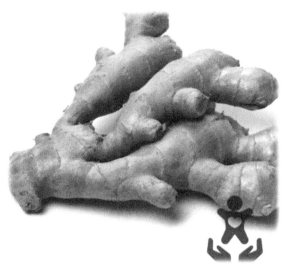

Ginger is used for minimizing pain and motion sickness. Ginger could decrease pain caused by pregnancy and chemotherapy. Surgery and motion-induced nausea are implicated in these areas under review. Gas, bloating, heartburn, and nausea are among the side effects identified

4) Wild Ginger

[Asarum]

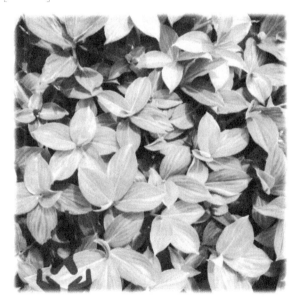

To treat earaches and ear infections, this herb is used by healers. They also found a gentle tea for the rootstock to stimulate the digestive system & reduce bloating, and it also aids in bronchial diseases and exhaustion.

6) Lavender

[Lavandula angustifolia]

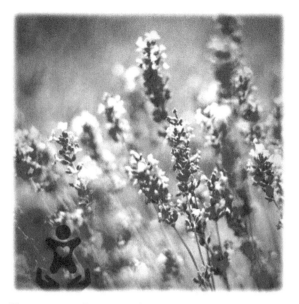

You can combine it with virtually every other oil in the market; you can use undiluted sparingly without side effects, and it can be used for a multitude of health reasons: dermatitis, earache, eczema, psoriasis, sunburn, muscle aches, asthma, bronchitis, whooping cough, colic, flatulence, nausea, flu, insomnia, headache, nervous tension, and dry scalp. That is just the shortlist.

7) Eucalyptus

[Eucalyptus Globules]

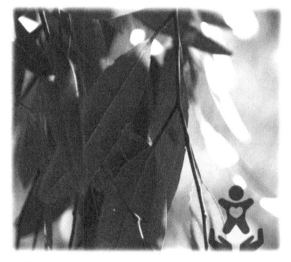

Well known for being used in vaporizers and other diffusion devices, eucalyptus has been used to open nasal passages and congested chests. It can also help treat insect bites, skin infections, ease muscular aches and pains, sprains, and throat infections. It is also effective in treating bronchitis, sinusitis, colds, flu, and measles.

8) Roman Chamomile
[Chamaemelum nobile]

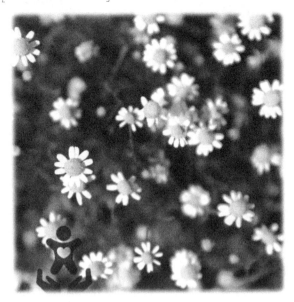

Roman Chamomile is a perennial flower originating in the Mediterranean region. It boasts many different colors, including white, yellow, pink, red, and purple.

The main use of this herb is in the treatment of anxiety and depression. It is also beneficial for stomach ulcers, and, like dill, it acts as a great anti-inflammatory agent. It has the same actions as lavender and ginger but with a stronger antibacterial effect.

Natives of America used chamomile in teas, flowers, sachets, and garlands to help treat colds, fever, inflammation, pain, indigestion, and headaches. Medicinally it was used to aid muscle spasms, nervous conditions, and insomnia.

It is also said to be very attractive for bees. However, many have reported that honey from Roman chamomile has a bitter taste.

Chamomile's main chemical components are bisabolol, flavonoids, and coumarins, such as chamazulene.

Roman chamomile is used in the form of extracts, ointments, capsules, and tinctures. It is also used to make teas and other beverages.

9) Yarrow
[Achillea millefolium]

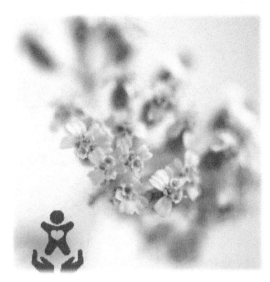

The restorative history of this herb is the length of the rundown of ills it can treat. The Greek saint Achilles is said to have utilized yarrow to treat the injuries of his stricken warriors. Native Americans likewise utilized yarrow for wounds, yet that was only the start.

Yarrow was frequently taken as tea for stomach issues and fever. It was used to make poultices for the treatment of rashes, eczema, dermatitis, and bug nibbles. Students of history gauge that 46 unique clans use yarrow for upwards of 28 issues, making it one of the most broadly utilized herbs. Present-day herbalists have made the rundown much more. Some suggest yarrow for hypertension, ulcers, interior and outer dying, liver issues, loose bowels, colds and influenza, bad-tempered bowel syndrome, Crohn's ailment, bladder contaminations, gas pains, hemorrhoids. It additionally goes about as a gentle narcotic and can help ease nervousness and a sleeping disorder. A juice produced using the leaves can help decrease the redness of ragged-looking eyes. Strategies for Use: the most intense pieces of the plant are the highest leaves and flowers, which are appropriate for making tea. A few herbalists prescribe making a poultice and applying yarrow straightforwardly to the skin. At times, it's even a bit to calm toothache.

10) Geranium
[Pelargonium Graveolens]

172

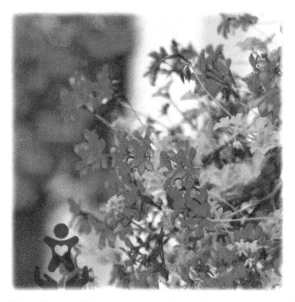

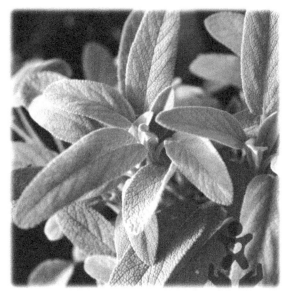

This floral oil has been used in the treatment of bruises, burns, congested skin, dermatitis, eczema, oily complexions, tonsillitis, sore throats, and nervous tension. Can cause dermatitis in highly sensitive skin.

11) Mandarin

[Citrus Reticulata]

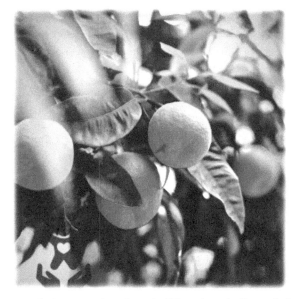

Mandarins are abundant in Vitamins A, B, and C, which are beneficial for avoiding infections, eliminating free radicals, and maintaining skin health. Vitamin C helps to prevent colds and keep your children's immune system operating correctly so you can fight off any unpleasant illnesses that come your way.

12) Clary Sage

[Salvia sclarea]

Sage is a perennial herb native to southern Europe, northwest Africa, and the Middle East. Its leaves are used in cooking for their unique flavor. Sage is also used in traditional medicine to help with respiratory problems, heartburn, and sore throats.

It is considered a food plant by some farmers because it has antimicrobial and insecticidal properties that deter pests from attacking crops like mint or oregano. It is a good remedy for coughs and sore throats, and it can also be used for treating indigestion. It will help if you know you can use the potent sage for numerous things. First, sage has a dominant aroma and intrinsic flavor, which is why it's typically used in small portions. Even so, the unique advantage is that it's stuffed with a mixture of crucial nutrients and composites. Sage is also used as a natural cleaning tool (and pesticide). This fresh, green herb is accessible fresh, dried, or in oil forms, and it will help if you know it has infinite health advantages (for both males and females).

13) Nutmeg

[Myristica fragrans]

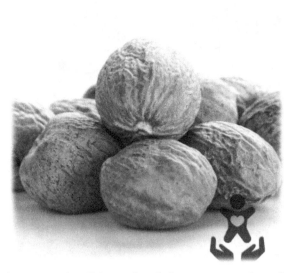

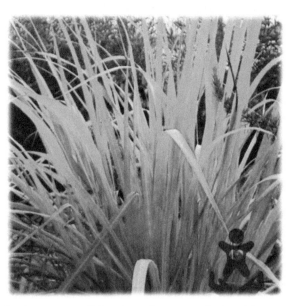

Its aromatic oil is used to help treat muscular aches and pains, flatulence, indigestion, nausea, and bacterial infections.

Its important oil has been known to help with acne, dermatitis, minor skin infections, scarring, facials, oily skin, dry skin, intestinal infections.

14) Palmarosa

[Cymbopogon martinii]

Warning

Don't use the remedies in the book to treat illnesses without proper medical support, especially when it comes to your children. Make sure always to see a specialist before commencing any treatment.

You must be seeing someone who can help you through the process of using herbal medicine properly, especially if you actually wish to use Ayurvedic medicine. You can usually find a specialist in your area, and they will help you actually to get through the process. Though, it will also be important that you talk to your regular doctor as well.

Your doctor may be able to actually give you a referral to help you get to an accredited specialistwho will help you through the process. Your doctor can also help you determine if you can actually use Native American medicinal herbs without interacting with any of the modern medicines you are taking, including over-the-counter medication. This means that you will need to list the over-the-counter medication you are currently taking.

CHAPTER 32:

HERBAL REMEDIES FOR YOUR CHILD'S HEALTH

Do you realize how important it is to have a stockpile of items on hand before you become a parent? When your child falls, gets a scrape while playing, develops a fever or pain, comes into contact with something extremely hot (such as a pet or an oven), develops a nasty sore, requires an immune system boost, and the list goes on, having an arsenal of natural treatments on hand would be beneficial.

Here are some of my best suggestions for some of the most common problems that could affect your kid. Let's go through them deeply, with the suggested remedies.

Immune Building Herbs For Kids

You certainly know that it's critical to maintain your child's immune system robustly throughout the cold and flu season. Below, I have listed the best remarkable herbs and supplements that are vigorous immune-builders and a do-it-yourself recipe for hand sanitizer that your children can use.

- Elderberry
- Echinacea
- Golden Seal
- Vitamin C
- Vitamin D
- Oregano Oil
- Black Seed Oils

Hand Sanitizer

Do you know how to develop a fantastic recipe for a potent hand sanitizer? Instead of wiping alcohol on your child's hands (which is less than ideal), why not make your own?

Ingredients:

- 3 oz. high-proof vodka
- 1 oz. pure aloe vera gel
- 5-10 drops lavender essential oil
- 30 drops tea tree essential oil
- ¼ tsp. flarnin e oil

Instructions:

1. Go ahead and mix essential oils in a small glass container. Then mix it.
2. Add alcohol and shake it.
3. Add aloe vera gel.
4. Shake mixture tenderly before using it!

Kids With Sleep Issues And Sleep Apnea

Did you realize that children may and do suffer from sleep apnea? If they suffer from this problem, you can know it when they snore loudly most evenings, or they may snort and halt breathing, gulp for oxygen, or they hesitate in their breathing. They could sweat much when sleeping. When it goes undetected and untreated, it may contribute to daytime fatigue and behavioral issues at school. According to a new study, children who snore loudly are twice as likely to struggle in school.

To compound matters, when kids experience a night of poor sleep, they are more likely to be hyperactive, have trouble paying attention, and show symptoms of attention deficit disorder. Sleep apnea in children may also be connected with slowed growth and cardiovascular problems.

If your kid has sleep apnea, be on the lookout for some of these signs:

- Trouble waking up in the morning
- Have headaches when they wake up and during the day
- Be sensitive, irritable, hostile, and experience distress
- Behavioral or social problems at school or home
- The kid has a nasal voice and breathes heavily through their mouth

Natural remedies for kids with sleep apnea

CPAP Mask. The most important thing to do is to take your child to a professional and have them tested. It may be that your kid needs their tonsils removed immediately, or other things may be blocking their airways. The specialist can also order a child-size mask to wear at night called CPAP (continuous positive airway pressure device).

You should attempt to learn to play the didgeridoo. This isn't something you have lying around the house. You may not have heard of it, but if your kid has sleep apnea, this strange wind instrument known as a didgeridoo may assist in the short term.

According to recent studies, 4-months of playing the didgeridoo worked well for modest sleep apnea victims, made for a better night's sleep, and decreased daytime drowsiness. How does it work, you may ask? You should know that playing the instrument will empower you by strengthening your child's upper airway and preventing it from narrowing as the child inhales. Hey! You should know, going the extra mile to learn to play a musical instrument to help with breathing and lung ability has been used for kids and grown-ups for several ages.

Petroleum Jelly And Listerine For Sores

Are you aware that sores (Blisters) hurt and might upset your child? Do you need an immediate solution? Listerine is an antibacterial as well as a breath refresher. On the other hand, Listerine may dry up any sores your children may have.

Apply the antiseptic on a cotton ball and apply it to your child's sores (blisters) two to three times a day until the sores dry up and the discomfort goes away. Furthermore, a recent study suggests utilizing petroleum jelly on a sore (blister) for short pain relief. The great news is that Listerine has been used for several years as a straightforward way to treat sores (blisters). If your kid has a blister, this common remedy works perfectly!

Lemon Balm To Treat Cold Sores

It is no longer a secret that lemon balm is one of the most efficient medicines available. Cold sores may be severe in young people and children. They're prompted by the FISV (Herpes simplex virus) that penetrates tissues in the body when a kid is growing; it is latent and might reappear as an adolescent later in life.

Sometimes cold sores are a result of:

- Too much vulnerability to the sun
- Respiratory diseases
- Emotional strain

It is high in polyphenols, which have antiviral properties, and it tastes and smells delicious. A recent study found that not a single cold sore recurrence happened once healed with lemon balm. Try lemon balm salve; It may also be used to treat chapped lips, wounds, small burns, scratches, and other minor injuries in children.

Ginger For Motion Illness

Are you going on vacation with your children? You'll need ginger, the most sought-after herb! Ginger tea, tablets, or syrup are all options. They are all effective for motion sickness or if your youngster is feeling unsteady.

You should know ginger is one of those remedies you want to keep in your pocket, kitchen, or even your home first-aid bag.

When traveling with your children, be sure to have ginger tablets for any motion sickness that may occur. If you wish to use it with essential oils, apply the ginger-infused oil to the skin.

One research found that ginger functioned better than anti-nausea medication for motion sickness. In addition, ginger was discovered to aid in the treatment of seasickness.

Using A Duct Tape For Warts

I know that's startling, but I can assure you that it works like a charm! Do you know that using duct tape to remove warts seems to be a myth? Nonetheless, it serves a purpose and performs better than freezing them off. According to recent research, duct tape eliminated overeighty percent of patients' warts in less than three months.

This' how to use it on your warts:

1. You should make sure the wart and surrounding skin are clean and neat.
2. Then go ahead and cut a piece of duct tape a bit bigger than the wart and press into the spot.
3. Go ahead and remove the tape every 3-days, rub the wart with a sandpaper board or pumice stone, and redo it unlit the wart is slopped.

Papaya For Smoother Skin

Do you know that children and young adults want flawless skin? Exfoliating dead skin cells may help, and papaya can work as a usual exfoliant for children's and young adults' skin! The energetic ingredient in papaya is papain, an enzyme that eradicates dead surface cells that give skin a matte, rugged look. Go ahead and try this fruity facial on your kids and young adults to relax, soften, and polish their skin:

1. Wash and peel ripe papaya.
2. Put two teaspoons in a food processor; blend thoroughly.
3. Add one teaspoon of withered oatmeal; mix into a paste.
4. Then apply to your freshly cleansed face and leave on for 10-15 minutes.
5. Remove the paste with warm water or a soaked washcloth.

You should know Papaya is a great fruit to help kids and young adults with trivial breakouts on their skin. If you want to try a blender, you can do this; blend the papaya until it is smooth, add some oatmeal, and put it on your face. It serves as a natural and safe exfoliator to eliminate lifeless skin that can clog pores and cause break-outs.

Egg White Parts, Mustard, And Lavender Oil For Minor Burns

Does your child or teen enjoy cooking or baking with you in the kitchen? If so, have some remedies prepared for the unavoidable minor burns that may occur:

Lavender essential oil
Did you know that Lavender essential oil may treat burns and agony in minutes? Any blistering will be killed if you apply Lavender essential oil to the burn as soon as possible.

The white pad of egg
If your child gets a burn, immediately take an egg, leaving the yolk and egg, and apply it to the child's skin. You may be confident that it will remove the burn, restore the skin, and relieve the pain. Egg white is a common and effective home treatment for treating small burns in yourself or your children. Simply massage the burn smoothly; it relieves pain and leaves no sores on the skin.

Mustard
When your child has a burn, go ahead and spread mustard on the burned skin. After an initial burn, the mustard will relieve the discomfort and stop hurting and blistering.

Remedy For Bites And Stings

You're likely aware that adolescence isn't complete without a few stings from wasps, bees, or insects. It will assist if you know that bites and stings may be severe, even fatal, to some children.

Some are so serious that they need medical attention. If a string or bite causes chilly skin, an itchy rash on the child's skin, or slow breathing, get them to a doctor as soon as possible! For lesser bites and stings, try these homeopathic solutions:

Poison ivy stings
Accept it or not, onions will kill the discomfort and inflammation (in kids) connected with poison ivy stings. All you need to do is this:

First, cut the onion in half and rub it on the afflicted area. Then wash the area with soap and clean water.

Lastly, use a paste of clean water and sodium bicarbonate on the area.

Bee stings

My mother used to use the following for bee stings on us kids when I was a little; mud and sodium bicarbonate (baking soda) mixed with a little water to make a paste. She put either the mud or soda onto the bee sting, and in a few minutes, the discomfort was gone, and the bee sting was barely noticeable. There is some disagreement about utilizing mud since it may include other substances (and can be messy). So, stick to sodium bicarbonate (baking soda).

Wasp stings

You must respond promptly if a wasp stings your kid as a mother. All you have to do is apply undiluted vinegar or lemon juice to the skin using a cotton ball. It will quickly neutralize the toxin.

Pure Essential Oils For Headaches

Do your kids often suffer from headaches?

Severe headaches often lead to children having difficulty speaking. If you suspect your kid has a headache, here are some common cures that make use of herbs or essential oils. However, some headaches are severe and need more than a cup of tea or essential oils. If you believe your child's headache is severe, contact your doctor right away.

Essential Oils:

The therapeutic-grade essential oils listed below are astounding for headaches and can be used with young kids:

- Rosemary
- Marjoram
- Peppermint
- Eucalyptus
- Lavender
- Grapefruit

My favorites are a lavender and peppermint combination. Here's how you should apply them to your children:

1. Apply three drops of lavender oil (or any of the oils listed above) to the temples on the side of your child's head.
2. Take another three drops and massage them into the kid's head's back (at the base of the head behind the ears).
3. Repeat this same procedure with peppermint oil. Peppermint oil will boost the strength of any oil you use

CHAPTER 33:

QUICK RECIPES TO TREAT THE MOST COMMON CHILDREN'S ILLNESSES

Children Of 12 Months To 5 Years

Chamomile infusion for insomnia

This infusion may also help your kid obtain the sleep he or she needs.

Ingredients:

- 1 teaspoon dried chamomile
- 1 cup boiling water

Instructions:

1. Combine the chamomile and boiling water in a teapot. Let the tea steep for 10 minutes. Allow the infusion to cool to lukewarm.

2. Pour 2 teaspoons into a sterilized bottle and give it to your baby to drink. Repeat once or twice a day as needed to relieve colic symptoms.

Dry rash

Because of their oil and wax composition, salves are emollient, particularly when a moisturizing oil, such as olive oil, is used as the basis. The soothing and anti-inflammatory properties of the herbs improve the emollient effect in this basic composition.

Ingredients:

- Licorice-infused oil—2 fluid ounces
- Beeswax—1ounce plus more as needed
- Calendula-infused oil— 3 fluid ounces
- Plantain-infused oil —3 fluid ounces

Instructions:

1. Prepare a salve as usual
2. Apply a thin layer at least twice a day

Marshmallow infusion for colds

The infusion in the jar is an effective cold remedy. You can add some glucose or other sweetener to make it palatable for the child.

Ingredients:

- Marshmallow root (dried)—28g
- Freshwater—1 liter

Instructions:

1. Wrap the marshmallow root in a cheesecloth
2. Tie up the bundle

3. Immerse the cheesecloth bundle in the cold water in a jar
4. Pull the tied end of the cheesecloth over the mouth of the jar.
5. Cover the jar with its lid nicely.
6. Let your jar rest overnight, or, at least, for 8hrs, during which time infusion will be taking place.
7. Pull out the bundle from the jar.

Elderberry thyme child spray for throat

This is used to make tea for the treatment of sore throats, coughs, colds, and general ailments. It can be made in a spray bottle.

Ingredients:

- Dried Echinacea leaves—1 tablespoon
- Dried Ginger leaves—1 tablespoon
- Dried Marshmallow root—1 tablespoon
- Dried Elderberry leaves—1 tablespoon
- Dried Thyme leaves—1 tablespoon
- Fresh boiling water—¼ cup
- Echinacea tincture—1 cup

Instructions:

1. Mix the ingredients in a mason jar.
2. Add in boiling water.
3. Add in the Echinacea tincture.
4. Cover the jar tightly with a lid.
5. Leave contents for 2 weeks or longer.
6. By then, your cold spray will be ready for your child.

Muscle relaxing massage

A massage mixture made with plants such as peppermint, sandalwood, and wintergreen oils is used to relieve muscle aches and pains.

Massage oil is made of equal portions of the above plants and applied to the child.

Ingredients:

- Peppermint essential oil—20 drops
- Wintergreen essential oil—20 drops
- Camphor essential oil—10 drops
- Sandalwood essential oil—10 drops
- Ginger essential oil—10 drops
- Juniper berry essential oil—10 drops

Instructions:

1. Combine all ingredients into a dark bottle to preserve the oils
2. Gently massage into affected areas of your child

Ginger-cinnamon infusion for colds

Ginger root is boiled in water. Cinnamon bark is also boiled in this mixture. It should be drunk every morning before meals to relieve cold symptoms.

Ingredients:

- Ginger (grated)—1 stick
- Cinnamon—1 stick
- Lemon zest—2 lemons
- Freshwater—½ cup

Instructions:

1. Mix the ginger, cinnamon, and lemon zest in a small pot
2. Add in the water and boil the contents for ¼hr.
3. Your infusion is ready for use. A teaspoon twice a day is generally good for a child with a cold.

Marshmallow-sage spray

This is used for treating sore throat, coughs, diarrhea, fevers, and nasal congestion.

Ingredients:

- Freshwater—¾ cup
- Sage leaf—2 tablespoon
- Marshmallow root—2 tablespoon
- Peppermint hydrosol—¼ cup
- Raw honey—1 tablespoon

Instructions:

1. Bring the water to a boil
2. Mix the sage and marshmallow and pour the hot water over the mixture.
3. Steep for ¾hr, then strain its contents.
4. Add in the honey and peppermint hydrosol.

Honey-ginger rinse

This is a great way to treat a sore throat, aching gums, and it can be used as a gargle for colds. It can help repair damage caused by untreated dental gum infections.

Ingredients:

- Organic ginger (grated)—1 tablespoon
- Boiling water—1 cup

- Honey—1 teaspoon
- Cayenne pepper—a pinch

Instructions:

1. In a saucepan of boiling water, add the ginger and stir for a couple of minutes.
2. Let the mixture cool a bit, and then add in the honey and cayenne pepper.
3. Assist your child to rinse

Cough syrup

It can help reduce the frequency of coughs and colds. This syrup can also be used for treating sore throats, itchy throats, and bronchitis.

Ingredients:

- Boiling water—1 cup 1 pound of honey
- Wild plum root—1 tablespoon
- Coltsfoot leaves—2 teaspoons
- Mullein leaves—2 teaspoons

Instructions:

1. Combine the above herbs in the boiling water; in a nonmetallic container, steep for half an hour, and strain
2. Add one pound of honey, heating, and stirring until the honey is dissolved; cool and store in a glass container.
3. One tablespoon as needed.

Carminative tincture

It is a strong and powerful diuretic and can help in clearing up tonsillitis and laryngitis. It also helps to reduce the inflammation of mucous membranes.

This combination warms the center of the body, activating the digestive organs and preventing the intestines from becoming sluggish. If peppermint isn't your child thing, try angelica instead.

Ingredients:

- Tincture of ginger— 1½ fluid ounces
- Tincture of fennel—1 fluid ounce
- Tincture of peppermint —1 fluid ounce
- Tincture of licorice— ½ fluid ounce

Instructions:

1. In a small bottle, combine the tinctures. Cap the bottle and label it
2. Give 1 to 2 drops to your child after each meal or whenever his or her guts feel uncomfortably stuck

Children Of 5 Years To 12 Years

Licorice root infusion for colds

This is used to make tea for the treatment of colds, coughs, and general ailments. It is made by boiling licorice root in water.

Ingredients:

- Piece of Licorice root
- Freshwater—1 glass

Instructions:

1. Place the licorice root in a small pot
2. Add in the freshwater
3. Place the pot on the fire and bring the water to a boil
4. Lower the fire and let the contents simmer for around 10 minutes.
5. Sieve the liquid that will serve as your child's cold infusion.

Lemon-honey-apple cider infusion

This is a great way to treat a sore throat and can help loosen congestion.

Ingredients:

- Apple cider vinegar—1 teaspoon
- Fresh lemon juice—1 lemon
- Raw honey—1 teaspoon
- Cayenne pepper—just a pinch
- Freshwater—1 glass

Instructions:

1. Heat the water first till it boils
2. Take the water off the fire
3. Add in half of the lemon juice
4. Add in the apple cider vinegar
5. Add in the honey too
6. Add in the cayenne pepper, or leave it out if the child is very young.

Sage-echinacea cold spray

This is a great all-around remedy against colds, allergies, and asthma. It can be sprayed on the throat and sinuses to help relieve all of these conditions.

Ingredients:

- Ground sage—1 teaspoon
- Ground Echinacea—1 teaspoon
- Freshwater—½ cup

Instructions:

1. Boil the water
2. Put the sage and Echinacea in a tiny jar

3. Pour in hot water and let contents steep for ½hr.
4. Strain the contents and store them in a tiny spray bottle.

Oregano-peppermint-thieves spray

This is for those with colds, sore throats, and bronchitis. The peppermint and oregano help to clear out mucus and calm a cough. This spray can also be used as a mouth wash.

Ingredients:

- Apple cider vinegar—1 tablespoon
- Freshwater—7 tablespoons
- Raw honey—1 teaspoon
- A blend of Thieves oil—8 drops
- Lemon essential oil—8 drops
- Peppermint essential oil—7 drops
- Oregano oil—1 drop

Instructions:

1. Mix the honey and the apple cider vinegar and stir to dissolve the honey.
2. Put the solution in a 4oz bottle.
3. Add in the oils
4. Under room temperature, the spray lasts 4 days, but if refrigerated, it can last 2wks.

Apple cider-sage gargle

This can be used to relieve sore throats, laryngitis, and swollen tonsils. It is very helpful to treat allergies.

Ingredients:

- Sage—1 teaspoon
- Apple cider vinegar—¼ cup
- Brown sugar—¼ cup
- Freshwater—1/8 cup

Instructions:

1. Mix the ingredients well, and the gargle is ready for use.
2. Assist your child to rinse

Baking soda rinse

This is a rinse for sore gums and can be used to help reduce inflammation in the mouth.

Ingredients:

- Baking soda—¼ teaspoon
- Warm water—1 cup
- Salt—1/8 teaspoon

Instructions:

1. Mix and gargle every 3hrs, helping your child to rinse

Flower decoction

Great to alleviate the symptoms of allergies such as pollen or dust allergies

Ingredients:

- One teaspoon of yerba santa leaves
- Three cups boiling water

- One teaspoon oxeye daisy leaf
- One teaspoon of pearly everlasting

Instructions:

1. Combine the herbs in a glass container. Cover with the water and steep for a half-hour before straining.
2. To use, give one-half cup a day to your child.

CONCLUSION

Do you know that most people feel herbal remedies are ineffective? I can tell you that several studies (from all over the globe) have shown the effectiveness of herbal medicines for a wide range of common and significant health issues.

Most herbal medications have a long track record of being safe when taken correctly. Herbs are a local alternative that is readily accessible to people all over the globe; although some natural herbal knowledge has been lost in certain places, the plants remain. We have just recently lost contact with these old-fashioned healing substances in favor of pharmaceuticals.

Most plants contain hundreds, if not thousands, of medicinal compounds. When these compounds are coupled, they function best and have the least amount of adversity.

Taking herbal remedies that utilize the whole therapeutic components of the plant, such as tinctures or teas, is always preferable to taking a single chemical isolated in a lab.

Herbs have a holistic impact, which means they cure the body from the inside. It may take a little longer for you to see a difference in your symptoms, but this is because they concentrate on the root cause of the problem rather than addressing a sign or combination of symptoms with a Band-Aid treatment.

In the following pages, I will focus on the best herbs to cure the most common diseases of children and recipes to make the best of these herbs.

Just like that! The herbs have positive effects also on our children; it is enough to have a little more attention in using them correctly.

BOOK 9

EVERY DAY HERBAL REMEDIES

A Special Collection of Natural Daily Remedies to Take Care of Yourself... And Not Only

Citali Galwen

INTRODUCTION

Plants are the building blocks of life as we know it. They grow and yield fruit; they supply the oxygen we breathe, the water we drink, and a variety of medications that help us recover. And, since polluted air and contaminated water endanger human health now more than ever, plant knowledge is more important than ever.

Certain plants have been shown in studies to be effective in the treatment of ulcers, rheumatism, malignant tumors, and a variety of other common disorders. There are many of these therapeutic plants in your area or even in your own home. The majority of these therapeutic plants may even be cultivated in your own garden. Some of them are so common that you can buy them at a grocery store or hardware store. Others are extremely rare and expensive.

Herbal medicines have been used by families for generations to treat common ailments for both adults and children. When American physicians were almost impotent to combat many of these ailments, many parents resorted to herbal medicines that had been shown to be successful in reducing the symptoms of these infectious diseases.

Nowadays, you may be more informed about how to protect your child from a variety of common, and not so common—illnesses than you were years ago. But, are you aware of which plants make good natural herbal remedies for a child's health? The older generations were well acquainted with them. Their forefathers had passed the knowledge of these herbs down from one generation to another for many centuries. And this information was written down and documented, in some cases, as early as the first half of the fourteenth century.

Herbal remedies are highly beneficial for your health and usually get a faster healing time. When used wisely along with modern medicine, with intelligence, or self-help programs, you may be able to heal almost totally on your own with just a few weeks of herbal healing.

CHAPTER 34:

BEST COMMON DIY HERBAL TEA RECIPES

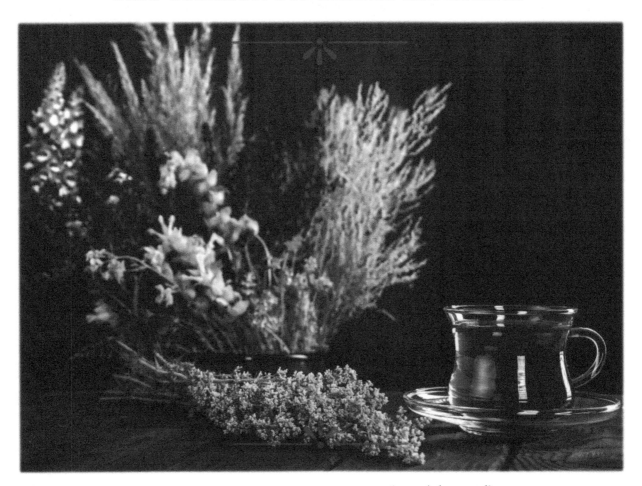

Anxiety

This is a great tasting tea to help with anxiety, and it can be used in a number of ways to soothe the nerves.

Anxiety relief tea #1

Ingredients:

- 1 tsp. hops
- 2 tsp. Betony dried flowers
- 1 cup distilled boiling water

Instructions:

1. Pour boiling water over the herbs mixture. Let sit for half an hour. Strain and drink throughout the day.

Anxiety relief tea #2

Ingredients:

- 1 tsp. hops
- 1 tsp. Betony dried flowers
- 1 tsp. Linden dried leaves and flowers

- 1 tsp. Ashwagandha root
- 1 cup distilled boiling water

Instructions:

1. Pour boiling water over the herbs' mixture. Let sit for thirty minutes. Strain and drink one cup per day.

Anti-Oxidant

This is a great recipe that has an important detoxifying effect and protects cells from free radicals, which can lead to severe health issues

Antioxidant tea #1

Ingredients:

- 10 Drops Cayenne Tincture
- 25 Drops Burdock Tincture
- 20 Drops Goldenseal Tincture

- 5 Drops Ginger (Root) Tincture
- 1 Cup Gingko Biloba Tea

Instructions:

1. Combine the tinctures in an amber glass bottle with a dropper lid. Label it. Add ten drops of the tincture mix to your Gingko Biloba Tea.

Antioxidant tea #2
Ingredients:

- ½ cup Gingko Biloba Tea
- ½ cup Ginseng Tea

Instructions:

1. Combine the two varieties of tea and drink it throughout the day.

Bronchitis
Bronchitis tea #2
Great to relieve bronchitis pain.

Ingredients:

- 1 teaspoon elecampane root
- 2 tablespoons nettle leaves
- 1 cup boiling water

Instructions:

1. Combine the above herbs.
2. Strain.
3. Sweeten with honey, if desired.
4. Take up to two cups a day.

Bronchitis tea #3
Great to relieve bronchitis pain.

Ingredients:

- 1 to 2 slices of fresh ginger root,
- 1 teaspoon pearly everlasting flowers or leaves,
- 1 teaspoon redroot,
- 1 cup boiling water

Instructions:

1. Combine the above herbs; steep in the boiling water for 30 minutes; strain.
2. Take one-half cup of tea three times daily.

Cold Sores
Cold sore tea
This tea is also very helpful in soothing and healing cold sores. Use the tea bag right on the sore for best results.

Ingredients:

- 1 teaspoon burdock root
- 1 teaspoon dried and powdered goldenseal root
- 1 cup boiling water
- Honey, to taste

Instructions:

1. Combine the above herbs in a glass container.
2. Steep for 30 minutes, calm, and strain.
3. You may want to sweeten with honey. Take up to one cup a day.

Anti-congestive tea
This tea is an effective anti-congestive known to help relieve congestion of the lungs.

It is also very helpful for relieving coughs.

Ingredients:

- 2 teaspoons black cohosh root
- 2 cups boiling water
- 4 teaspoons ginkgo Biloba leaves

Instructions:

1. Combine the overhead herbs in a non-metallic vessel, then pour the boiling water over them. Immerse for 30 minutes, calm, and strain.
2. Take up to six times a day, take two to three tablespoons at a time.

Cold And Flu
This is a great way to cure colds and flu. It is made from the following: Ginger, rose hips, garlic, elecampane, thyme, and elderberry.

Decongestant tea
This tea can be brewed and consumed to help to relieve congestion and mucous.

Ingredients:

- 2 slices fresh ginger
- 2 teaspoons pleurisy root
- 1 cup boiling water

Instructions:

1. Combine the herbs in a glass container, steep for 30 minutes, calm, and strain.
2. Take up to two cups each day, a tablespoon at a time.

Lung-lubricating tea
Makes 2¾ cups dried herb mix.

This tea is used for all sorts of respiratory problems, including the common cold.

Ingredients:

- 1 cup dried marshmallow root
- 1 cup dried mullein leaf
- ½ cup fennel seed
- ¼ cup dried licorice root, or to taste
- Honey, for extra soothing (optional)

Instructions:

1. Mix all the herbs. Store in an airtight container.
2. Make a cold infusion: pour in cold or room-temperature water and steep for 4 to 8 hours.
3. Strain the liquid and serve it immediately, or warm if preferred.
4. Add honey (if using) for extra soothing.

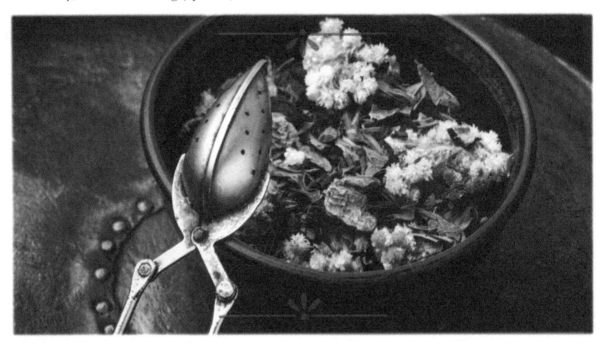

Constipation

Purifying digestive tea

This tea is great for relieving diarrhea and other digestive issues, such as nausea and bloating.

Ingredients:

- 2 teaspoons cascara sagrada
- 3 to 4 slices ginger root
- 1 teaspoon cayenne
- 1 teaspoon Oregon grape root
- 2 cups boiling water

Instructions:

1. Take one tablespoon at a time, up to two cups per day.

Diarrhea

Soothing diarrhea tea

This tea is also known as "carrot chamomile." if you have diarrhea, this tea can help reduce the amount of water that passes through the bowels, improving symptoms. You can use it to treat diarrhea or to dilute

a remedy to ease the symptoms if your diarrhea is caused by a problem with your bowels.

Ingredients:

- 2 teaspoons alumroot
- 2 teaspoons blackberry leaves
- 2 teaspoons angelica seeds
- 1 teaspoon Oregon grape root
- 2 cups boiling water

Sweet relief tea

This tea is great for relieving diarrhea, dysentery, and bloating. It also soothes the stomach and helps to control nausea.

Ingredients:

- 1 tablespoon raspberry leaf
- 1 teaspoon white willow bark
- 2 cups boiling water

Instructions:

1. Combine the above herbs and cover with boiling water; steep for 30 minutes; strain.

2. Take as needed.

Fever

Fever relief tea

This is one of my favorite teas, especially when I am feeling under the weather.

The use of barberry berries, angelica root, and dried yarrow create a wonderful tea with both antibacterial and anti-inflammatory properties.

Ingredients:

- 1 teaspoon angelica root
- 1 teaspoon ground ivy leaves
- 1 teaspoon barberry berries
- 1 teaspoon peppermint leaves
- 2 teaspoons blue vervain leaves
- 1 tablespoon dried yarrow
- 1 teaspoon catnip leaves
- 1 cup boiling water

Instructions:

1. Combine the above herbs.
2. Place one tablespoon of the mixture in a cup; steep for 30 minutes; strain.
3. Take up to one cup a day.

Food Intolerances

Gut-heal tea

This digestive herb mix has all of the functions required to restore healthy function to the stomach, intestines, and liver. It is the single most frequently recommended formula in our practice and is open to a wide degree of individual customization.

Ingredients:

- ½ cup dried calendula flower
- ½ cup dried plantain leaf
- ½ cup dried chamomile flower
- ½ cup dried tulsi leaf, cup dried marshmallow leaf
- ¼ cup dried ginger
- ¼ cup dried licorice root
- ¼ cup dried yarrow leaf and flower, ¼ cup dried St. John's wort leaf and flower

Instructions:

1. Add 2–4 tablespoons of the herb into one cup of boiled water and steep for 10–15 minutes.
2. Drink 1 cup as needed.

Quick-acting flatulence tea

This tea eases intestinal gas and general flatulence. It is good for bloating and diarrhea and can help expel parasites.

Ingredients:

- 1 teaspoon catnip leaf
- 1 teaspoon grated ginger root
- 2 teaspoons dandelion leaves
- 2 cups boiling water

Instructions:

1. Combine the herbs and cover with boiling water; steep for 20 to 30 minutes; strain.
2. Take as needed.

Hangover

No-fuss hangover tea

This tea is said to help with headaches and t hangover.

It's also a great remedy for anyone who gets an upset stomach from drinking too much alcohol.

Ingredients:

- 1 teaspoon ripe barberry berry
- 2 cups boiling water
- 1 teaspoon Oregon grape root

Instructions:

1. Combine the herbs in a non-metallic vessel, then cover with boiling water; steep for 30 minutes; cool and strain.
2. Take up to one cup a day. Dilute in an adequate amount of cool water.

Headache

Soothing headache tea

This tisane is said to be helpful for relieving headaches and tension.

Ingredients:

- 1 teaspoon catnip leaf
- 2 teaspoons feverfew leaves
- 1 to 2 cups boiling water

Instructions:

1. Combine the catnip and the feverfew in a glass container
2. Steep for 30 minutes. After this strain it
3. Take a tablespoon at a time, up to one cup each day.

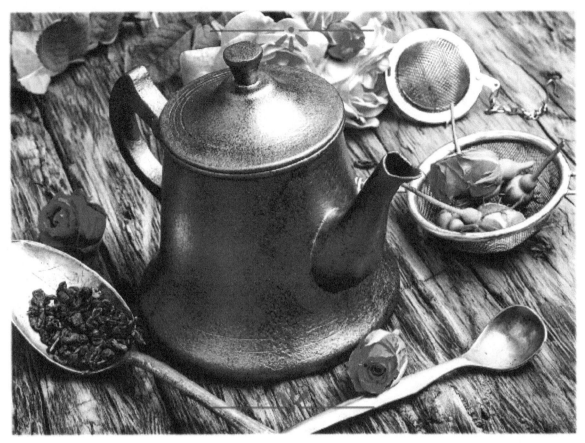

Heartburn

Quick-acting heartburn tea

Sip a cup of this calming tea before a big meal to help relieve the pain of heartburn.

Ingredients:

- 1 teaspoon dried angelica root
- 1 cup boiling water
- 1 teaspoon crushed juniper berries

Instructions:

1. Combine the herbs in a non-metallic vessel, then cover with boiling water; steep for 20 to 30 minutes; strain.
2. Take a tablespoon at a time, as needed.

Soothing heartburn tea

This tea helps relieve the discomfort of acid reflux

Ingredients:

- 1 teaspoon catnip leaf
- 1 teaspoon oxeye daisy herb
- 1 cup boiling water

Instructions:

1. Combine the herbs in a non-metallic container and cover with boiling water; steep for 30 minutes; strain.
2. Take a tablespoon at a time, as needed.

Indigestion

Digestive tea

This tea is used to treat ulcers, gas, colic, indigestion, and pain in the abdomen.

- 1 teaspoon blue cohosh root
- 1 cup boiling water
- 1 teaspoon coneflower root.

Instructions:

1. Combine the herbs in a glass vessel.
2. Steep for 30 minutes; cool and strain.
3. Consume as needed, up to one cup a day.

Quick-acting digestive tea

This tea effectively aids in digestion and is effective for nausea, diarrhea, vomiting too.

Ingredients:

- 1 teaspoon licorice root
- 2 cups boiling water

- 1 teaspoon peppermint leaves

Instructions:

1. Combine the herbs in a non-metallic vessel, then cover with boiling water; steep for 15 to 20 minutes. After this strain it.
2. Consume as needed, up to one cup per day.

Menstruation

These teas are all alleys to soothe menstrual issues like cramps; they soothe and relieve pain during the menstrual period

Stomach cramps soothing tea
Ingredients:

- 1 tsp. St. John's Wort leaves
- 1 tsp. Raspberry leaves
- 1 cup distilled boiling water

Instructions:

1. Pour boiling water over the herbs mixture. Let rest for half an hour. Strain and drink throughout the day.
2. Warning: do not use in case of pregnancy. It definitely should not be the case because you would not have menstruation, but in any case, the substance contained in this tea can cause damage to the uterus if taken during pregnancy

Dysmenorrhea rescue tea #1
Ingredients:

- 1 tsp. Black Haw Root
- 1 tsp. Black Cohosh Root
- 1 tsp. Crampbark (bark)
- 1 cup distilled boiling water

Instructions:

1. Pour boiling water over the herbs mixture. Let rest for 30 minutes. Strain and drink throughout the day.
2. Warning: do not use in case of pregnancy. It definitely should not be the case because you would not have menstruation, but in any case, the substance contained in this tea can cause damage to the uterus if taken during pregnancy

Dysmenorrhea rescue tea #2
Ingredients:

- 1 tsp. black haw root
- 1 tsp. passionflower
- 1 cup distilled boiling water

Instructions:

1. Pour boiling water over the herbs mixture. Let rest for half an hour. Strain and drink one cup per day, two or three tablespoonfuls at a time.
2. Warning: do not use in case of pregnancy. It definitely should not be the case because you would not have menstruation, but in any case, the substance contained in this tea can cause damage to the uterus if taken during pregnancy

Stable flow tea
Ingredients:

- 1 cup nettle dried flowers and leaves
- 1 cup goldenrod dried leaves and flowers
- ½ cup dandelion dried leaves and flowers
- 1 cup heal-all dried leaf
- ½ cup angelica dried root

Instructions:

1. Mix the herbs in a mason jar for easy storage. Put 1 tbsp. of the mixture in 1 cup of distilled boiling water. Let rest for half an hour. Strain and drink 1 cup per day.
2. Warning: do not use in case of pregnancy. It definitely should not be the case because you would not have menstruation, but in any case, the substance contained in this tea can cause damage to the uterus if taken during pregnancy

Bleed on tea

To induce menstruation, drink this tea for three days to 1 week before the expected start of your next period. Drink this tea scalding to make the most of it. Reheat as needed and consume a quart or more throughout the day. For a more substantial effect, take a drop of angelica tincture together with each cup of tea.

Ingredients:

- 1 cup of chamomile flower, dried
- 1 cup of tulsi leaf, dried
- 1/3 cup of goldenrod leaf and flower, dried
- 1/3 cup of ginger, dried
- 1/3 cup of angelica root, dried

Cramp relief tea
Great for relieving the pain of cramps

Ingredients:

- 1 teaspoon St. John's wort leaves
- 1 teaspoon raspberry leaves

Instructions:

1. Drink as needed to relieve cramps

Muscular Cramps

Cramps are involuntary muscle contractions that can lead to pain and the temporary impossibility to move the affected muscle.

Root causes for cramps can be many: from excessive muscular fatigue to dehydration and poor diet, which affect the number of electrolytes in our body (mediators used for muscular neural signal transmission). More rare causes can be pregnancy, menstruation, or gastroenteritis.

Cramp tea
Ingredients:

- 1 tsp. Ashwagandha root
- 1 tsp. black cohosh root
- 1 cup distilled boiling water

Instructions:

1. Pour boiling water over the herbs mixture. Let rest for half an hour. Strain and drink throughout the day.

Nausea

The causes can be infinite: from psychosomatic, to food poisoning, to pregnancy (*Morning Sickness*), to serious diseases like viral or bacterial infections.

The teas will relieve any nausea symptoms

Nausea stop tea #1
Ingredients:

- 1 tsp. catnip leaves and flowers
- 1 tsp. chamomile flowers
- 1 cup distilled boiling water

Instructions:

1. Pour boiling water over the herbs mixture. Let rest for twenty minutes. Strain and drink two or three tablespoonfuls each hour until you do not feel the nausea sensation.

Nausea stop tea #2
Ingredients:

- 1 tsp. lizard tail root, powdered
- 1 tsp. powdered ginger root
- 1 tsp. peppermint dried leaves
- 1 cup distilled boiling water

Instructions:

1. Pour boiling water over the herbs mixture. Let rest for half an hour. Strain and drink throughout the day.

Nausea-soothing tea
This is a very effective and time-tested treatment for morning sickness and upset stomach.

It is also used as a useful alternative medicine for women's monthly cycles.

Ingredients:

- 1 teaspoon catnip leaf,
- 1 teaspoon chamomile flowers

Instructions:

1. Boil water and add the herbs to boil for 10 minutes. Let it cool, and drink 1 cup of warm tea if you have any symptoms of nausea.

Calming tea
The herbs in this blend will help to soothe the stomach and calm nausea.

It can also help relieve vomiting.

Ingredients:

- 1 cup dried catnip leaf and flower
- 1 cup dried chamomile flower
- ½ cup dried peppermint leaf
- ½ cup fennel seed
- ¼ cup dried ginger

Instructions:

1. Mix all the herbs. Store in an airtight container until cool enough to drink.
2. Consume a cup carefully in little swallows. If the nausea is extreme, just sit for a few minutes and smell the aroma coming from the hot tea.

Relax
Sleep-time tea
This evening tea is a decent decision for quite a long time when everybody is excessively drained or experiencing difficulty slowing down. You can utilize tea instead of water when making gelatin for a sleep-time dessert.

Ingredients:

- 1 cup (235 ml) water
- 1 teaspoon passionflower
- 1 teaspoon chamomile
- 1 teaspoon lemon salve
- Yield: 1 cup (235 ml)

Instructions:

1. Consolidate the water and herbs in a pot and bring to a stew. Expel from the warmth and let steep.

Sinusitis

Sinusitis is the inflammation of the sinuses. It causes nasal congestion, headache, and a feeling of heaviness around the eyes. The inflammation can also lead to fever, cough, and frequent sneezes.

The causes can be allergic or due to the presence of a bacterial/fungal/viral infection in the sinus cavities.

Mucus-freeing tea

This tea is great for relieving stuffy noses, coughs, congestion, and sore throats.

Ingredients:

- 1 teaspoon bayberry root
- 1 teaspoon white willow bark
- 2 cups boiling water

Instructions:

1. Combine the above herbs in boiling water.
2. Drink one warm cup in case of any symptoms as above

Unclogging decoction #1

Ingredients:

- 1 tsp. white willow bark
- 1 tsp. bayberry root
- 1 cup distilled boiling water

Instructions:

1. Boil the bark and the root for half an hour in the indicated proportion. Strain, wait a few minutes, and drink hot.

Unclogging decoction #2

Ingredients:

- 1 tsp. Echinacea root
- 1 tsp. goldenseal root
- 1 tsp. lizard tail root
- 1 cup distilled boiling water

Instructions:

1. Boil the roots for half an hour in the indicated proportions. Strain, wait a few minutes, and drink hot.

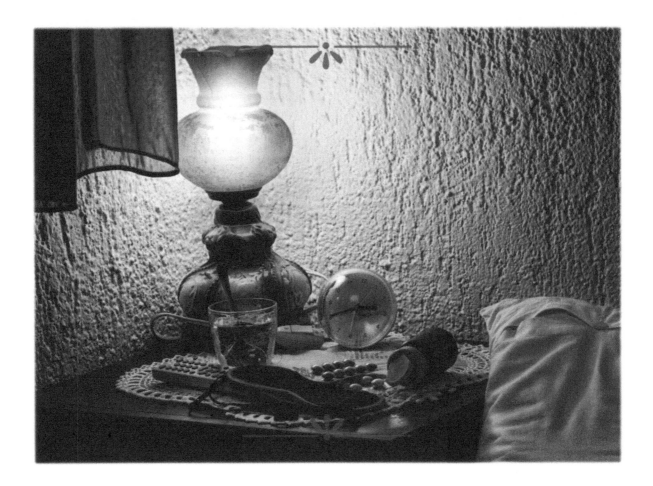

Sleep and Insomnia

Insomnia is defined as any difficulty in having restoring sleep.

It may happen in the form of fighting to fall asleep, or infrequently interrupted sleep, or in the incapacity to sleep for sufficient time.

It can be due to stress, poor diet, or excessive caffeine intake.

In addition, many studies highlighted the fact that exposure to bright, artificial light (such as TV or phones) in the evening may affect the circadian rhythm of our body and indeed cause insomnia, so my first go-to advice when dealing with sleep issues is to avoid them starting from 18:00.

Insomnia relief tea

This recipe is a simple formula made from the most effective herbs for insomnia. These herbs will relax you and help with stress, making it easier to fall asleep at night. This is a simple recipe that anyone can make at home, with ingredients available from almost any local grocery store.

Ingredients:

- 1 teaspoon chamomile flower
- 1 teaspoon hops
- 1 teaspoon valerian root
- 1 cup boiling water

Instructions:

1. Combine the above herbs.
2. Drink warm, as needed, half a cup at a time.

Sleep time tea

This tea can be used to help cure insomnia, being especially helpful for people who often wake up during the night and are not able to sleep more than 3 hours in a row

Ingredients:

- 1 cup (235 ml) water
- 1 teaspoon passionflower

- 1 teaspoon chamomile
- 1 teaspoon lemon salve
- Yield: 1 cup (235 ml)

Instructions:

1. Consolidate the water and herbs in a pot and bring to a stew. Expel from the warmth and let steep.

Goodnight tea #1
Ingredients:

- 1 tsp. dried hops
- 1 tbsp. chamomile flowers dried
- 2 tsp. passionflowers dried
- 1 cup distilled boiling water

Instructions:

Pour boiling water over the herbs mixture. Let rest for ten minutes. Strain and drink before going to bed.

Goodnight tea 2
Ingredients:

- 1 tsp. dried hops
- 1 tbsp. chamomile flowers dried
- 1 tsp. valerian root powdered
- 1 cup distilled boiling water

Instructions:

1. Pour boiling water over the herbs mixture. Let rest for half an hour. Strain and drink throughout the evening.

Stress

This is a good way to treat a mild anxiety disorder. It helps the person relax and promotes better sleep. It is made by boiling valerian root, ginger, and pleurisy in water.

Calm down tea
Ingredients:

- 1 teaspoon powdered ginger
- 1 teaspoon powdered valerian root
- 1 teaspoon powdered pleurisy root
- 2 cups boiling water

Instructions:

1. Mix the herbs in a non-metallic container, cover them with boiling water, and let infuse for 30 minutes; cool and strain.
2. As needed, take 1 tablespoon at a time, up to 2 cups per day.

Sore Throat

The medical term for *Sore Throat* is Pharyngitis. It means throat pain and normally indicates an inflammation status to the pharynx due to a viral or bacterial (mainly streptococcus) infection. Other causes of pharyngitis may be exposure to irritants or substances that cause an allergic reaction.

This condition causes pain when swallowing, and sometimes is accompanied by cough, fever, and mucus secretion in the nasal cavities.

Sore throat tea 1
Ingredients:

- 1 tsp. slippery elm bark
- 1 tsp. echinacea root
- 1 cup distilled boiling water

Instructions:

1. Pour boiling water over the herbs mixture. Let rest for half an hour. Strain and drink throughout the day.

Fatigue

Pick-me-up tea
This pick-me-up is a great antidote for those days when you feel like giving up and letting the chips fall where they may.

This is a great tea to drink right before you do anything, such as exams or social events, as it helps give you the extra burst of energy you need.

Ingredients:

- 1 teaspoon ginkgo Biloba leaves
- 1 teaspoon dried mirabilis root
- 1 teaspoon dried ginseng root
- 1 teaspoon pulsatilla herb
- 1 teaspoon Gotu kola leaves
- 1 teaspoon St. John's wort leaves

Instructions:

1. Take as needed.

CHAPTER 35:

DIY PERSONAL CARE HERBAL RECIPES

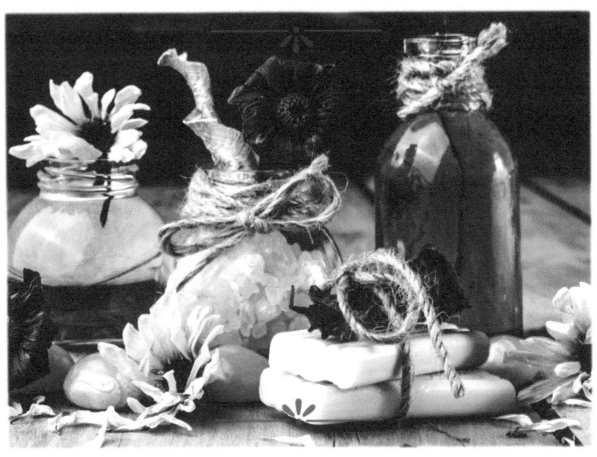

Haircare

Rosemary-infused oil

Great for strengthening hair.

You can use this infused oil for a hair mask and in balms and salves.

Ingredients:

- Rosemary leaves
- Carrier oil (like olive oil)
- Tools:
- Quart jar
- Cheesecloth
- Glass bottles

Instructions:

1. This method doesn't have specific measurements; it's okay to eyeball it.
2. Rinse your rosemary, making sure to dry completely. Put the herbs in a quart jar with 1–3 inches of space on top. For a multipurpose infusion, olive oil is a great choice.
3. We've seen formulas that let the rosemary infuse for up to a month. If the sun is really hot, you can cover the jar with a paper bag. When infusion time has passed, strain the oil through a cheesecloth into a cup or bowl. With a funnel, pour into clean glass bottles. On the label, write "Rosemary oil with olive oil" and the date.

Rosemary conditioner

Makes 1 cup.

This straightforward antifungal treatment mixes a natural, odorless conditioner tailored to your hair type with rosemary essential oil, which is highly concentrated and delightfully aromatic. If you don't have rosemary essential oil, a tincture will be fine.

Ingredients:

- 1 cup odorless natural herbal conditioner, such as stonybrook botanicals
- 40 drops rosemary essential oil

Instructions:

1. Combine the conditioner and essential oil in a large container, stirring thoroughly with a fork. Transfer it with a funnel to a BPA-free plastic bottle with a squeeze cap.
2. After shampooing, apply a nickel-sized dab of conditioner to your scalp. Wait for 2 to 5 minutes before rinsing with cold water to remove the conditioner. Hair should be styled as normal. Use it on a daily basis for the best result.

Precautions: if you have epilepsy, avoid using rosemary.

Facial Care

Acne is a common skin ailment that manifests with the inflammation of the hair follicle and the related sebaceous gland.

It occurs when the sebum (which is produced by the sebaceous gland to lubricate the skin) clogs the skin pore, and a small bacterial infection takes place.

It is very common in the teenage years due to the strong hormonal activity, but it can occur also in adolescence due to many causes such as the use of antibiotics, allergies, wrong diet, food poisoning, genetics.

Tonic for skin
Ingredients:

- 8 oz. Apple cider vinegar
- 8 oz. witch hazel water extraction
- 8 oz. rose water

Instructions:

1. Combine the ingredients in a container. Avoid any metal to come in contact with the mixture to prevent any oxidative reaction that can cause the liquid to contaminate with metal.
2. Apply once a day on clean skin without scrubbing. Double the frequency in case of persistent acne. Be consistent, and the results will come.
3. Note: Adjust the proportion of the mixture according to your skin type (i.e., for dry skins, reduce the apple cider vinegar).

Facial steam
Ingredients:

- ¼ cup dried chamomile flowers
- ¼ cup dried sage
- ¼ cup dried thyme
- ¼ cup dried yarrow
- 32 oz. water

Instructions:

1. Before steaming, gently clean your face with water and soap.
2. Mix the herbs. Bring the water to a boil, remove from heat and place the pot on your kitchen table (be sure to use a trivet). Put ½ cup of the mixture in hot water and use a towel to make a tent with your head at the apex. Steam your face for 10 to 20 minutes max.

Acne-reducing tea
Ingredients:

- 1 cup Oregon grape root tea
- 2.5ml yellow dock tincture

Instructions:

1. Drink the tea mixed with the yellow dock tincture. One cup throughout the day is the recommended dosage to avoid any side effects of the Oregon grape root.

Lotion for acne
Ingredients:

- 1 cup horsetail tea
- 1.5ml gotu kola tincture

Instructions:

1. Gently rub the mix of the two ingredients on the skin three times a day.

Skincare

Calendula salve

Great to treat skin irritation, dried skin, eczema, wound healing.

Calendula has antifungal, antibacterial, and anti-inflammatory properties. A salve made with this herb is great for chapped lips, dry hands, cuts, scrapes, and bruises.

Ingredients to make the calendula oil:

- Calendula flowers, dried
- Coconut oil

- Vitamin E oil

Ingredients to make the salve:

- 4-ounces calendula-infused oil
- ½-ounces chopped beeswax

Directions for the oil:

1. In case your coconut oil is solid, warm it very gently until it turns into a liquid.
2. Put dried calendula flowers in a glass jar (leaving about ¼ of it empty) and fill with oil so the flowers are covered.
3. Label your jar. Place your jar in a sunny windowsill and gently shake every 2–3 days. After at least 3 weeks, the oil will be thoroughly infused.

Directions for the salve:

1. In a double boiler, add your infused oil and beeswax.
2. Heat and stir so the beeswax melts and mixes in smoothly with the oil. Remove from the heat and funnel into a glass jar or tin. Let the salve cool before closing the lid.
3. Label the container remembering to write down the date. Store in a cool, dry, and dark place. When using the salve, don't scoop out with your finger, as this increases the risk of contamination. Use a swab. When stored properly, this salve can last up to 3 years.

Chickweed tincture

Great to treat skin irritations, acne, scrapes, bumps, bruises.

This tincture can be applied to irritated skin, acne, scrapes, and any other area where you need skin healing. A standard dose (20–75 drops) can also be added to tea for digestive issues like constipation.

Ingredients:

- ¾ cup chickweed, fresh, chopped
- 1 cup 80/100 proof alcohol (like vodka)

Instructions:

1. Put your chickweed in a clean jar. Pour vodka over the herbs so they're completely covered. Seal and label the jar.
2. When the steeping time is up, line a sieve with cheesecloth and strain the tincture. Funnel into a dark-colored glass dropper bottle.

Rose beads

This is a great way to make your own rose water, which can be spray-cleaned in case you don't have access to clean water.
It's also a good way to make your own perfume!

Ingredients:

- 1 tablespoon finely powdered flower petals (the most profound shading you can discover is ideal)
- 1/4 teaspoon gum tragacanth powder
- 1/2 teaspoon red or pink earth
- 1 tablespoon (15 ml) rose water, or more varying

Instructions:

1. In a bowl, mix the powders and include the rose water. The consistency ought to take after demonstrating earth. Fold the dots with your fingers into the size and shape that you'd like, and string them onto a thick wire. I utilize botanical wire from the specialty store, the thickest accessible. Leave around 1/2 inch (1.3 cm) between globules.
2. Wrap the wires of dots over a case or bowl so that there is a course underneath the dabs. Tenderly pivot the dabs on the wire every 8 or 10 hours. Contingent upon the size of the dabs you make, they may be dry the following day, or it could take a few days.

Dry rash salve

This salve is good for dry skin and can help soothe the skin and protect it from infection.

Ingredients:

- 3 fluid ounces calendula-infused oil
- 3 fluid ounces plantain-infused oil
- 2 fluid ounces licorice-infused oil
- 1-ounce beeswax, plus more as needed

Instructions:

1. Place the oils in a boiler and heat them, then add the beeswax. Stir to melt.
2. Make the consistency soft and pour in a jar.
3. Apply a teaspoon amount on the rash when needed

Rose milk bath

This bath can help with dry skin, eczema, and acne. The rose water can also help with cellulite, and it's a great way to relax and relieve stress.

Ingredients:

- 2 cups flower petals (the most fragrant you can discover)
- 2 cups violet leaves
- 2 cups (240 g) milk powder
- 1/2 cup (40 g) cereal

Instructions:

1. Pour all the ingredients in a water/airproof container. To utilize, place around 1/4 cup of the blend into a material sack and mix it in simply bubbled water for 10 minutes while the shower runs. Pour the tea (and the pack) into the tub and drench your considerations away. It's soothing to dry or desolate skin.

Plantain skin care

This is great stuff for all sorts of skin care needs. It helps with dry, cracked lips, sunburns, bug bites, and even burns. It also makes an excellent tincture that can be used as a salve or ingested to help with conditions such as gout or arthritis.

Ingredients:

- 3 tablespoons (45 ml) plantain-mixed oil
- 1 tablespoon (14 g) cocoa butter
- 1 tablespoon (14 g) beeswax

Instructions:

1. In a pot, heat all the ingredients delicately over low warmth until liquefied. Mix together and fill tins.
2. Let cement before putting tops on the tins. In the event that you need a demulcent that is fewer firms, utilize less beeswax.

CHAPTER 36:

DIY HERBAL REMEDIES FOR PETS

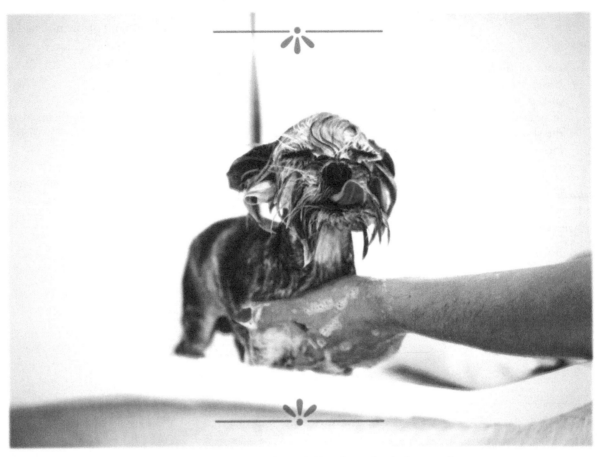

The following recipes are applicable for all our four-legged friends, so both dogs and cats.

Skin Diseases

Grooming shampoos and soaps

All-natural aromatherapy starts with the addition of essential oils to all-natural shampoo or soap base. All the ingredients have to be natural. Don't add high-quality essential oils with a synthetic chemical soap. Buy a truly all-natural shampoo, or create your own one. Here following, you can find a foaming, gentle soap, shampoo base for your dog grooming needs:

Ingredients:

- Distilled water 4.5 oz. (135 ml)
- Decyl Polyglucose 3.2 oz. (95 ml)
- Xanthan Gum Powder
- Cider Vinegar ½ tsp.
- Grapefruit Seed Extract (GSE) 1 ml
- Rosemary Antioxidant Extract 1 ml

Instructions:

1. Combine these ingredients to make an all-natural shampoo base for your dog and for yourself. This recipe makes 8 oz. or 240 ml of unscented shampoo base. You can use dried and fresh herbs such as chickweed, coltsfoot, horsetail, nettles, marshmallow root, slippery elm, calendula blossoms, comfrey root, oat straw, or chamomile flowers in the water phase of the shampoo. The herbs provide supportive and synergistic effects and increase therapeutic value.

2. It takes a lot of plant material to make a small quantity of essential oil. So it won't change the balance of the mixture. Start off with hot water, infuse the herbs. Add the GSE, cider vinegar, decyl poly glucose, and rosemary antioxidant and mix completely. You can use a stick blender to blend all the ingredients; while the mixture is still very warm, add the xanthan gum powder and blend until totally combined. Let the mixture cool, add

essential oils, and your very special, all-natural shampoo is ready for use with your dog.

Itchy skin and allergies
Add the following essential oils to 240 ml/8 oz. all-natural shampoo base:

Ingredients:

- Carrot Seed—2 drops
- Roman Chamomile—1 drop
- Lavender—6 drops
- Rosewood—6 drops
- Geranium—2 drops

Tip: Blend in 1 tablespoon of finely ground oatmeal to provide additional relief.

Skin infections and small wounds
Caused by insect bites, minor scrapes, and nicks.

Add the following essential oils to 240 ml/8 oz all-natural shampoo base:

Ingredients:

- Lavender—3 drop
- Helichrysum—1 drop
- Labdanum—2 drop
- Ravensara—4 drops

Skin infections and small wounds (for calming effect)
Add the following essential oils to 240 ml/8 oz. all-natural shampoo base:

- Sweet Orange—2 drops
- Sweet Marjoram—3 drops
- Petitgrain—4 drops
- Vetiver—2 drops
- Valerian—3 drops

Flea and insect repelling
Add the following essential oils to 240 ml/8 oz all-natural shampoo base:

- Lemon—4 drops
- Peppermint—8 drops
- Citronella—2 drops
- Clary Sage—4 drops

Tick repelling
Add the following essential oils to 240 ml/8 oz. all-natural shampoo base:

- Bay Leaf—1 drop
- Opoponax—2 drops

- Myrhh—2 drops
- Lavender—3 drops
- Rosewood—2 drops
- Geranium—2 drops

Calming effect for puppies
Add the following essential oils to 240 ml/8 oz all-natural shampoo base:

- Petitgrain—5 drops
- Roman Chamomile—2 drops
- Geranium—5 drops

- Ylang Ylang—2 drops
- Rose—2 drops

Deodorant
Add the following essential oils to 240 ml/8 oz all-natural shampoo base:

- Bay Leaf—3 drops
- Black Pepper—3 drops
- Caraway—5 drops
- Cinnamon Leaf—5 drops

Repel Flea

Use 4 oz. Of any base oil or 240 ml or 8 oz. all-natural shampoo as a base. Add 5 to 7 drops of Peppermint (scientific name: Mentha piperita), 4 drops of Citronella (scientific name: Cymbopogon nardus), 2 to 5 drops of Clary Sage (scientific name: Salvia sclarea), and 2 to 4 drops of Lemon (Citrus limon).

Make a fragrant flea collar by putting a few drops of this blend on the bandanna or cotton collar of your pet dog. Use as a flea repellent by applying some drops of the blend on your dog's tail, legs, back, chest, and neck.

Tick Repellent

Ticks simply cannot withstand lavender, bay, and geranium. Use this knowledge to concoct a tick repellent using the essential oils of the aforementioned plants and keep those ticks at bay.

To 120 ml or 4oz of base oil, add the following: 6 drops of Lemon Eucalyptus (scientific name: Eucalyptus Citriodora), 8 drops of Geranium (scientific name: Pelargonium graveolens), and 10 drops of Lavender (scientific name: Lavandula angustifolia). Apply some drops to your dog in areas most susceptible to ticks—tail, legs, chest, back, and neck.

CONCLUSION

Of course, nature has not always been regarded with suspicion. Much as when they were angry, the spirits of animals and other facets of nature could be dangerous, but they might also be beneficial when they were happy. For one, the Native Americans believed that herbs and even animals' organs were full of enormous healing powers. During their various curing rituals, they also called on the spirits of animals for help. It was believed that various species had special characteristics and qualities, such as cunning, intellect, and courage. During healing rituals, Native Americans may call for individual animal spirits, asking each in return to share their special gifts with the person being healed. Still, of course, doctors are unlikely to consider calling on the spirits of eagles and bears to regulate blood pressure or cure arthritis but depending on how it is handled, they are very mindful of nature's ability to cure or hurt.

Native American medicine included the use of many different herbal remedies and sometimes bones, feathers, and other parts of animals as well. Some of them were used to treat infections and ulcers, while other herbs were considered powerful contraceptives or even aphrodisiacs. It was also believed that certain animals could cure the sick or provide protection from harmful spells. Cherokee medicine is famous for using bear grease to treat open wounds.

BOOK 10

ESSENTIAL OILS

A Beginner's Guide to Essential Oils to Improve Your
Well-Being with Homemade Techniques and Recipes

Citali Galwen

INTRODUCTION

Essential oils have been available since ancient times, and early Egyptians were given credits when essential oils were used for cosmetics, perfumes, and embalming purposes. For example, sandalwood, peppermint, lavender oil, citronella oil, and eucalyptus, etc. are essential oils. The essential oil is named from the plant material in which it was extracted, depending on the given an example.

Primary oils are produced in various ways. Most of these are made through distillation (steam distillation). Distillation is a mechanism by which liquids with different vapor pressures are separated. In chemistry, we have learned that the higher vapor pressure substance has a lower boiling point. This process is illustrated in the next paragraph. The plant material is therefore kept in a pressing material or stored in a particular container where liquids can evaporate. Liquid substances are first distilled in plants with low boiling points, while liquid material with higher boiling points remains as in essential oils. However, other essences (essential oils) are so difficult to extract that they have to undergo a complex process. Examples are jasmine and rose oils. They undergo a strict distillation process by first washing a mixture of process-derived essential oils into a sea of osmotic material (supercritical hexane or carbon dioxide). The concrete must then be subjected, using alcohol-based materials, to a second stage in the distillation process and effectively insulate various volatile (absolute) oil from the distilled contents.

Not all of the essential oils will get into your bloodstream and evaporate as soon as they reach your skin. Since carrying oils have a large molecular structure, some of the essential oils remain mixed with a carrier oil on top of your skin. This offers you more benefits. Not only can you get the essential oils that penetrate the skin, but your skin's oil has many medicinal advantages as well.

CHAPTER 37:

ESSENTIAL OILS. THE HISTORY

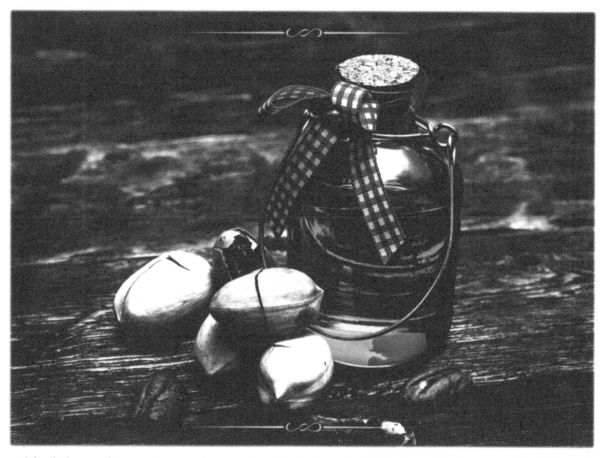

Essential oils have a history that can be traced as far back as the biblical age. In fact, essential oils have been mentioned several times throughout the Bible in various passages. It is easy to dismiss these traditional treatments and remedies as old wives' tales, something that isn't as effective as modern-day medicine is. However, sometimes, what you find in nature can hold a cure that is more powerful and effective than any medicinal drug can ever be.

Essential oils were used as a form of ancient medicine because the early humans back then could literally find anything they needed to cure their ailments within nature. The options were vast, and the side effects were less worrying the way modern medicine is. The results even lasted much longer too. For thousands of years, these oils were very much an integral part of people's lives. Throughout the Bible, several essential oils were mentioned in different passages. Within the Bible, these oils were referred to in terms such as ointments, perfumes, aromas, fragrances, odors, and even sweet savors.

Hyssop, frankincense and myrrh, and rosemary were some of the common oils used in the Bible for the anointing and healing of the sick. In the Old Testament, it is pointed out that Moses and other important figures used essential oils when they were anointing leaders and kings. Priests were also mentioned to use these oils for healing purposes. The most infamous story in the Bible, the one which told of Jesus' birth in the manger, also points out how the three wise men came from afar to offer several gifts to the King, including frankincense and myrrh as the anointing oils. In historical times, it was frankincense oil—due to its anti-inflammatory properties—which was often rubbed on children to help minimize any swelling and provide immunity protection for them. Myrrh, on the other hand, was a natural antiseptic oil, which helped to heal tissues and balance out the body's hormone levels.

These wonderful, natural resources were how people throughout history had kept their health and well-being in optimal condition. The Ancient Egyptians also had a great love for essential oils, and these were frequently used in the embalming and mummification process. Essential oils, which included juniper berry, spikenard, cedar wood, cinnamon, and myrrh, were used to help preserve the bodies, especially of Pharaohs and other royalty, as they were prepped and prepared for the afterlife. When King Tut's tomb was uncovered by archeologists back in 1923, among the discoveries were alabaster jars that contained essential oils.

Ancient Egyptians were also famous for burning incense when they honored their gods because they firmly believed that the aromatic smoke emitted from the incense would go up to the heavens. Along with it, the smoke would carry all their prayers which they wanted to be answered. There were temples used for producing and blending essential oils that have been recorded throughout history in Egypt. Oil recipes could even be found written in hieroglyphics on the walls of these temples. That was how significant essential oils were at the time. Egyptian women were famous for bathing themselves in these essential oils to help keep their skin rejuvenated.

Ancient Chinese were also firm believers in the power of essential oils as ancient medicine. Shennong's Herbal, the oldest Chinese text in existence, dating back to 2700 B.C., written by Shennong, who was considered a mythical sage ruler in prehistoric China. It was reported that he actually consumed hundreds of herbs during his time to test out their medicinal value. The ancient Chinese used essential oils along with other ingredients as an advanced form of holistic healing, tapping into the power of these essential oils and their healing properties to help sustain their health for thousands of years.

Essential oils have even shown up in ancient Greek, where it is believed that Hippocrates, whom many credit as the '*Father of Western Medicine,*' documented over 200 different types of herbs during his lifetime. He believed that these plant-based medicines were the first key to saving lives and that any form of surgery should only be seen as a last resort measure.

In the 1800s, pharmaceutical companies started to emerge, many of whom are still in existence today, including Abbott and Parke-Davis. Companies like Pfizer, Johnson & Johnson, and Merck would later go on to become the mainstream drug companies that we know today. Back then, these companies were still using plant-based medicines as synthetic drugs began gaining momentum and popularity.

Native Americans And Their Aromatherapy

herbal oils have long been used by Native Americans and ancient civilizations in their everyday routines and spiritual and domestic rituals. They have a deep admiration for Mother Nature and utilize only natural products in their daily lives. They think that herbal oils, with their potent scents, may ward off evil spirits while also improving their overall health. For example, aromatic oils and herbs are used in Native American cleaning rituals. Aromatic herbs such as Sage, Sweetgrass, Cedarwood, Juniper, Pine opinion spikes, and others help purify and rid the air of bad energies and bring positivity into life. But why would we discuss Aromatherapy in the Native American tradition? It is simple, practical, primal, and very natural. Americans have a broader understanding of Aromatherapy than other aromatherapists, and they recognize which oils or plants to use to combat strong emotions, mental turmoil, and other negative energy in life. The majority of the Natives' herbs and oils are widely available and obtained at Aromatherapy shops and online stores. They employ herbs in their most pure and natural state as aromatic plants with fragrances rather than making appealing combinations (as many aromatherapists do).

CHAPTER 38:

INTRODUCING ESSENTIAL OIL THERAPY

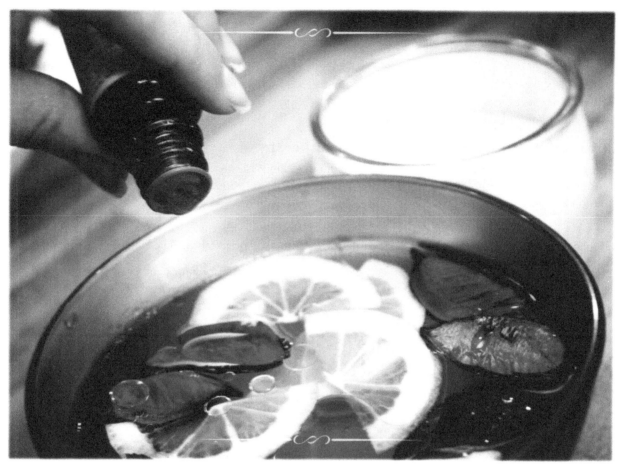

Essential oil therapy is becoming increasingly more popular in America each year and is a great way to keep your home healthy. A Native American herbalist has created a line of essential oils that are said to be the purest in the world. The Essential oils are made from all-natural ingredients and are safe for use with anyone, including pets. Many people have found relief using these oils for their ailments such as sinusitis, anxiety, depression, and more.

Native American Herbalist's essential oils not only works to treat the symptoms of health problems but has also been used for many other purposes. You can use essential oils in your bath, massage, or as an inhalant vaporizer to relieve tension and stress. It is also excellent for general wellness and may just be the thing that you need to help you relax during finals week!

Essential oils are made from all-natural ingredients and are safe for use with anyone, including pets. Many people have found relief using these oils for their ailments such as sinusitis, anxiety, depression, and more.

Essential Oils Impact On The Body

Native American herbalists have been using plant essential oils for healing purposes since ancient times. Some Native American herbalists use pure essential oils, while others take a more holistic approach and make their own formulas by blending various herbs with other natural ingredients such as plants, flowers, roots, stones, or water. This blend of herbs and natural ingredients can vary depending on the idea that each has a different function to enhance its healing properties. The popularity of these types of blends is steadily increasing into this century because the oils do not only heal the body but also help to nourish it with antioxidants to provide a sense of vitality and well-being.

A very common blend used by many Native American herbalists is known as "fresh feet." The origins of this blend are unknown, but it has been used for many years by Native American herbalists and healers. Fresh feet can be used to treat a variety of ailments caused by bacteria or viruses in the body, such as colds, flu, sore throat, infection, and other bouts caused by germs or toxins in the body. Most commonly, it is administered through steam inhalation to the upper respiratory tract, where it can relieve sinus congestion due to infections. It can also provide relief from bronchitis caused by temporomandibular joint dysfunction and cough associated with asthma and other lung conditions. It also soothes skin irritations such as insect bites, burns, rashes, or sunburn.

To prepare fresh feet, place equal amounts of eucalyptus essential oil, pine essential oil, and peppermint essential oil into a small bowl. Inhale the vapors from this mixture through a towel placed over your head and around your neck to help relieve sinus congestion. Also, add several drops of this mixture to an aroma diffuser to help increase the effects of your inhalation therapy treatments.

Advantages Of Essential Oils And Aromatherapy

Aromatherapy and essential oils can help you feel better in all kinds of ways. Whether you're having trouble sleeping or just want to unwind, these oils can help bring a little calm into your life. In fact, the use of scents has been quite common for centuries!

Essential oils are not only good for your mood but also have many other uses. They're amazing natural cleaners, and they make great perfumes, lotions, and cosmetics, even in food preparation! The list goes on and on.

Essential oils have been used as therapeutic agents for ages, both for minor injuries and even major ones. They can help boost the immune system, relieve migraines and many other conditions. Essential oils and aromatherapy can also help with sleep, depression, anxiety, and many other issues. It's important to understand that essential oils are strong and should be used in small amounts due to allergies (especially if you have sensitive skin).

How To Mix And Match Essential Oils

Mixing essential oils can be a delightfully therapeutic experience—or it can be a headache-inducing nightmare if you don't know what you're doing. In this article, we'll give you some tips on how to mix and match essential oils with confidence.

Where To Store Essential Oils

You may be tempted to keep your essential oils in the kitchen cupboard or in a bathroom cupboard. If you do, however, don't follow that idea too literally. The lighting is different from there than it is within the front room of your house; bacteria can thrive in these conditions. It's better instead to store essential oils in a cool dark place, preferably away from direct sunlight.

How To Select Essential Oils

There are probably hundreds of essential oils from which to pick. Choose your personal favorites or those that can help you meet a health issue. Keep some on hand for everyday use and others for special application when you're feeling under the weather.

Take a sniff first—a potent blend may be just what you need! But before you buy, ask if it contains any synthetic ingredients, like petroleum, which can be absorbed by the skin and may cause irritation or other conditions.

How To Mix Essential Oils

Carrier oils include jojoba, olive, peanut, sesame, and avocado oils. Some essential oils can be mixed directly with others without dilution; this usually depends on their chemical composition and the percentages of each chemical within the blend.

On the other hand, some essential oils should be mixed with a carrier oil so that they can be absorbed by the skin. Lavender, for example, is a skin sensitizer and may cause irritation when applied without dilution.

For this reason, it's best to begin by mixing a dilution of 1 part oil to 5 parts carrier oil. Mixing with a mortar and pestle or even an empty eggshell can also work—just keep in mind that it requires more effort. An electric blender is also a good method for making blended oils. The oils should be mixed into the water-based base entirely before blending and will churn as they mix together.

Essential oils can be very concentrated. New brands of essential oils contain less than 2 percent phenols, which are the chemicals that make an essential oil its distinct nature. For this reason, some people recommend diluting essential oils when mixing them. If you're new to mixing your own blends, it's best to start with a low dilution and work your way up to a higher one until you're comfortable with the recipe.

How To Apply Essential Oils

You should apply diluted blends sparingly to the skin or take them internally only under medical supervision. Be sure to follow the instructions on your bottle.

Some essential oils are heat-sensitive. For example, peppermint is a remedy for colds when applied to the chest and throat but can cause irritation if exposed to direct sunlight. If you want to use a freshly mixed blend in the middle of summer, it's best to store it in a cool dark place until time for use.

How Do Essential Oils Accomplish All These Benefits?

How essential oils work to promote health

The primary mechanism of action for essential oils is through the olfactory receptors in the nose that send messages to the limbic system in the brain. The limbic system is responsible for regulating emotions, which means that inhaling certain scents can result in emotional changes, which can affect a number of other physical aspects of our being. Essential oils work in the body by either stimulating, blocking, or altering the effects of the olfactory receptors involved.

How do you know what oil to use?

Aroma: This is obviously the primary characteristic of essential oils that associate them with their health benefits. Most people will almost immediately recognize that a particular oil has a specific aroma because we are familiar with just about all food and spice scents. The way this works is that different aromas tend to result in different types of reactions in our bodies, which can lead to very distinct health conditions. For example, the scent of cinnamon for a lot of people produces an adrenaline response, which is to say that it can boost mental alertness. This pushes our heart rate up, and our adrenal glands release hormones that increase our blood pressure. In some cases, this may result in raised blood pressure, and it may be important to be careful when using cinnamon as a treatment for hypertension or even for treating insomnia if you are naturally anxious.

CHAPTER 39:

HOW TO PREPARE ESSENTIAL OILS DIY

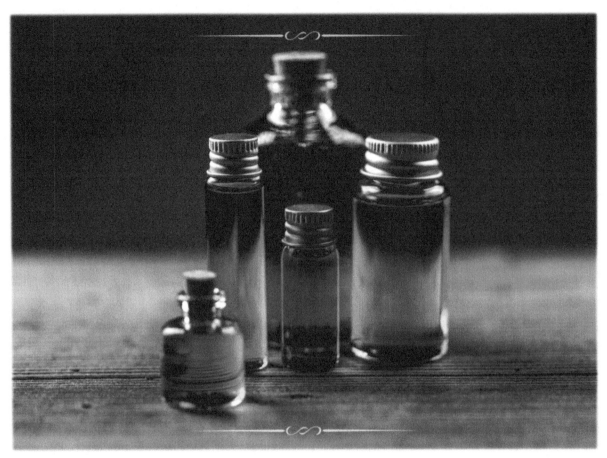

Although it is easy to buy essential oils from your local drug or grocery stores, they can be a bit on the expensive side. You can instead make these oils at home by extracting them directly from raw materials such as herbs, flowers, and fruit peels.

Depending on the degree of concentration and purity, three types of methods to extract essential oils can be used. The most widely used method is known as the distillation method, in which a special oil extraction device called a distiller is used. This particular method is most preferred as it gives off the strongest and most concentrated results. Carrier oil and infusion are the other two types of oil extraction methods.

Let's have a look at each one in detail.

Distillation Method

The distiller is an apparatus that is used to extract oils from herbs, flowers, and fruits. The basic mechanism that a distiller employs to extract the oil involves the heating and cooling down of the raw materials in close succession and ultimately collecting the oil.

A distiller has three components—a heating device, a steam carrier tube, and a collector. The heater is a vessel that helps in heating up the raw materials in boiling water to allow them to release their oil. The heat then escapes in the form of steam along with the essential oil.

The steam-containing oil is then passed through copper tubing that is immersed in ice-cold water. The cold water helps in condensing the steam and turning it into liquid, with the oil still intact. The water is then collected and further allowed to cool. After it cools completely, the oil collects at the top and can be easily skimmed off.

Distillers are available in most hardware stores and can also be bought online. A standard oil distiller can cost anywhere between a few hundred to several hundred dollars, depending on quality and size.

As expensive as it might sound, a distiller is a great investment as it can be used to extract any amount of essential oils from any number of raw materials, making it cost-effective in the long run. But if the price is a factor, then a distiller can easily be made at home.

The quality of oil output might differ and not be as high as store-bought oils, but homemade distillers can help in extracting good quality essential oils. The process of building a distiller might be simple, but you will be required to conduct several trial-and-error methods to arrive at the right way of extracting the best concentration and quality of the oil.

Building A Distiller

A distiller can easily be built at home with raw materials purchased online or from hardware stores. If it is difficult to find a pressure cooker, then it can be substituted with a tea kettle.

Here are the raw materials needed to build a distiller:

1. Standard pressure cooker—1
2. 10 mm copper wire—10 meters
3. Plastic tube—2 inches
4. Large plastic tub—1
5. Large glass jar—1

Method:

- Prepare the lid of the pressure cooker by blocking all other valves and keeping only the steam valve open.
- Bend the copper wire in such a way that it coils one fold in the middle. You can either do it yourself by wrapping it around a mini cylinder or have a metal worker do it for you.
- Place the rubber tube over the steam valve so that it fits perfectly and no steam can escape. You can also further secure it using a waterproof sealant.

Your distiller is now ready. The correct method of using the distiller to extract oil is as follows:

- Place the cooker on top of the gas stove.
- Collect a substantial amount of your raw materials (orange peels, lavender flowers, and more) and place them inside the cooker so that only an inch of space remains at the top.
- Pour water from a recently boiled kettle over the raw materials, making sure to use three parts of water to one part material.
- Place a large tub of cold water next to the cooker and immerse as much of the copper tube in it as possible.
- Place the open end of the copper tube inside a glass jar which will act as the receiver of the oil-containing water.
- Once the jar fills up, or you have collected a satisfactory amount of oil, switch off the gas and allow the collected water to cool down.
- After it cools, the essential oil will float at the top and can be easily skimmed and collected.
- Place the oil in a small glass bottle marked with the name of the oil.

Your essential oil is now ready to use.

Note: the collected oil might be extremely concentrated so, before applying to the skin, it should be diluted with a carrier oil such as coconut or olive oil. The ratio of carrier to essential oil will depend on the concentration level of the latter.

Carrier Oil Method

Essential oils can also be extracted without the help of a distiller. The results might not be the same, but it is an easier and cheaper method of extracting the oil.

No special apparatus will be required for this process, and only a few household items will be needed.

The following items are required for the carrier oil method of extraction

1. Large utensil for boiling—1
2. Rose petals or any other raw materials—1 cup
3. Carrier oils (coconut, almond)—½ cup
4. Vitamin E oil—2 drops
5. Fine cloth strainer—1
6. Dark glass bottles for storage

Method:

- Place the flowers or fruit peels inside the utensil along with the carrier oil.
- Add in the vitamin E oil, and give it a good mix.
- Place on low heat for four hours.
- Do not bring the mixture to a boil, and maintain a gentle heat supply.
- Switch off the heat, and let the mixture cool down before passing it through a fine cloth sieve.
- Collect it in glass jars and allow it to mature for a couple of days.

The essential oil collected through this method is generally less concentrated as compared to the oils made through the distilled method and can be used as-is for cosmetic purposes.

Infusion Method

The infusion method is an even simpler method that can be employed to make essential oils at home. The resultant oil will probably be the least concentrated but will still serve as a great alternative to expensive store-bought oils.

The infusion method will require the following materials:

1. Carrier oil (coconut, sunflower, olive)—½ cup
2. Oil raw materials (flower petals, fruit peels, herbs)—1 cup
3. Glass jar—1

Method:

- Place the carrier oil along with the raw materials in an air-tight glass jar and give it a good mix.
- Let the oil infuse with the raw materials for a minimum of two weeks.
- Strain the mixture and collect it in a second jar.

The oil is ready to be used.

Regardless of which method is employed to make the essential oils, they will always be better options than store-bought products as they will be free from any form of chemicals. Also, the costs to make them will work out to be much less than the cost of commercial oils.

Important safety measures

- Be sure to use only glass bottles for storing the essential oils as any other materials such as plastic can react with the oils and modify their composition.
- Always mark your oils with their date of creation. Essential oils come with shelf lives and it will not be safe to use them after their expiration dates.
- Store them in dark rooms away from direct sunlight so that their potency and shelf life can increase. Using dark color glass bottles also helps.
- Cleanse the distiller thoroughly after every use and discard any residual fragrance and oil from previous processes as to not interfere with subsequent usage.

CHAPTER 40:

ESSENTIAL OIL BENEFITS

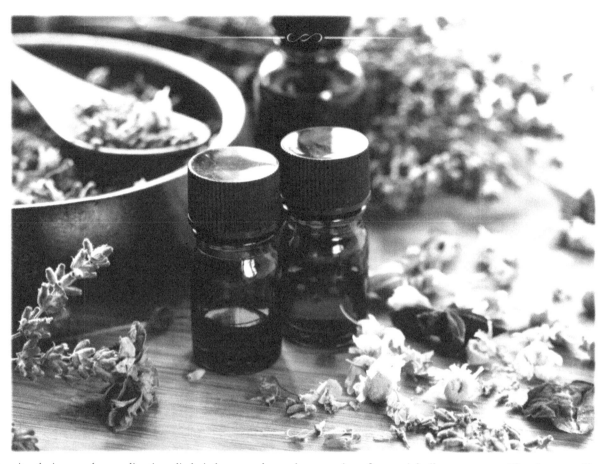

Despite their popular application, little is known about the capacity of essential oils to cure specific ailments. Here's a look at the research supporting the use of essential oils and aromatherapy to treat some of the most prevalent health problems.

Stress And Anxiety

It's expected that 43% of persons with stress and anxiety use unusual therapy to help them cope with their symptoms. Initial aromatherapy research has been fairly positive. Many studies have shown that the aroma of certain essential oils may help cure stress and anxiety in addition to regular therapy. Unfortunately, due to the fragrances of the chemicals, blinded trials are difficult to conduct, and biases are difficult to rule out. As a result, numerous studies on herbal oils' stress and anxiety-relieving properties have come up short. Using essential oils during a rubbing and massage, for example, may help ease stress, albeit the special effects may only persist for the duration of the session. Aromatherapy was also found to be effective in the treatment of anxiety.

To Kill Bacteria

Native plant extracts kill bacteria and might have served as a useful remedy for the Native Americans. For bacterial infections, white sage, black sage, and sagebrush would be useful medical therapies. In addition, compounds of these essential oils may be valuable in developing new forms of medicinal therapies that could save lives.

Migraines And Headaches

In two small studies conducted in the 1990s, it was observed that applying an ethanol mixture and peppermint oil to the foreheads and temples relieved headache discomfort. Recent research has also discovered that applying lavender oil and peppermint to the skin relieves headache pain.

Additionally, it has been suggested that headaches and migraines can be treated with a blend of chamomile and sesame oil applied to the temples. This is a traditional Persian headache remedy. More high-quality research is, however, required.

Sleep Or Insomnia

Lavender oil has been demonstrated to improve sleep quality in women after delivery and heart disease patients. An analysis of fifteen studies on essential oils and sleep looked at the findings. The majority of research found that inhaling the oils, particularly lavender oil, improved sleep habits.

Reducing Inflammation

Essential oils are recommended as a possible aid in the fight against inflammatory disorders. According to some test-tube research, they have anti-inflammatory properties. In one mouse trial, consuming a mixture of oregano and thyme essential oils helped induce colitis remission. Caraway and rosemary oils produced similar benefits in two rat experiments. However, the effects of these oils on inflammatory ailments have been studied in only a few human trials. As a result, their efficacy and safety are unidentified.

Antibiotics And Antimicrobials

The emergence of antibiotic-resistant germs has reignited interest in finding new ways to combat bacterial illnesses. Tea tree and peppermint essential oils have been studied comprehensively in test tubes for their antibacterial effects, with some promising results. While the outcomes of these test-tube studies are intriguing, they do not always reflect the impact of these oils on your body. For example, they don't show that a specificessential oil can treat microbial infections in people. Essential oils may provide a variety of health benefits. However, a further human study is required.

Use As A Pesticide

Essential oils can act as a natural insecticide. Certain oils have been demonstrated to have a range of deterrent effects on pests, notably insects and certain arthropods, in case studies. Pests that ingest the oil may be repulsed, have their digestion slowed, have their growth stunted, have their reproduction rate slowed, or die due to these consequences. The chemicals in the essential oils that induce these effects, on the other hand, are typically non-toxic to animals. Because of the unique reactions of the chemicals, these green pesticides can be used widely without causing harm to anything but pests. Rose, lavender, thyme, lemongrass, eucalyptus, and peppermint, are some of the essential oils that have been studied. Essential oils offer the potential for agricultural, urban pest control, or indoor plant protection and marketed insect repellents and bug spray, even if they aren't a perfect replacement for all synthetic pesticides. Some essential oils have been found in trials as efficient as, if not more effective than, DEET, the most potent insect repellent now on the market. Although essential oils are efficient as insecticides when applied topically, such as a mosquito repellant, they are only effective when vaporized. Polymers and cream combinations are utilized to extend the vapor phase of effective repellent because this stage is relatively short-lived. Using essential oils as green—pesticides instead of synthetic insecticides - has environmental benefits in any form, including reduced residual activities. Furthermore, as the essential oil market expands and popularity grows among organic produced farmers and ecologically conscious consumers, expanded usage of essential oils as pest management could have ecological and economic benefits.

CHAPTER 41:

USING ESSENTIAL OILS

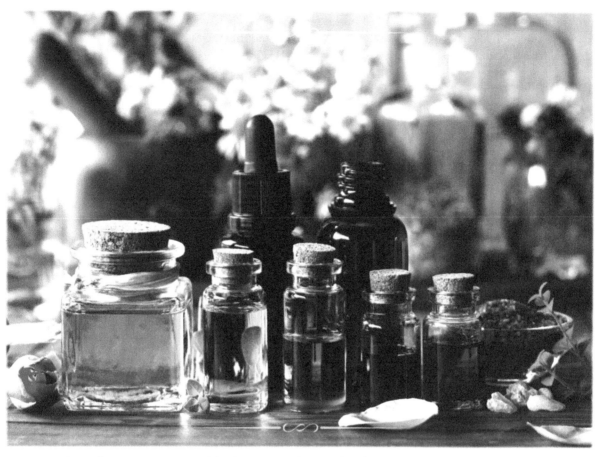

There are a variety of ways to use essential oils. You might even be able to come up with a few on your own.

Just remember to be alert for signs of sensitivity whenever introducing a new oil to your regimen. And, of course, avoid consuming the oils!

Use a method of administration that works for your situation:

1. **Inhale the scent directly.** This is the easiest way to get started. Place a couple of drops of essential oil on a tissue or paper towel. Hold the tissue close to your face and inhale through your nose.
2. **Bath.** Just 5 drops in one ounce of carrier oil, such as almond oil, can be added to your bathwater. Ensure that you're choosing an appropriate essential oil.
3. **Inhale via steam.** Boil two cups of water and then transfer the water to a bowl. Add approximately five drops of essential oil to the water. Keep the bowl close to you and enjoy the scent. Stop if you experience any discomfort.
4. **The room method.** Follow the previous method, but use 10 drops of essential oil. Place the bowl near the center of the room.
5. **Massage.** Add 10–20 drops of essential oil to 1/8 cup of carrier oil. Almond or jojoba oil are acceptable carrier oils. Ideally, have a partner massage the oil into your skin. Keep away from the eyes and mucous membranes.

Try all the different methods and see which works the best for you.

There's no method that is universally superior to another. Keep an open mind and experiment. You'll likely find one method that you prefer over the others.

Diluting Oils

Essential oils are very powerful. They can make breathing easier, relieve pain, and even combat cancer. You'll want to dilute them in some kind of carrier oil before applying them to your skin in order to provide a barrier between the delicate membranes of your body and the potent oils.

We are often asked, "How much oil should I put in my blend?" As a general guideline, we recommend using 1 to 2 teaspoons of essential oil per 10 ml of the carrier. Keep in mind that this is only a guideline, and some oils can be used at higher concentrations.

Topical Use

Oils can be rubbed or massaged into the skin or into clothing. They can also be dispensed through a dropper, but that is more difficult.

For external use only—not for ingestion! Do not use essential oils directly to your eyes. If you are allergic to any of the oils, do not use them topically. Essential oils are very concentrated, and if you apply too much, they could burn your skin or cause an adverse reaction.

When using essential oils on the skin, always dilute the oil before applying it. The easiest way to do this is to place your carrier oil in a bowl and slowly add the essential oil, making sure it is well mixed before adding more—this will prevent clumping of the carrier oil at the bottom of the bowl. The preferred method by most people is to add about 10 drops of essential oil to 1/4 cup (60 ml) of a good quality carrier oil.

Diffusion

The aroma of an oil blend will be affected by the amount of air that comes into contact with the oils. Some oils diffuse very easily, and some can take hours or even days to fully release their fragrance. It's best to keep your blends in a glass bottle or a stainless steel atomizer to prevent evaporation.

We recommend that you perform your blends in a well-ventilated space if possible. You'll want to work with a fan or an oscillating fan going at high speed. If you don't have a fan, set your burner on low, but never leave your home without ventilation.

Bottles of spice oils are very effective for diffusion, and they come in small bottles that can easily be tucked into a handbag. The oils will dissolve and disperse into the air, and people around you will breathe in the therapeutic benefits of the essential oils that you've blended.

Inhalation

The aromatic benefits of the oils are most effectively absorbed through the mucous membranes of the sinuses. Simply inhale the aroma of your blend for a minute or two, and you should feel some immediate benefits. If you feel light-headed, stop immediately and take deep, even breaths until you feel better.

For children, place a few drops on a tissue and let them breathe in slowly to smell the fragrance.

Inhaling oils can be very relaxing, and many people like to add 1 or 2 drops to a hot bath before getting in for 20 minutes. This is an excellent way to benefit from essential oils while soaking in a tub of hot, soothing water.

Internal Use

Before ingesting essential oils for internal usage, they must be diluted in a carrier oil. Follow this ratio for internal use:

3 drops of essential oil per teaspoon (5 ml) of carrier oil.

Essential oils should never be swallowed undiluted. Keep out of the reach of children and pets.

Shake well before each use to disperse the natural essential oils that might have settled on the bottom of the container. Avoid heat, light, and air as much as possible to preserve your essence.

Makes 24 capsules with 100 mg each:

- Put the gelatin capsules in a bowl of hot water for 5 minutes to soften them. Once they are soft, drain the water out of the bowl. You can use a small funnel to pour in the contents of your bottle if you would prefer not to shake all the oil out.
- Gently shake out as much of the carrier oil as possible without shortening the life of your capsules by breaking them open and spilling their contents into the gelatin capsules.
- Add the drops of essential oils, be sure to shake the bottle first, and fill each capsule with your blend.
- Once the capsules have been filled with an even amount of oil on each one, you can use a wet toothpick to scrape away any excess oil from the opening on the top of each capsule. This will help them from sticking together in storage. Cap tightly and place into a cool dark place until ready for use or into a bottle for daily use or into another container of your choice for storage—I like to use old film containers with lids.

You may also create your own roller bottle by using an empty 10 ml glass bottle and a roll-on cover.

Safety Measures Using Essential Oils

Safety tips for internal use

It is usually advised not to ingest essential oils. In fact, the International Federation of Aromatherapists strongly advises that essential oils should not be swallowed.

The reason for this directive is the concentrated nature of the oils. When taken in the absence of adequate supervision, they could damage the internal organs and may even lead to the destruction of the digestive tract. In addition, any food that is ingested is first processed by the liver. In the case of essential oils, the concentrated nature of the product can damage the liver.

Furthermore, metabolism releases the toxicity in essential oils. The prevalence of this toxicity is increased when the product is ingested. It is advised that if you, of necessity, have to use products high in such substances as ethers or phenols, it should be used only in small doses and only for short periods. This will help minimize the risks associated with the ingestion of essential oils.

Generally, for whatever reason, you have to use the essential oils; make sure you do not use them on a daily basis. Because of how dangerous the internal use of essential oils can be—it is actually the most dangerous of the three modes of application—it has been advised that ingestion should only be a last resort. It should only be resorted to when every other form of application has failed or when the situation is very dire. Ingestion should never be done for the fun of it; that is one sure recipe for disaster.

If you have any need to ingest any essential oils, make sure you are under the supervision of a licensed caregiver. Under no circumstance should children who are less than 6 years old be given the oils to ingest. The same also applies to pregnant women.

Safety tips for topical use

If you intend to apply directly on your skin, the most relevant advice is that the product should be diluted. Always make sure you dilute before use.

Also, there may be cases of irritation of the skin from the use of essential oils. This mostly depends on the nature of your skin and may range from mild irritation the first time it is used to actual allergic reactions. Irritation is usually of a temporary nature and is evidenced by itching and redness around the particular area. Usually, it gets resolved after a while as your body gets used to the product, especially if that was your first time ever applying the oils.

Some people also experience phototoxic reactions as well as sensitization. Sensitization is often of a longer period than irritation. Sensitization occurs as a result of the immune system fighting this 'unknown' substance used on the skin. Thus, it may not even be noticed till the second or third time of use of the product.

Some of these cannot be avoided but can be managed when the product is properly diluted before use.

Essential oils usually cause irritation when they have oxidized. Oxidation occurs when the product is exposed to direct sunlight or air. Thus, there is the need to store the product carefully to make sure there is no risk of it oxidizing.

Furthermore, conduct patch testing at every point. To conduct patch testing, rub the oil on an area of your skin for a short while, then look out to notice if you would have any irritation.

You must dilute the product first because it would hardly make sense to conduct patch testing with undiluted oil. The area you rubbed the product should be left dry for a period, maybe up to 24 hours.

Some of the properties of the oils make it are more likely to be more irritating than others. This irritation may occur immediately after the product is first used, or in some cases, it could occur as the product is used over a period of time. These kinds of oils are best used in their diffused state i.e., it would be ideal to use them as sprays, etc. But even this could result in irritation of the mucus membrane, thus it is advisable to always look for alternatives if this is the situation that you are in. If it isn't possible to find an alternative, then apply such oils sparingly. Also, make sure that if you are to use them on your skin that they are diluted more than you would any other ordinary essential oil.

General Safety Precautions

1. Storage: Essential oils are famous for being volatile. They can be damaged when exposed to heat or sunlight or any other adverse conditions. Ideally, essential oils come in opaque containers to prevent the penetration of sunlight. Always ensure that the cap is securely screwed on your every time you use it. The cap of the bottle should be arranged in such a way as to allow the dispensing of accurate measures of the oil. This is particularly important when you may try to dilute the oils.
2. You should also ensure to keep the product out of the reach of children. If you have a shelf, you may consider placing the bottle at the top of the shelf or cabinet where they would not readily access it.
3. Always read the review of others before purchasing any essential oil. As a matter of fact, this should be done for any product you are purchasing. A quick surf on the internet would tell you what previous users think of that particular essential oils. Also, some specific essential oils have particular precautions associated with them. Do make sure that you research the ingredients used in the production of that specific essential oil to be sure that it has no side effects that would affect you.
4. Use the least possible quantity possible: this is one of those situations where less is more. Make sure that it is only one drop that would bring the desired result, then stick with using just that drop. Resist the temptation of increasing the drops in order to increase the effects, which may be potentially dangerous. Some sales reps may advise that you use any quantity that you desire. It is in their interest when you do so because you would be purchasing more of their products. Find out what quantity works for you and make sure you do not exceed it during any application.
5. If you intend to use the essential oils for aromatherapy, make sure that it is suitable for such: People often make the mistake of thinking that every essential oil can be used for aromatherapy, that is not so. For some products specifically, it should only be qualified aromatherapists who should use them for aromatherapy because they would be more equipped to handle whatever issues that may arise. Examples of such oils include wormwood, wintergreen, rue, and bitter almond.
6. Do not use the same blend you use for yourself on your dog or any other pet: many people may want to share the product with their pets, but it may not be wise to do so. If you must use essential oils on your pet, then make sure you get the right blend for them. Find out from your resident vet which would be suitable for application on them.
7. Essential oils can be quite inflammable, do not put near open flame.

CHAPTER 42:

7 MUST-KNOW ESSENTIAL OIL REMEDIES

Inflammation

Inflammation is the body's way of protecting itself from infection. In some diseases such as arthritis, this defense system triggers an immune response when no threat of infection exists, causing pain and swelling. If essential oils do not bring relief, see your doctor.

Neat basil treatment

Basil essential oil is both an anti-inflammatory and antispasmodic, making it an excellent muscle relaxant. When muscles are tired, inflamed, or cramping, basil essential oil promotes rapid relaxation. If you are sensitive to basil or have sensitive skin, dilute the basil essential oil to as low as 1 part essential oil to 4 parts carrier oil. Massage it into the affected area, then relax comfortably. Taking a hot bath or shower before the application will intensify the effect.

Infection

Swelling, redness, pain, heat, and the presence of pus are among the most prominent infection symptoms. Small, localized infections typically respond well to treatment with essential oils; systemic infections or large infected wounds are considered medical emergencies and require a doctor's intervention.

Neat clove treatment

Clove essential oil is a powerful antibacterial, antiviral, and antifungal agent. Besides addressing the infection, it numbs the pain. Use the smallest amount of clove essential oil possible to treat each infection, and apply it neatly. Dilute clove essential oil with an equivalent quantity of carrier oil if you have sensitive skin.

Insomnia

Insomnia is characterized by trouble sleeping or staying asleep. Some sufferers often wake up during the night and have difficulty going back to sleep. Some have trouble falling asleep even though they are tired, and some wake up early in the morning and can't get back to sleep. Almost all insomnia sufferers are chronically exhausted. If your insomnia does not respond to natural treatments, visit your doctor to rule out an underlying medical condition.

Neroli-spikenard bedtime massage
Makes 12 treatments

Both neroli and spikenard essential oils have strong sedative properties and are ideal for inclusion in bedtime routines, particularly for those who have a tough time falling or staying asleep. For extra benefits from this treatment, be sure that your bedroom is quiet and dark; watching TV or using electronics right before bed can disrupt sleep.

Ingredients:

- 3 ounces carrier oil
- 24 drops neroli essential oil
- 12 drops spikenard essential oil

Instructions:

1. In a dark-colored glass bottle, add the carrier oil along with the neroli and spikenard essential oils, and shake well to blend.

2. Using your fingertips, apply 1 tablespoon of the blend to the body just before getting into bed.

3. Repeat this treatment once a day at bedtime until normal sleeping patterns resume.

Acne

Acne may be mild, moderate, or severe; in all cases, it is caused by sensitivity to androgenic hormones, which are primarily produced during the teenage years. This sensitivity, coupled with the presence of bacteria, dirt, and oil on and beneath the skin, produces blackheads, whiteheads, cysts, bumps, and nodules. Seek medical treatment if acne fails to respond to natural remedies.

Geranium spa facial mask
Makes 1 generous treatment

Geranium essential oil combines with spa facial clay, yogurt, and honey to soothe the inflammation that accompanies acne.

Ingredients:

- 1 tablespoon honey
- 1 tablespoon plain yogurt
- 1 tablespoon spa facial clay
- 6 drops geranium essential oil

Instructions:

1. In a small glass bowl, add the honey, yogurt, clay, and geranium essential oil, and stir to combine.

2. After cleansing the affected areas, use your fingertips to apply the mixture, avoiding the eye area.

3. Leave the mask in place for up to 1 hour, then rinse it off with warm water.

4. Repeat this treatment every 2 to 3 days until symptoms subside.

Bronchitis
Bronchitis is an inflammatory respiratory illness that affects the respiratory system, causing inflamed bronchial tubes, excess mucus production, and coughing. Acute bronchitis is often caused by a virus and may occur in conjunction with an upper respiratory tract illness such as a cold or the flu. It can also occur due to the aspiration of liquid or food into the lungs or following exposure to irritants such as heavy smoke. Cases of acute bronchitis typically last two to three weeks. See your doctor if symptoms do not respond to treatment, as bronchitis symptoms can be an indicator of a more serious underlying disease.

Diffuse eucalyptus
Eucalyptus essential oil helps open constricted airways and ease coughing. If you do not have a diffuser, the eucalyptus scent can be inhaled directly from the bottle or used in an aromatherapy pendant, or a few drops can be added to bathwater. If eucalyptus essential oil is not available, you may substitute rosemary essential oil, which also eases bronchitis symptoms. Diffuse eucalyptus essential oil in the area where the sufferer is spending the most time.

Eucalyptus-lavender rub
Makes 12 treatments

Lavender, eucalyptus, and tea tree essential oils have antibacterial and antiviral properties that help prevent bronchitis from getting worse. They also soothe inflamed airways. Rosemary essential oil can be substituted for eucalyptus essential oil if desired.

Ingredients:

- 2 ounces carrier oil
- 20 drops eucalyptus essential oil
- 20 drops lavender essential oil
- 20 drops tea tree essential oil

Instructions:

1. In a dark-colored glass bottle, add the carrier oil along with the eucalyptus, lavender, and tea tree essential oils, and mix well to combine.

2. Using your fingertips, apply about 1 teaspoon of the blend over the chest area, and massage it into the skin before relaxing.

3. Repeat this therapy up to 4 times a day until symptoms subside.

This humble and inexpensive extract is so effective against bacteria and viruses that it, and a derivative called eucalyptol, are used extensively in modern medicine. You'll find it in many OTC remedies, including cough drops, mouthwashes, and antifungal body powders.

Canker Sore

Canker sores are small ulcers of the mouth. They are usually round and are typically gray to white in color with red borders. They are often accompanied by tingling, burning, and soreness. Most respond well to natural treatments with essential oils and often heal within three to seven days. If sores are persistent, large, or numerous, or if they are accompanied by swollen lymph nodes, a fever, or physical sluggishness, be sure to see your doctor, as they could be symptomatic of an underlying disease.

Neat clove treatment

Clove essential oil stops the pain and itching that accompany canker sores, and it is a strong antiseptic that promotes healing. Using a cotton swab, apply 1 drop of clove essential oil to the canker sore 3 times a day. If you are sensitive to the essential oil, do not apply clove oil neat; instead, dilute it with a small amount, up to half with a carrier oil, or add 1 drop to 1 tablespoon or more of water and use it as a mouth rinse.

CONCLUSION

Herbal medicine is the central focus of complementary and holistic medicine, which has acquired growing popularity across the globe in recent years and is steadily streaming towards integration into the established healthcare systems. Herbalists prefer to use extracts from sections of plants, such as the leaves or roots, assuming that plants are sensitive to natural stresses and therefore establish tolerance to hazards such as reactive oxygen species, microbial attack, and radiations, offering protective phytochemicals for use in herbalism.

The medicinal and herbal wisdom of the Native Americans has been overlooked by history for so long. This book aims to introduce their medicinal experience and deep knowledge of natural supplements back to life.

With this book on the shelves, you have at your hands a proud tradition of herbal craftsmanship and herbal culture. Medicinal plants are a good way to get the good stuff out of the ground and into your body. Medicinal plants can help with everything from relieving muscle pain to improving brain function. Many medicinal plants can be used to treat various skin conditions. For example, don't forget about the healing and skin-beneficial properties of aloe vera.

Medicinal plants and essential oils are an important part of any natural medicine cabinet. They have been used for centuries by humans to help with ailments and diseases.

After implementing some of the information found in this book, I hope that you will find that anyone can use the healing essential oils and some of the other techniques described in this book, and they can become a regular part of your life.

Live a healthy and fulfilling lifestyle. Be happy and smile a lot. If you feel stressed out, take a deep breath or go stay alone by the sea. Remember, herbs work with nature. Therefore, as you consume them, they rely on your connection with nature to be able to work effectively. Give yourself time to recover and never hurry herbs. You can achieve the ultimate health desire that you want as long as you follow the right instructions, listen to your doctor and pay attention to your body.

All the best to your good health!

BOOK 11

HERB GARDENING
FOR BEGINNERS

Easy Guide to Start Growing Herbs at Home Today

Citali Galwen

INTRODUCTION

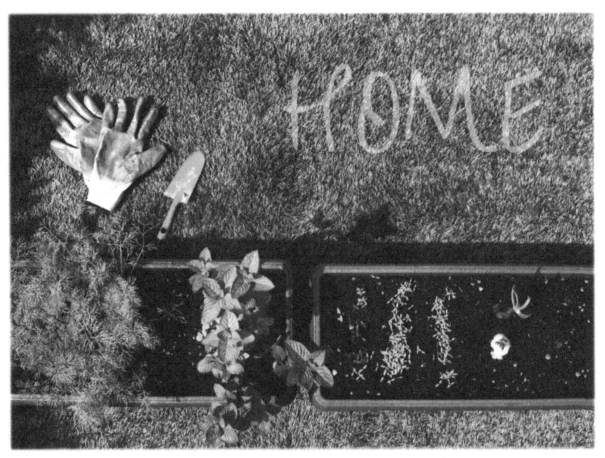

If there is one thing we can learn from our history, it is that plants have always been necessary for human existence and evolution. They have been used as both remedies and food throughout our whole existence, proving the usefulness of the nature that surrounds us. Without them, our evolution would have been completely different. However, natural selection taught us during this time that it would always be better to harvest our crops than to go out into the wild to seek them. Not only because it helped us stay in the safety of our homes and avoided predators, but because it was the only way of making sure we were consuming something completely healthy, instead of a poisonous herb that looked a lot like a harmless one.

y Surely, nowadays, we have come to a point where we don't need to risk our lives for plants, but that doesn't mean we no longer need these plants in our lives. Instead, now we can enjoy the task of growing our gardens, not only for their usefulness but also for their flavor and beauty. We still need plants to survive as a race, but now they can help us improve additional aspects of ourselves.

The times are changing. Humans have gone past the stage of history where we need to seek our survival at all costs. We have built a safe community around us, securing safety and long life for most of us. With these changes, there comes a new revelation. We don't need to own the world. Instead, we can live in a harmonious partnership. Growing your garden not only helps you improve your lifestyle and yourself both physically and mentally, but it also helps the earth. Have you ever wondered what kind of impact you could have on the world? Well, let me tell you, you can do quite a lot.

Maybe you have an unoccupied windowsill in your kitchen or a space in your garden for herbs. Whatever it is, it is plenty of space to start growing your herbs. Don't let the location of your garden, or that ugly corner in your home, hold you back, and we can figure it out together.

I will focus on how to grow herbs in planters and pots, just because it's easier for a beginner and it's convenient for numerous reasons. They are easier to look after, and there is a lesser chance of weeds and critters affecting them.

Moreover, if you would like to grow them outside, pots are an amazing solution, either for your balcony, terrace, or whatever outside space you have to place them.

But then there are a few aspects you need to consider if you would like them to flourish well. Learn the basics, and you are sure to get a green thumb soon. So here comes this easy-to-follow guide about how to go about it all year round for annual and perennial herbs.

CHAPTER 43:

SIMPLY HERBS

This is a beginner guide, so let's start from the beginning. The first thing is that you should have a clear idea about why you should consider growing plants. Well, if you are reading this, you probably already know what herbs are, but let's have a little brush-up anyway in case you have any small gaps.

So, what are herbs? In the culinary arts, the term 'herb' refers to any green or leafy part of a plant that can be used for your medical remedies, season your dish or flavor a recipe, and other amazing things such as essential oils, pomades, and so on.

You may be wondering if herbs are used to flavor or season a dish without it being the main ingredient; aren't they the same thing as spices? Well, that's a very valid question, and the truth is that no, they are not the same. Their difference lies in the part of the plant they come from. In fact, spices are made from plant parts such as roots, seeds, twigs, dried bark, and more. For example, cinnamon is the bark of a tree, and cloves are dried flower buds. Notice that spices are often used in dried form, while herbs can be used both dried and fresh.

So, why should you grow herbs at home? As we have already established, growing your garden at home can be physically and mentally beneficial for you. It can turn into a beautiful, healthy hobby that you can teach the people around you to help them improve their lifestyles. It is something on which you can focus your mind, and it can bring you closer to nature and the many possibilities it offers you. Expert growers assure that herbs are hands down the easiest plants to grow. Also, they simply look beautiful. Don't they? They can turn your garden or your empty home spaces into a piece of work art with their wonderful colors.

In conclusion, herbs are not only an amazing addition to your cooking, but they also have great health benefits that can help you live a healthier life, not to mention the great psychological effect an indoor garden like this can have on you, being able to visualize and appreciate the product of your hard work, right at your fingertips. Other members of your family and your friends can see them too, and they can learn from your experience.

We will continue to list out the benefits an indoor herb garden can offer you, but as of now, we hope you can see the wonders these little plants can give us beyond their rich flavors and fragrances. So how about starting a new hobby today? One that can help you improve your life, both mentally and physically!

CHAPTER 44:

ANNUAL AND PERENNIAL HERBS

You should first differentiate between annual and perennial herbs before proceeding with the rest of the information.

First of all, annual herbs germinate, bloom, produce, seed, and complete their life cycle within a year, no matter the season. These herbs have a shorter lifespan than perennials. An excellent example of an annual herb is parsley, which grows and goes quickly. On the other hand, perennials can live for several years and flower or yield fruit year after year. Regular harvesting is essential for these herbs to prevent flowering. An example of a perennial herb is rosemary. Secondly, annuals are best grown from seeds, whereas perennials are better off by starting with seedlings from stores or cuttings. The latter type takes a long time to grow from seed and become bigger in size compared to annuals. Furthermore, most of them get wilted or go dormant during the winter month. However, they come back from the root, and therefore you wouldn't have to regrow them.

With the knowledge you gained about annuals and perennials, you now need to take on the next phase of our gardening journey, wherein you need to decide which herbs to grow. For this, you need to consider the purpose for which you will be using the herbs. Is it for medicinal purposes, or is it for culinary purposes, or is it for attracting beneficial insects to your outdoor garden? If you are utilizing herbs for culinary purposes, you should grow those you would be using every day. Gardening for freshness and flavor is indeed exciting.

Sure, if you are here, your purpose is clearly for medical usage, but if you have read the previous pages carefully, you will certainly have understood that I consider food to be the first medicine we ingest on a daily basis. So here we are, the culinary purpose merging with the medical one.

Whatever the purpose is, if herbs are given the correct soil, adequate sun exposure, and an apt amount of water, they flourish. Most herbs need direct sunshine to thrive indoors, so giving them a sunny, warm place is a priority. Sunny window sills, patios, etc., are familiar places where they are usually grown. The next essential ingredient is soil which shouldn't be soggy or saturated. Instead, it should drain well so that the soil is moist. And finally, they should be consistently watered.

CHAPTER 45:

GROWING HERBS AT HOME: FUNDAMENTALS

Sunlight

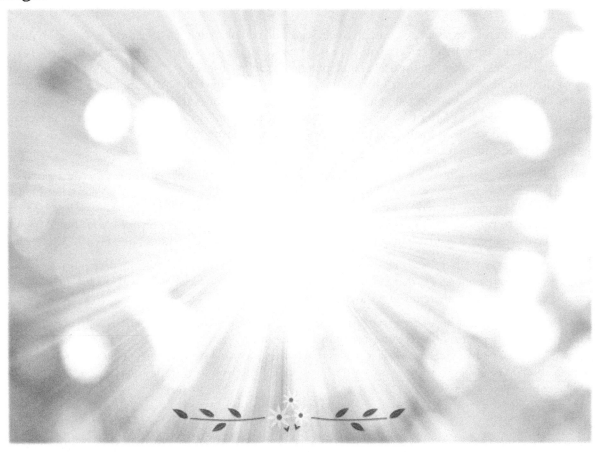

An adequate amount of sunlight ensures enhanced growth for the herbs. Most of the herbs require six to eight hours of sunlight. Place them in those areas where they get the brightest light. For example, most indoor herbs would prefer a south-facing wall to get the optimal amount of sun's heat and light. The more sunlight you can provide to the herbs, the better will be the herbs' flavor. The taste is influenced by the intensity of the light. Those grown in solid sunlight areas will be sure to have the best taste. However, if you are staying in a hot climate, it would be better to keep them in the shaded area during the hottest period of the day.

On the other hand, growth will be slower in winter, during which you should consider investing in grow lights if you live in an area where winters are particularly harsh. They are available at most gardening supply stores. These lights can mimic direct sunlight and are an additional source of the same during the wintertime. The ideal temperature from these lights would be 18 to 21 degrees Celsius.

If the plants are not getting adequate light, some of the warning signs would be stems that grow unusually long between the leaf sets and leaves, which are smaller than usual. At times, you will even be able to notice leaves that are yellow and are abnormally pale. If any of these are seen, change their location immediately.

Grow lights
Sometimes it may be necessary to invest in grow lights in order to provide your indoor herbs with enough light and heat., especially when you don't have places that provide full sunlight throughout the day.

Grow lights can aid you in cultivating those herbs for which you have set your mind by providing sufficient light and heat at any time of the year. They are considered a substitute for natural light while providing the proper conditions for photosynthesis and a color spectrum where the plants will thrive and flourish.

Most of the grow lights are LED as they are more efficient while providing the right amount of light without causing as much heat as fluorescent lights. Based on the herbs you have chosen, your budget, and the light conditions of your home, you can choose between various types of grow lights. One of the most popular ones is the clips-on grow lights that you can clip onto the edge of tables or desks. Or else, you can select grow lighting fixtures that can provide light and heat for multiple plants evenly at the same time, though they tend to be on the expensive side. Based on your consideration, you can choose the right one for you.

Choosing Containers

You may use any container for growing herbs as long as it has enough drainage and is not too large. Plastic pots, clay pots, unglazed ceramic pots, and even terracotta pots are all acceptable options. Each kind of pot has its advantages and disadvantages.

For example, ceramic pots will hold in more water, whereas clay pots will dry up faster. On the other hand, terracotta pots are the popular choice as they are permeable, allowing water and air to flow easily. This feature is beneficial since it helps avoid root rot, which happens when there isn't sufficient air and ventilation available for the plant roots. One crucial step you need to undertake before using terracotta pots is to be soaked in water overnight and then dry for 20 minutes before planting. This safeguards the moisture. In the soil, it supports the moisture from the plants. If you grow Mediterranean herbs like rosemary or thyme, then a clay pot would be a better choice as they like to be watered well and allowed to dry in between.

Likewise, you can choose any size, but it is always better when you match the container size to the size of the full-grown plant you are growing. A good rule to follow here would be to choose a pot or planter that is at least one-third tall as a whole grown plant and about half to three-fourths of its width. If the container is too big, the herbs will concentrate more on growing their roots, and it will be more challenging for the sail to be evenly moist. On the other hand, if the planter is small, the herbs will be root-bound because of the cramped space. This, in turn, will affect their growth and nutrition, which can ultimately kill them off.

As herbs do not have large roots, they can be grown even in small containers. The smaller the containers, the lesser the soil there is. Consequently, there is a smaller margin of error with too much or too little water. But then, you will have to report soon if they are too small. For example, even mason jars can be used for growing herbs. They would be too good to look out for, but they might not seem an apt option in the long run. Self-watering containers are another option. Herbs requiring constant moisture levels such as chives, parsley, marjoram, and mint are good candidates for these containers. Furthermore, you wouldn't have to worry more about whether you are watering it more or less.

To understand whether the container's drainage is suitable or not, you can check by pouring water into it before adding soil to it and observing how fast or slow the water drains from the bottom. If the water is draining little by little, you can add a layer of pebbles so that the herb's roots are not standing in water,

Fertilizers

Most of the herbs do not require much fertilizer. Adding fertilizer once or twice wouldn't hurt, though, as it supplements the feeding when the herbs are confined indoors. Perfect for indoor herbs, fish emulsion is one of the standard fertilizers on the market. Or else you can go for seafood extract. Both these fertilizers have a higher nitrogen content in them, leading to an increase in the growth of leaves. This fertilizer application can be made once a week in summer or once a month during winter.

Sometimes, you may see a white residue around the rim of the pot in the long run. This is the result of the fertilizer accumulation and the residue left over from the use of tap water. If this is left as it is, it will cause a problem for the herbs gradually. You can take one measure to place the pot over the sink and thoroughly water it until the water runs from the pot's bottom portion. It would help ensure that water had been drained off well before keeping it back in the same position. Do the above procedure every three to four months to prevent the scenario mentioned above.

Soil

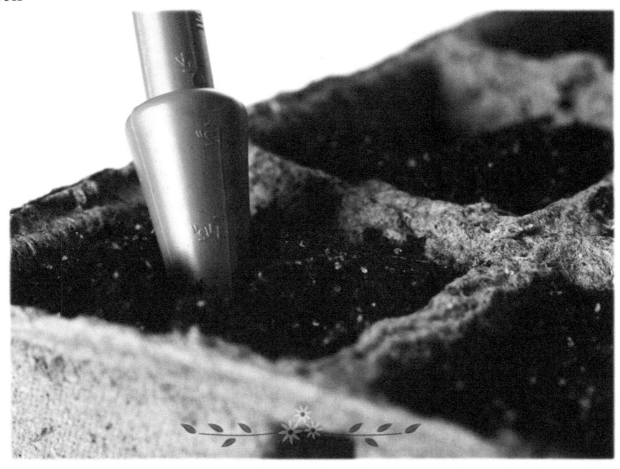

Along with suitable containers, another essential ingredient for the herbs to grow well is a high-quality potting mix. A good quality potting mix has the capacity to efficiently ventilate the air and drain the water. Both the soil and container can prevent accidental drowning of the herbs.

There are potting mixes and potting soil available in the market. Potting soil is coarser, unlike the potting mix, which is lighter and contains compounds like perlite that act as an aerator. For indoor herbs, the potting mix would be the better choice.

Once you have the soil, digging them up with a fork would be the first step as it would allow the water to drain well and make space for the roots to go down into the soil. You can even add compost to the topmost layer, which makes drainage easier while being a fertilizer. Work this layer of the soil to the top portion before planting. Instead of compost, you can also use coarse sand. Coconut coir is another element that can be added to keep the soil moist. Alongside, the coir can improve the drainage and aeration capacity of the soli.

Furthermore, its pH is neutral, and plants prefer this kind of soil because it allows them to absorb nutrients more effectively. Taking outdoor soil for the indoor plant is considered as unfavorable as its drainage properties would change. On top of that, as it is riot sterilized, it can introduce pests and larvae into the herbs.

For most of the herbs, while potting them, they require at least this much space.

- 3-4 feet - Rosemary, Sage, Mints, Oregano, Marjoram
- 2 feet - Basil, Thyme, Tarragon, Savory
- 1 foot - Cilantro, Chives, Dill, Parsley

Watering

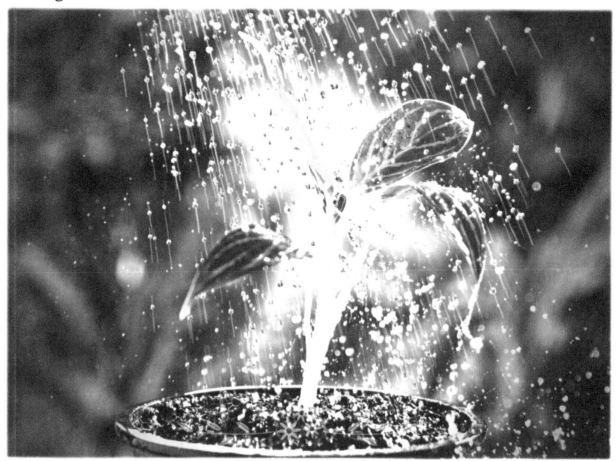

Watering the plant properly and regularly is critical since it directly affects the plant's overall health.

Before watering, you need to make sure the plants need water. Place one of your fingers into the container and stick it down till your second knuckle tests the container moisture. If the soil surface appears dry to your fingertips, then you need to water it. Most of the time, you will need to water around an inch of water approximately every week for the growing season once the transplanted plant is established. Moisture levels can change rapidly across the day as the container may seem moist in the morning and become dry by mid-afternoon. Therefore, check on them often. Overwatering can cause it to rot quickly or lead to poor growing conditions. Overwatering is often more problematic for herbs than under-watering.

Similarly, we need to make sure that you are watering it deeply and slowly. When you water the plants, you should see water running from the containers' drainage holes. If you don't see this, it means that you have not watered sufficiently. Deeply watering helps with the development of a strong root system and the provision of greater nutrients to the plant. The surface soil may seem dry at the top portion, whereas it will be moist in the lower sections. Hurriedly watering the plants can result in the water running fast through the pot and coming out of the drainage holes without providing the soli with a chance to absorb it.

According to one of the studies published in Horticulture Magazine, it was found that watering plants in the morning makes the plants more receptive to it than watering them in the afternoon. The reason is that morning watering can provide sufficient moisture to the plant that lasts throughout the day, and there is less evaporation caused by wind and heat, which allows the plants to dry out only by night. Conversely, when you water during the evening, the plants don't get enough time to dry out by night. Wet foliage can cause diseases from fungi like mildew etc.

Another point to reflect on is that you should be watering only the soil rather than the foliage, as it might quickly cause the plants to become susceptible to -fungal diseases. If the leaves have begun to wilt or turn yellow, reduce the amount of watering.

Transplant Herbs

When you buy starter plants from nurseries, make sure to move them to bigger pots within 7 to 14 days so that they have sufficient space to grow. When the plants are to be shifted, the soil should be moist. The soil should clump together when held together rather than having water dripping from it.

Harvesting

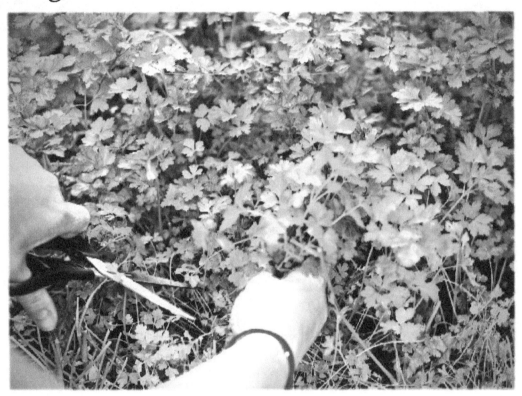

The rule of thumb is to snip and pinch back as necessary. It encourages the herbs to branch and fills out when you harvest consistently, improving your overall harvest. When done correctly, it prepares the plant for new growth. Consider harvesting based on your growth pattern and avoid cutting more than one-third of the plant during the growing season. When more than one-third is cut, the plant will take a more extended period to recuperate and produce new ones.

Snip the plant's leaves from the top to flourish by branching out while getting bushier at the bottom. Similarly, cut close to the leaf intersection so that they can regrow quickly. When you pinch them from the bottom, there is a chance for the base to become like the tree's trunk. You can snip items out either by using kitchen shears or with your hand. When you snip the herbs, it also prevents the herbs from becoming leggy.

Try to harvest during the early morning and, if possible, harvest before they bloom if possible.

CHAPTER 46:

HOW TO PLANT HERBS IN A CONTAINER

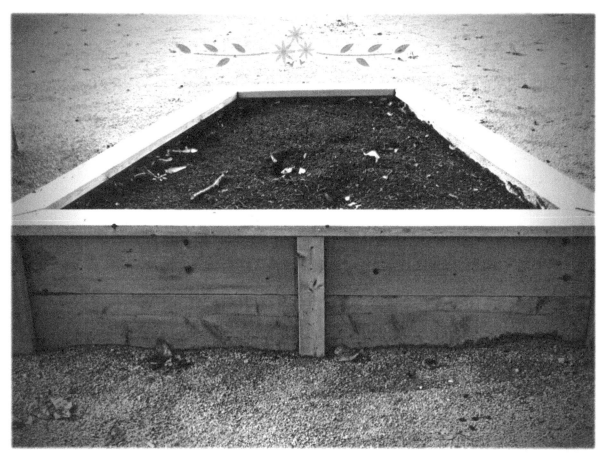

Check that the container is big enough for your situation and needs.

Then fill it with potting soil mix and dig it well with a fork. Now, pour water into the mixture until the soil seems damp down. Next, dig the exact place where you need to place the plant. The hole's size should be roughly twice the width of the root ball of the plants to be held in it. Release the plants from the starter bag by turning them upside down and tapping them gently from the bottom. Gently pull until it comes out of the container. Then, place the plant in the hole you dug and press the soil gently around it to fill. Water the plant immediately. Place the pots or containers in a saucer or a plastic protector to protect the surface underneath.

The best time to plant a new one would be during the morning or late in the afternoon, as it will prevent the transplanted plant from wilting in the midday sun. You can use either seeds or cuttings. Cuttings are branches of an existing plant cut at the node and soaked in water until new roots appear. When you notice the perennial herbs are growing well, you can dig them up with a fork and pull the roots apart by hand or divide the root mass into several pieces. Once you see the roots appearing out of the holes, it is time for the plant to be replanted as the growth will otherwise become stalled or flop over. Make sure you do not overcrowd them while planting them.

Once the plant flowers and becomes a seed, the seasonal growth cycle for that herb is done, it will no longer put out new growth.

Pests To Look Out For

Pests must be checked on a regular basis. Aphids, spider mites, and scales are some of the common ones you can find in herbs. Aphids and scales make sticky drops alongside the plant, whereas spider mites make a web between the leaves.

As soon as you detect them, wash the plant with insecticidal soapy water to remove them off the plant.

CHAPTER 47:

TIPS FOR GROWING AND MAINTAINING HERBS

1. Having individual containers for each plant would be the perfect scenario. When two different herbs are grown in the same container, you must make sure they have similar requirements. For example, some require more sunlight, whereas some need more water. If they are not identical in their needs, both the herbs' growth would be affected negatively.

2. Do not use regular garden soil for herbs growing in containers as they will not drain well. Potting soil is lighter and porous, whereas garden soil is dense and traps water inside. Furthermore, there will be tiny bugs and parasites in the garden soil that we wouldn't want to bring inside.

3. The root is one of the primary causes of the death of plants. It happens when the roots are standing in water or oversaturated soil for an extended period. The soil should be damp but not wet at all times.

4. Plant perennials on one side and annuals on the other side so you can replant them quickly if you are growing both annual and perennial herbs.

5. The soil in which perennial herbs are grown should be replaced every three to four years. You can stir in a layer of compost around these herbs each time during spring.

6. Ensure that there is good air circulation within your herb garden. If the herbs are kept close to one another, diseases can spread quickly and cause airflow scarcity between them. In contrast, sufficient air circulation encourages the plant to absorb more nutrients and water from the soil without fungus and mild dew setting in. The herb garden must be rotated frequently. The air should never be stagnant around your plants.

7. Your containers should always have a sufficient number of drainage holes. To check the drainage capacity of the containers before planting the herbs, you can fill them with water and observe how fast or slow the water passes through the pot. If you observe that it is slow, you could consider adding pebbles at the bottom so that the water does not submerge the roots, which can cause root rot later.

8. I always recommend keeping saucers or protectors or drain pans under the pots. These are readily available in nurseries to protect the surface where the pots or containers are kept, as it might otherwise cause a mess each time the plant is watered. Choose plastic or rubber ones, as clay ones would let moisture pass through. Also, make sure to drain the saucers when excess water accumulates.

9. Though specific smaller containers might look good and pretty, always consider the total size of the herb you will be growing. If you riot, you will have to repot it again, which can cause unwanted stress for both you and the plant.

10. The herbs can grow well only when they receive proper sunlight. During the winter season, when it is hard to get full sunlight, consider the case of investing in grow lights if required. The amount of sunlight received and the flavor of the herbs is directly proportional. Those herbs which get the most sunlight will be the ones with the most robust flavor.

11. Keep a lookout for signs to ensure that the herbs are growing well. For example, if the plants are not receiving proper sunlight, the most common symptom would be poor growth. Apart from that, if the size of the leaves is smaller or if the sterns are unusually longer between the sets, then insufficient sunlight can be the reason behind them.

12. Transplant the herbs at the right time. Understanding the plant's requirements and providing the same will ensure that all goes well. When you notice roots coming out of drainage holes or when the plants are flopping over, it is the right time to change to a bigger pot. If not, their growth might get stalled.

13. When watering the plant, make sure to water it slowly. If it is done quickly, water will instantly come out of the drainage holes without giving the soil the chance to absorb the water. Slow, thorough watering is the best course while sticking to a routine. Based on the moisture condition of your home, you can come up with a pattern. Based on the state of your herb, you can supplement their growth with fertilizers. Initially, it would be a better option to start with half the required amount. Once noted, you can add more if needed. The herbs would have a more concentrated flavor when fewer fertilizers are used. If the plant seems to be limp and struggling, you can add more fertilizers, whereas if it is a lot of wispy growth, you can reduce it.

14. Always check out whether the herbs are getting affected by drafts and wind through the windows. It can lead to creating dry conditions around the herb, which would be detrimental to their growth.

15. It is not necessary to water your herbs at the same time every day with the same amount of water. You have to water them, considering the moisture condition of the soil and your home temperature. Otherwise,

to confirm if your herbs need water, you can stick your finger to the soil's surface, and if it is starting to dry, then you can water them. Most of the time, you wouldn't have to water the herbs every day. Most of the time, the lower level would be damp. You can also purchase a soil moisture meter, which helps us understand whether you have underwatered or overwatered your herbs.

16. Rotating the pots on all sides can ensure the consistent growth of the herbs as they will naturally gravitate towards the sun normally. If not turned, then the plant will lean towards one direction and can give an uneven shape.

17. Mulching the plants needs to be done when you need to maintain the plant's moisture and discourage the growth of pests. Mulching means covering the open surface with a layer of external growth. The material used for mulching is known as mulch.

18. If you wish to dry the seeds of the herbs from your indoor garden, the best step would be to place them on a dry paper cloth; once it starts drying out, nib them between your palms to remove the dirt. Now return them to the dry cloth and dry them again.

19. If the leaves seem dense, then it means that it is time to harvest.

20. You can also grow herbs in water indoors without soil. With the cuttings that you have of the chosen herb, trim them first into about 6-inches. Next, remove the leaves from the bottom portion and cut the stern at an angle to absorb more water. Now, fill the container with water and place the herb stems in it. Place them in a sunny location and harvest them when each leaf has grown to full size.

21. Trimming the leaves every week can ensure that the plant is growing. When trimming is done, it will keep the flowers from flowering and ensure that the plant grows well.

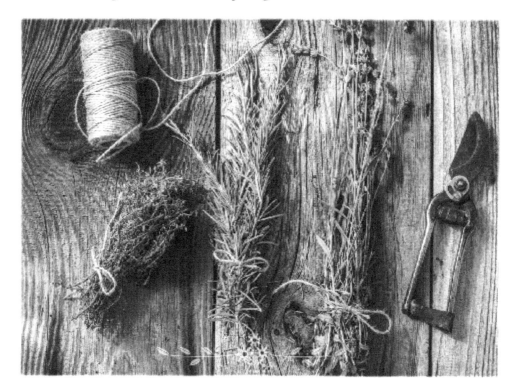

CHAPTER 48:

7 BEST HERBS TO GROW AT HOME

Rosemary

Rosemary is a typical Mediterranean herb that gives an intense fragrance to food. For this reason, the 'upside-down' herb with purple flowers is used in salad, roasted vegetables, and even in tea. Alongside, the stiff and spiky texture of the plant with its needle-like thread leaves gives it a gorgeous appearance and thus imparts a natural charm to the interiors wherever they are placed.

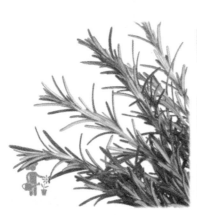

Plant type	**Perennial herb**
Sun expose	**Full sun**
Soil type	**Loam, well-drained**
Soil pH	**Neutral to acidic**
Bloom time	**Summer**
Flower color	**Whiter pale blue**
Mature size when grown indoors	**12-14 n. tall and 6-12 in. wide**

- **Plant Type**: Rosemary is a summer-loving perennial herb.
- **Sunlight**: They prefer excellent conditions with at least 6 to 8 hours of direct sunlight. Therefore, place them near the brightest window of the house as poor sunlight is often cited as one of the main reasons the herb tends to die quickly indoors. When the herbs are brought indoors, make sure they are acclimated to the change in the light as it requires light throughout the day. One good tip would be to place the starter herb on a sunlight diet before being brought inside to function smoothly. Thus, it will get used to four to six hours of indirect sunlight instead of the direct light provided in the former state.
- **Soil:** Sandy or loamy soil is preferred since the water does not sit on the ground. The type of the soil should therefore be gritty and sharply drained. The herb can rot in moist soil since it prefers dry soil, similar to the Mediterranean outdoors.
- **Watering**: Rosemary is a drought-resistant herb. Because of its upside-down structure, it can even receive moisture from the air through its foliage. Therefore, it is always better to make a mistake in underwatering the herb rather than over-watering, which causes many problems, including root rot. The soil should get dried in between the watering but should never be completely dried out.
- **During winter:** the growth will be less and, therefore, would require much less water. Misting the herb is an option to consider then. By observing the color of the leaves, you would understand whether the herb is thriving or not. If leaves are turning yellow, it means insufficient water. Cut the other hand, and if it turns black, the environment is not humid enough for the herb.
- **Humidity and Temperature:** Rosemary is sensitive to powdery mildew as high humidity, and poor air circulation are the main culprits behind this dusty white appearance of the leaves. To avoid this, place it under the fan to improve the air circulation or those areas with open-air circulation like windowsills. Or you can apply a fungicide concerning temperature. It flourishes well at a temperature between 50 to 80° F. Under no conditions should it be placed in bathrooms where there is an excess amount of humidity.
- **Pot or containers**: It requires well-draining terracotta or clay pots with adequate holes at the bottom.
- **Germination:** Rosemary grows well from cuttings. As it is a slow-mowing plant, it takes a long time to germinate from seeds.

- **Harvesting:** Rosemary tastes better before the plant blooms. Usually, the growing season is during spring which continues until the fall period. When used as a culinary treat, it is advisable to use organic fertilizer or compost to enhance soil fertility.
- **Mature size**: the herb can grow to a substantial extent. Therefore, while repotting, decide whether you would want the plant to remain the same size or not. If yes, you would have to root prune in the same pot with fresh soil by 1/31,1 to stunt its growth.

Parsley

An anti-oxidant-packed herb, parsley is much more than a garnish. These bright-green-colored triangular plant leaves can instantly bring out the brightness in any dish. Because there are two types of parsley, curly-leaved and flat-leafed, you should determine which variety to use depending on your needs. Alongside, growing parsley indoors is easy as they do not require much space to produce.

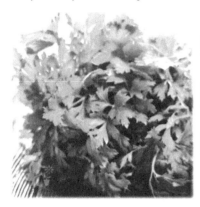

Plant type	**Annual Herb**
Sun exposure	**Full sun**
Soil type	**Moist and well-drained**
Soil pH	**Slightly acidic to neutral**
Bloom time	Summer
Flower color	**White, pale blue**
Mature size when grown indoors	**6 to 12 in. tall and 6-12 in. wide**

- **Plant Type:** Parsley is a biennial herb and needs to be replanted every two years. It is not pruned after the first year; it tastes bitter than the first time.
- **Sunlight**: It prefers full sunlight but can grow in partial shade. In warm places, they benefit from afternoon shade protection. Curing winter, the herb would benefit from wowing under the light.
- **Soil**: It requires rich, slightly damp soil or loam soil but not water-logged. If the soil becomes dry, the parsley will wilt. To boot, the herb wows steadily when the soil is rich in organic matter.
- **Watering**: Water until the soil is moist. Ensure that the soil is never dried out completely as it does not endure drought well and can wilt soon.
- **Humidity and Temperature**: They require steady moisture and can withstand temperatures ranging from 7O to 80 ° F. If it is too hot, providing a bit of shade can help grow.
- **Containers**: Terracotta and clay pots are the best options for parsley as they can wick the excess moisture from the soil.
- **Germination**: as parsley is a slow-growing herb, it takes time to grow from seed. It takes about 14 weeks to harvest them. On the other hand, when grown from seedlings, it takes about six weeks.
- **Harvesting**: Harvest by pinching off from the base intersection as the new ones come from the center. If the older ones are not removed, the new ones wouldn't be able to grow correctly. Do not shave off the top portion of the stem as it affects the plant negatively, and the shoots from the soil level.
- **Mature Size**: Parsley can grow up to 12-inches tall. To encourage growth, gather whole sterns from the bottom of the herb. Once it becomes relatively bushy, you can harvest them. And under no conditions should more than 1/3"1 of the leaves be cut for harvesting as it will hamper the growth clue to the stress from extra pruning.

Thyme

With its anti-bacterial properties, this aromatic, earthy herb gives the best of itself added to vegetable and grain dishes to produce essential oils or make infusions. Furthermore, the shrub appearance and needle-like leaves make it a delight to see it grow indoors. It is relatively easy to grow thyme indoors, especially for beginners, as it is a low-maintenance herb that requires only bare attention.

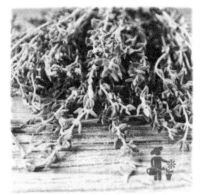

Plant type	**Perennial herb**
Sun exposure	**Full sun**
Soil type	**Sandy, well-drained**
Soil pH	**6.0 – 8.0**
Bloom time	**Summer**
Flower color	**Purple**
Mature size	**6-12 in. tall, 6-12 in. wide**

- **Plant Type**: Thyme is a perennial herb.
- **Sunlight**: Requires full to moderate sunlight for around 7 to 11 hours and is slightly tolerant of shade. The plant prefers those spots wherein they can get full sunlight throughout the day. It is a known sun-lover herb,
- **Soil**: Requires well-draining alkaline soil, which is sandy and on the dry side. The presence of the sand ensures that the water drains quickly without causing any root rot or waterlogging.
- **Watering**: Finding the right watering cadence for thyme is critical. Minimal watering is always better than overwatering for thyme water when the surface is dried.
- **Humidity and Temperature**: the herb grows optimally in temperatures ranging from 50° to 80° F. If possible, avoid growing them in bathrooms as moisture tends to be high in those areas.
- **Pots and Containers**: Thyme grows well when in terracotta or clay pots. It will allow the soil to dry between waterings and avoid wet soil. Similarly, select pots that have a lot of drainage holes.
- **Germination:** It grows best from cuttings and can reach a height of "I 5-inch tall. You can also raise them from seeds, but thyme takes time to wow from seeds.
- **Harvesting**: Once they have grown well, you can harvest them anytime by snipping them off scissors. To encourage new growth, the woody stems must be cut off. Woody sterns usually appear after three to four years when you need to repot them into new pots. Similarly, removing the lowers can also increase the growth of the herb leaves.
- **Mature Size**: Rosemary can wow and spread up to 4 feet tall.

Oregano

This herb was called the "joy of the mountain" by the Greeks. It is used for its spicy, savory, and slightly bitter taste, making it suitable for use in sauces and soup. If you provide the spice with proper sunlight, then this culinary plant grows well indoors.

Plant Type	**Perennial herb**
Sun Exposure	**Full sun**
Soil Type	**Well-drained potting mix**
Soil pH	**6.5 to 7.0**

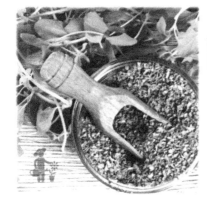

Bloom Time	**Summer**
Flower Color	**Blue, white, pink**
Mature Size	**Two ft. tall, 18 in. wide**

- **Plant Type:** Oregano is a perennial herb and is excessively easy to grow indoors.
- **Sunlight**: Requires full sunlight for at least 6 hours and grows best in sunny and warm places like the south-facing window side.
- **Soil**: They prefer fast-draining ordinary soil, which is mixed with sandy, chalk, or loam soil which is airy and light. This, in turn, aids in increasing the drainage capacity of the soil. No special fertilizer or compost needs to be added for oregano.
- **Watering**: Water when it seems dried out, but don't allow it to dry. Oregano is a drought-resistant herb and therefore thrives well with minimal care. Be careful of overwatering, though, as it can cause numerous problems for oregano.
- **Humidity and Temperature**: the temperature should be around 50 to 80 ° F for this herb to thrive. The plant might take a hit with the dry conditions of winter. Therefore, give them an extra dose of moisture or humidity during the wintertime. It can be completed by placing the pot in a tray filled with pebbles kept mist during winter.
- **Pots and Containers**: Terracotta and clay pots are the best options for oregano as they can wick the excess moisture from the soil. One point to be noted, though, while planting oregano is that the pot should be at least 12 inches in diameter as the growth of this herb is prolific.
- **Germination**: It grows best from cuttings. Cut it out during the summer and root it in water. It grows well from seeds also.
- **Harvesting**: Pinch back the herb regularly once it reaches 4 to 5-feet to keep it compact and blooming. If the flower buds are allowed to flower, the oregano leaves lose their taste and flavor. Similarly, once the plant reaches three to four years of age, its potency will start reducing.
- **Mature Size**: Oregano can grow up to 2 feet tall while spreading up to 18 inches.

Basil

This herb with a distinctive spicy aroma is used in many dishes and infusions with its tiny leaves. It originates from the tropical central regions of Africa and the Southeast of Asia.

Plant Type	**Annual herb**
Sun Exposure	**Full Sun**
Soil Type	**Moist but well-drained**
Soil pH	**Neutral to acidic**
Bloom Time	**Summer. fall**

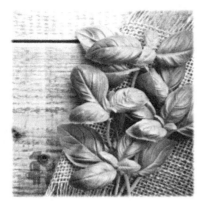

Flower Color	White. pink, purple
Mature Size	12-24 in. tall r 12-24 in. wide

- **Plant Type**: Basil is an annual herb.
- **Sunlight**: It requires full sunlight and heat for about 6 to 8 liars to thrive and flourish. As basil is a sun-lover plant, you can harvest it throughout the year if the place allotted for the herb comes with ample light.
- **Soil**: the herb requires rich, moist, well-drained soil, sand, or loam. It requires richer soil than the other herbs, and therefore, adding compost to your potting mix before planting basil would be an excellent idea.
- **Watering**: the plant requires plenty of moisture to hydrate and plump up its fleshy stems and tender leaves. Once the top portion gets dried, you can water it. You can understand that the plant is less on the water when it wilts and fades down quickly. Water it on, and it will bounce back as it was. Since it requires a bit of humidity to grow, misting the plant occasionally can do good for the herb.
- **Humidity and Temperature**: Since the herb is entirely concerned with the temperature, it doesn't do well in temperatures below 40° F. Basil prefers temperatures of 70° F or higher. As the herb is susceptible to mildew, it must require sufficient airflow, which can prevent the same.
- **Pots and Containers**: Clay and terracotta pots are excellent options to consider. Select those with adequate drainage holes as the herb is highly susceptible to water stress.
- **Germination:** They are best started from seed or seedling. It is effortless to root in water, primarily when they are grown from cuttings. Usually, they take less than six to seven days to germinate from seeds. The lower the temperature, the more time it will take to grow. Since it doesn't last much longer, not more than a few weeks, it is better to plant a new group of seeds every few weeks. And if it is only for culinary purposes, you would only need to grow one or two.
- **Harvesting:** They should be harvested regularly, and their flower buds should be removed but not cut back all the way. If the flower buds are allowed to flower, they lose their taste and flavor. Pinch the tops, as in entire side branches at the intersection, which will yield bigger leaves all summer.
- **Mature Size**: Basil can grow up to 18-inches tall. It needs plenty of air circulation and shouldn't be crowded.

Mint

With an unmistakable fresh and spicy taste and flavor, mint can be added to all kinds of dishes and infusions. It's very easy to grow indoors.

Plant Type	Perennial herb
Mature Size	12-13 in. tall, 113-24 in. wide
Sun Exposure	Full. partial
Soil Type	Loamy, moist, well-drained

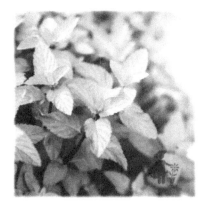

Soil pH	**Acidic, neutral**
Bloom Time	**Summer**
Flower Color	**Purple, pink, white**

- **Plant Type**: Mint is a perennial herb.
- **Sunlight**: They require moderate indirect sunlight and are okay in medium shade. Rotate the plant every few days as it usually leans towards the light, giving it a lopsided shape. The herb prefers a warm and sunny location with 6 to 8 hours of sunlight. If the site is too bright, there is a possibility of the plant getting droopy leaves.
- **Soil**: Rich, moist soil such as sand, clay, chalk, or loam soil would be an excellent choice. Before watering, the soil's surface doesn't need to be dry, as it is with the other herbs. Evade waterlogging of the soil as it can cause root rot.
- **Watering:** the soil should be moist most of the time but should not be soggy. If the soil surface seems dry, water them immediately. Furthermore, drenching them in the morning can also be suitable for the plant.
- **Humidity and Temperature**: the ideal temperature for the herb to thrive would be between 60 to 70 F. Alongside, ensure adequate air circulation for the optimal growth of the herb.
- **Pot and Containers**: It grows intensively fast both indoors and outdoors in unglazed clay pots. As a result, wide and shallow clay pots or planters would be an excellent choice because they will allow the excess moisture to escape.
- **Germination**: Mint grows best from young plants. Spearmint is an excellent option to start.
- **Harvesting**: Pinch out cower buds to encourage proper growth and to avoid the stem becoming leggy. For tastier leaves, pinch off the leaves when the buds are developing as they taste best during that time. Do not trim more than one-third of a plant at this time, as it will hamper the herb's growth.
- **Mature Size**: Mint can grow up to 3-feet tall.

Sage

An evergreen subshrub with wooly textured leaves and sturdy sterns, sage can be grown indoors with little difficulty, provided it receives proper direct sunlight. The herb is also known because its aroma helps to improve concentration.

Plant Type	**Perennial herb**
Sun Exposure	**Full**
Soil Type	**well-drained**

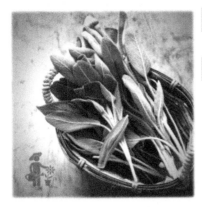

Soil pH	**Acidic, neutral to acidic**
Bloom Time	**Summer**
Flower Color	**Blue, purple, white, pink**
Mature Size	**1 -2 ft. tall, 2-3 It. wide**

- **Plant Type**: Sage is a perennial herb that needs to be replanted every three to four years.
- **Sunlight**: It needs full to moderate sunlight for six to eight hours.
- **Soil**: They require moisture in the soil but should be well-drained and sandy. Clay or loam pots could be an option to consider. It requires dry soil as it is more or less drought-resistant. There is a chance for mildew to appear when the soil is too moist.
- **Watering**: as the herb is drought-resistant, you don't need to water it frequently. When the soil becomes waterlogged, there is an increased choice for root rot.
- **Humidity and Temperatures**: Sage thrives in temperature of 70 F or higher. If possible, look out for those areas wherein you can have sufficient humidity.
- **Pot and Containers**: Clay pots are excellent to grow sage indoors as they can aid in proper drainage.
- **Germination**: They grow best from cutting, as it is hard to emerge from seeds.
- **Harvesting**: Pinching and pruning are necessary to prevent the herb from becoming woody. Therefore, harvest consistently but avoid doing the same during winter and fall to discourage recent growth.
- **Mature Size**: Unlike other herbs, sage's flavor doesn't decrease with flowering. It is more or less throughout the year, but then, the larger it grows, the more will be the flavor.

Chives

Chives is well known for their anti-bacterial and anti-oxidant properties.

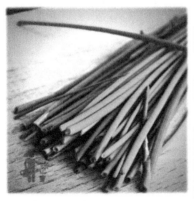

Plant Type	**Perennial herb**
Sun Exposure	**Full sun, light shade**
Soil Type	**Loamy, sandy**
Soil pH	**Slightly acidic to neutral**
Bloom Time	**Early summer**
Mature Size	**10-15 in. tall, similar spread**

- **Plant Type**: Chives is a perennial herb that grows year after year.
- **Sunlight**: for growth, it requires bright light for around 4 to 8 hours. They consistently thrive when the pots are turned periodically.
- **Soil**: Requires rich, moist soil, which needs to be well-watered. Soil can be sand, clay, chalk, or loam.
- **Watering**: the soil should be moist throughout. However, the water shouldn't sit at the bottom of the pot. You can water the herb when the top portion of the soil is dry to touch. The leaves will start turning yellow when the plant is dry.

- **Humidity and Temperature**: the ideal temperature for the herb is between 70 to 80° F. As they require humidity to grow well, misting them can do good. On the other hand, you can place a tray filled with pebbles and water.
- **Pots & containers**: All kinds of pools are suitable for growing chives.
- **Germination**: the herb grows best from the plant rather than seeds. You can cut a portion from an already grown plant. It doesn't take more than two weeks for the plant to germinate when produced from the plant. On the other hand, when grown from seed, it will take at least two months.
- **Harvesting**: Harvest them at the base but not more than 1/3rd at a time. Leave at least 2'inch growth above the soil. Their pots can get overcrowded fast because of the herb's clump-forming habit. Clumps form when the small bulbs multiply below the soil and clump together. Therefore, dividing the clump regularly can ensure proper growth.
- **Mature Size**: Chives can grow up to 10 to 20-inches high. To avoid the plant going to seed, you can cut off the flower. If not, the herb will self-seed freely and come up with new plants.

Cilantro

A delicious addition to spicy food, cilantro is one herb with many uses in the culinary and medicinal fields. Because of its anti-oxidant properties, the plant can reduce the number of free radicals in the body. The herb's green stem and flat leaves are called cilantro, while its seed is known as coriander.

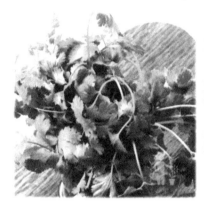

Plant type	**Annual herb**
Sunlight Needed	**Full sun with partial shade**
Soil type	**Loamy, well-drained**
Soil pH	**Neutral**
Bloom time	**Late spring, early summer**
Flower color	**White, light pink**
Matured size	**24 inches tall and 13 inches wide**

- **Plant Type**: Cilantro is an annual plant
- **Sunlight**: Keep the herb in a location where you get 6 hours of full sunlight and then partial shade. It doesn't need much high-noon sunlight as it can cause the leaves to get burned and baited easily.
- **Soil**: Cilantro requires fast-draining, well-drained moist soil. Too much moisture in the soil can make the plant bolt fast. Bolting refers to the process wherein the plant resorts to the reproductive mode when the weather becomes hotter than 65° F and above. When this happens, the leaves become thin and lose taste and flavor. On top, flowers and seed pots start appearing, which affects harvesting.
- **Watering**: when the soil's surface seems to be dry, water it. When the topsoil has lost more than 15% of its moisture, you can water the cilantro.
- **Humidity and Temperature**: the plant grows well when the temperature is between 50 to 80° F. Too much humidity does not go well with cilantro.
- **Pots and Containers**: Cilantro can be easily grown in terracotta pots. These pots help the soil keep moisture while not allowing light to pass through, which prohibits the growth of algae.
- **Germination**: the herb grows better from the large seeds rather than from cuttings. It takes time to germinate, and therefore you need to sow seeds every few weeks. But then you harvest within a month of planting it.
- **Harvesting**: Harvest consistently once it reaches 6-inches tall or within a month. You can snip them by pinching the rear portions of the upper stem, encouraging more growth. When it is not grown correctly, it will produce flowers and seeds instead of leaves. Do not cut more than one-third of the plant at a time.
- **Mature Size**: It needs plenty of space as it grows fast. The plant can reach up to 12 to 20-inches tall once grown.

Dill

With its delicate buttery and lemony flavor, dill's flavor gets accentuated in fish and egg fares, making them more delicious. Furthermore, this herb is full of anti-oxidants. They are used widely while making pickles and sauces. The taste of the spice is a cross between celery and fennel.

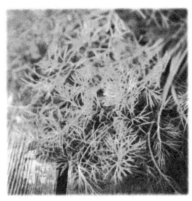

Plant Type	**Perennial herb**
Sun Exposure	**Full sun**
Soil Type	**Rich, well-drained**
Soil pH	**5.6-6.5 (acidic)**
Bloom Time	**Late summer, early fall**
Flower Color	**Yellow**
Mature Size	**3-5 ft. tall, 2-3 ft. wide**

- **Plant Type**: Dill is an annual herb.
- **Sunlight**: They require full sunlight of around 6 to 7 hours for proper growth.
- **Soil**: Soil can be clay, loam, or sand but should be rich, well-moist, and well-drained.
- **Watering**: the soil should be moist throughout and should not be allowed to dry completely. When that happens, the seed can get bolted prematurely.
- **Humidity and Temperature**: the optimal temperature for the plant to thrive is between 50 to 70° F. But then it can also withstand a temperature of less than 25° F.
- **Pots and Containers**: Unglazed terracotta pots are the best ones to grow dill. But then you need to make sure the pots are at least 12-inches deep and 8-inches in diameter, as dill has taproots that help them to anchor into the soil.
- **Germination**: the herb grows best from seed rather than through cutting. Once the taproots are developed, it is better not to disturb the plant by transplanting it. The new plant will be up within two weeks. And if you wish to get a continuous supply of dill, then it is advisable to sow the seeds every three weeks.
- **Harvesting**: You can start harvesting in the second month. Once the flowers are up, the plant concentrates more on seeds and less on producing foliage. Therefore, cutting back on flowers is done to encourage leaf production.
- **Mature Size**: the mature size of the dill plant can be up to 2 to 4 inches.

Fennel

A Mediterranean herb, fennel is best known for its crisp and robust anise flavor and taste and for its effectiveness in treating digestive issues.

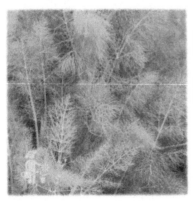

Plant Type	**Perennial herb**
Sun Exposure	**Full sun**
Soil Type	**Rich, moist, well-drained**
Soil pH	**5.5-6.8 (acidic)**
Size	**4-6 feet tall; 18-36 inches wide**

- **Plant Type**: Fennel is a perennial herb, but in those regions where the temperatures go below 15° F, it is grown annually.

- **Sunlight**: Requires full sunlight for at least 6 hours while being okay with partial shade. When the herb doesn't get the required sunlight, the plant can become leggy and woody. Similarly, it requires an adequate amount of air-circulation.
- **Soil**: It requires moist, fertile, and well-drained soil. Adding natural compost to the soil would be an excellent option for the herb to thrive well. Dig them deeply for them to germinate. The potting should never be allowed to dry completely and should remain moist at all times.
- **Watering**: watering can cause more problems for fennel than underwatering. Watering should be done regularly.
- **Harvesting**: You can start harvesting them from the stem when it becomes ripe or about 10-inches tall.
- **Germination:** It is best grown from seed. Fennel is a self-sowing seed plant, and therefore, it thrives on its own every springtime. For the new plant to come out, it will take about 10 to 14 days.
- **Pots and Containers**: You can grow fennel in any kind of container, provided it has an adequate depth and size to fit its roots.
- **Mature Size**: Fennel can reach a mature size of 5-feet tall.

Lemon Grass

With its solid lemony flavor, this tropical herb is best used in teas and soups. Furthermore, they are pretty rejuvenating and are used widely in Asian cuisine because of their calming properties. Because of its fragrance, lemongrass leaves and oil can repel insects, especially pest varieties like mosquitos. Moreover, the herb has anti-bacterial, anti-microbial, and antiseptic properties, which makes it a great natural ingredient to make personal care products such as shampoos and body lotions.

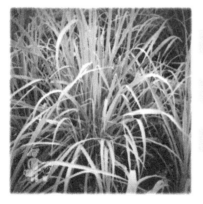

Plant Type	**Perennial herb**
Sun Exposure	**Full sun**
Soil Type	**Rich and loamy**
Soil pH	**Neutral (6.8 – 7.2)**
Bloom Time	**No flowers**
Flower Color	**None**
Mature Size	**2-4 feet**

- **Plant Type**: Lemongrass is a perennial herb
- **Sunlight**: Requires full sunlight for around six hours and prefers a hot sunny climate.
- **Soil**: Grows well in rich, fertile, well-drained loamy soil. Consistent moisture is needed as the roots should never dry out. Do not water more than required as it might lead to waterlogging, which is detrimental to the herb's growth. For the proper development of the herb, it is advisable to add nitrogen fertilizer to it.

- **Watering**: the soil should be moist throughout but should not cause waterlogging. Once the herb has grown, it is considered drought resistant. When the climate becomes too hot, misting it frequently can be an option.
- **Humidity and Temperature**: the plant thrives well when the temperature is between 40 to 70° F. A bit of moisture is okay.
- **Pots and Containers**: Terracotta and clay pots are the best choices for pots. The primary point to be noted, though, is that the pot should be big enough, at least 12-inches deep, so the herb fits in perfectly.
- **Germination:** the herb can be grown from cuttings or seeds, though the former would be better. When growing from seeds, the possibility of getting a fungal disease is high.

- **Harvesting**: Harvest frequently by cutting it off from the soil's surface once the plant has reached 1-foot tall or after two to three months. This will encourage the proper growth of the herb. Since it is a self-propagating herb, it will grow one after the other without much difficulty. Lemongrass comes in dense clumps when it grows well. Many stalks come out of the leading extensive stern base, further divided and replanted in different pots.

CHAPTER 49:

BENEFITS OF GROWING MEDICINAL PLANTS

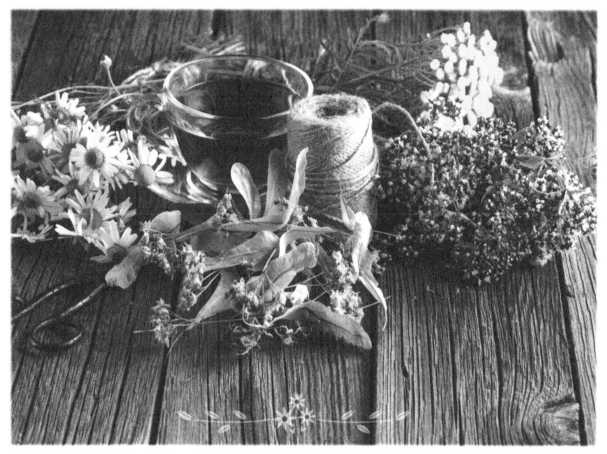

Growing medicinal plants provides numerous benefits to humans, plants, and the environment. The following are some benefits of growing medicinal plants in your garden.

Herbal Medicinal As Foods

As earlier mentioned, most of the plants we have come to depend on for food also have medicinal values. The food part, in some cases, differs from the therapeutic part—for instance, it's often the blackberry root bark that is used for medicinal purposes. But in most cases, it's the edible part of the plants that we consume as food, balancing and toning the body while adding spices to our meals, like peppermint, ginger, fennel, and cayenne, (a common digestive and circulatory system tonic). We ought to integrate such herbs more regularly into our diets and discover their use more formally when the need arises. For example, we could infuse fennel to stimulate appetite, digestion or treat colic.

Herbs Could Be Used To Prepare Other Foods With Medicinal Effects.

During the ancient periods, various herbal plants such as berries, elderflowers, St. John's wort, licorice, wintergreen, ginger, and yarrow were used to flavor and preserve ales and beers. Vegetable oils and vinegar can be infused with herbs such as cayenne, garlic, and rosemary and served on salad and other meals to improve our health. Mead, a fermented drink made from honey, has medicinal values but could also be prepared with herbs like heather to boost its medicinal richness.

Herbs To Boost Insect Diversity

Experienced homesteaders know that managing insects isn't killing them but allowing even more insect diversity, mainly by growing plants flowers all through the growing seasons. Numerous common herbal medicines-such as Echinacea, yarrow, calendula, fennel, peppermint, and chamomile are flowering plants and have the value of providing food and shelter to their beneficiaries. Growing flowering plants and herbs is more effective at boosting our insect allies when integrated with the crops to be protected instead of planting them separately.

Herbs As Fertility Plants

Clever homesteaders are also aware that we can grow more of our soil fertility. Fortunately, a number of the best fertility plants also possess medicinal properties. Comfrey-used for healing broken bones and wounds-and nettle are rich in protein and could be used to "spark" a compost heap or as nutritive mulch. Yellow dock and dandelion are deep-rooted active collectors that mine mineral deposits from the sub-soil and offer them to more shallow-rooted crops.

Herbs As Fodder Crops

A significant variety of medicinal herbs and plants serve two purposes: they provide dry feed for our animals and provide fresh green for us. Yellow duck and dandelion, I discovered, remain green deeper into winter cold than other forage plans. I gather them and feed them to my flocks. Oats could be used to feed livestock and also make an excellent nerve tonic. Either self-harvested or cut and fed green.

CONCLUSION

Having herbs around you, whether inside your home, on your balcony, or in your garden, is a truly refreshing, healthy, and entertaining experience. Gardening has taken center stage in the present-day world across the globe in an unprecedented manner, especially during this pandemic time. Their popularity and reach are increasing with every passing year. The calming and neutralizing effect that one feels when taking care of plants cannot be explained but should be experienced.

I wish you a world of happiness and good luck with your gardening journey!

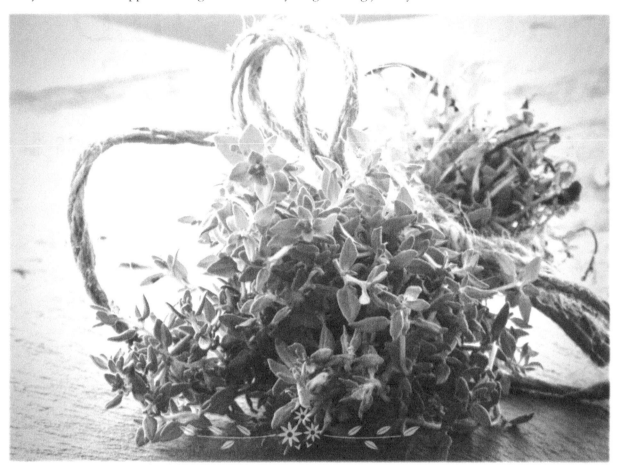

BOOK 12

FORAGING WILD EDIBLE PLANTS

A Beginner's Guide for Organic Wild Foods

Citali Galwen

INTRODUCTION

Foraging and harvesting are a way of life for the Native Americans in the Pacific Northwest. They committed to it because they understood that they had to provide for themselves while respecting nature.

Foraging and harvesting are two of the mainstays of Native American life. Native Americans would carefully choose which plants they collected, identifying them by taste, smell, and sight. They would then prepare them in dishes with other ingredients like wild game or fish. Here are some tips for identifying plants that can help you start your journey and see how the natives lived!

It is a skill that all Native Americans need to know. Foraging can be dangerous, so you should always have a full stomach before going out foraging. You should be with someone who knows what to do if you get lost or something terrible happens.

Foraging was also one way for the Native American people to learn about their environment and become more spiritually connected. For example, the plants in the area were used for almost every need. The Native Americans used plants like cedar and spruce for clothing and blankets and to make baskets, mats, and clothing. They used bark from trees to build shelters or to cover themselves at night. The berries were used for food and medicine; they had properties that kept animals away or killed parasites. Even in the Pacific Northwest, it was essential for their survival to know how to use what nature gave them.

It is among the most essential and sacred tasks of Native Americans to put in the necessary time and effort to harvest plants for food, medicine, and other purposes. Spring through fall is some of the best times of the year for gathering many types of plants. People of all ages participate in harvesting plants, and it is often a family project.

The plants harvested by Native Americans include many kinds of berries, such as pokeberry and blackberry. Native Americans also harvest grasses such as Indian ricegrass for their food value. The juice from the stalks of Indian ricegrass can be squeezed into a cup or bowl to make a nutritious drink. The crinkle-seed plant roots can be dug up, cleaned, and eaten raw or dried, and used as flour for making bread or cakes. Nettles can be picked and cooked with other greens as a tasty side dish.

It is essential to acknowledge this evidence of the people's ability to adapt, contributing to their survival for so many years. It allows us as a society to make a connection with the Native Americans and what they have had to endure.

CHAPTER 50:

FORAGING

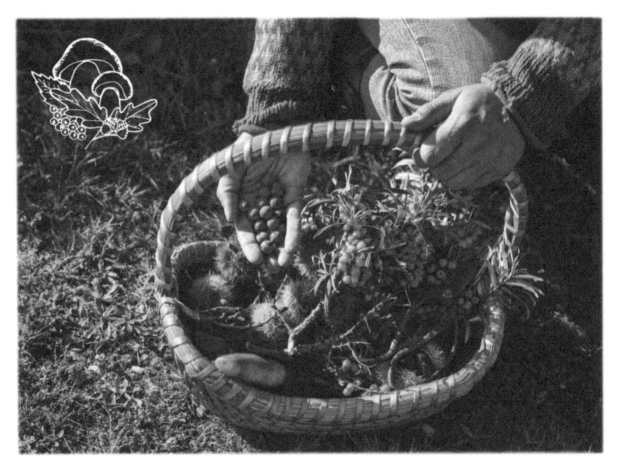

Foraging is characterized as the demonstration of scanning the wild for plants, spices and growths that are valuable to us. While the underlying meaning of the word was expected uniquely for looking for wellsprings of food, it is now applied to the demonstration that includes looking for plants for wellbeing and prosperity other than food. Searching is by and large connected with setting up camp and journeying across the woodlands of the world. In reality, even using a wild plant growing at the end of your street can be considered as foraging.

Our progenitors have utilized plants and mushrooms that are viewed as in the wild since the beginning phases of human existence for their endurance. A considerable lot of these contain minerals and different mixtures that can be utilized for relieving specific sicknesses or even work on the wellbeing of an individual overall. The vast majority of these plants have been named as weeds due to their capacity to develop anyplace. The main piece of scavenging is having the option to accurately recognizing a plant and to sort out in the event that it is palatable or helpful and not noxious to people. To do this, an individual needs a ton of direction and experience. Foragers throughout the most recent years have reported the plants that they have run over and their purposes to people. Mushrooms are the most broadly concentrated on growths in the wild, to decide whether they are palatable as well as to check whether they can fix or decrease human ailments.

What Is A Forager?

A forager is a person who sources and gathers edible foods from nature. What foragers also know is that time spent hunting for delicious greens, herbs, berries, or roots or finding useful, medicinal plants have satisfaction all its own. Connecting with nature through foraging is a calming, peaceful practice with many benefits as a hobby (aside from the tasty plants themselves). There is no better antidote to a busy, stressful day than heading out into nature to discover what treasures await the patient and observant forager.

Learning to identify edible wild plants is a critical step in learning how to forage. Many people will tell you that it's important not to eat a plant unless you're 100% certain of its identification; learning how to identify edible wild plants is a big subject and one that will take years of practice to master. However, that doesn't mean you can't start foraging now! Just make sure you do some research and start small.

Foraging for edible wild plants is a skill that takes time to develop but can easily be taught to almost anyone. To start with, you will want to find a walk in the woods that is relatively secluded and quiet, without any nearby roads or buildings. You want to find areas with a diversity of plants and lots of different terrain types. And finally, you want a place that isn't going through a lot of change - not going from drought to wet will help your ability to identify plants.

The best locations to look for wild edibles are

- Local parks
- Camp grounds
- National Parks
- Hiking trails
- Forests and woodlots

When you're out in the woods, it's best to go for a nice leisurely walk. Stop now and then and look around, take a good look at the plants you see. The more you look, the more you'll notice yourself recognizing plants - after a while, you'll start to see plants from your neighborhood or ones right outside your house in your favorite hiking spot. To begin learning how to forage, begin with plants that are reasonably easy to identify. If you're beginning, however, it's best to start looking for young plants - don't touch anything that has already flowered, and avoid any areas where more giant shrubs or trees are growing. Use your senses to gather details about the plant - look at the leaves and stems, feel the leaf textures between your fingers - then try a bite.

CHAPTER 51:

WHAT ARE WILD EDIBLES?

Native Americans were the first to invent and use wild edible plant herbs as a staple in their diet. These plants were used for food, medicine, and for other uses. They have been grown continuously from prehistoric times to the present day by native peoples, although there are only about 2–3 species of edible plants that are commonly used.

The majority of these plants grow naturally or near natural settings, so Native Americans normally ate them rather than cultivated them for human consumption. Thus, these plants were sought out and gathered from nature.

Native Americans spent a great deal of time and energy looking for and utilizing the wild edible herbs, as these plants were an integral part of their diet. They would use different senses and tools such as trees and boughs to locate the wild edible herbs. They would dig them out with their hands, use wooden tools to open the roots; sometimes, they would even chew on them to extract useful compounds from their leaves or roots, or they would boil or smash them before eating them. Universal symbols such as the sun (yellow) and moon (white) were also used as way-finding devices for navigators in the wintertime because wild edible herbs grew near lakes.

The use of these edible plants helped them to sustain themselves by providing them with much-needed nutrients and carbohydrates. They also used wild edible herbs as a source of income to trade for other goods that they wanted or needed.

What Methods Do Foragers Use To Gather Wild Edibles?

Solitary Foraging
This foraging approach involves seeking medicinal herbs and plants on your own through manual exploitation or by use of some specific tools. Solitary foraging allows you access to enough resources because there is minimal amount of competition so you are able to get as many plants as you want and exploit the rich environment to the fullest.

Group Foraging
Group foraging is when more than one person goes in search of edible plants and medicinal herbs. Every member of the group is essential to the success of this method. Group foraging can be grouped into two; dispersion economy and aggregation economy.

- **Dispersion Economy**: In dispersion economy, members of the group are not committed to a specific gathering plan. Although they all go out to gather food as a group, members of the group are on their own and choose what to pick and what not to pick.
- **Aggregation Economy**: Aggregation economy on the other hand is when the group is committed to a specific plan and tries to achieve a pre-determined goal. Members of the group may be assigned specific nutritional needs, which they have to cater to so that at the end of the day, the whole group shares what they have gathered amongst themselves.

CHAPTER 52:

THE FUNDAMENTALS OF FORAGING

Ethical Foraging

Until now, you were introduced to a list of wild edibles fit for consumption and wild plants to be avoided. Before you start foraging or call yourself a forager, you must understand certain things about the activity itself. The idea is to get a better understanding of nature and not harm it.

From interacting with nature to increasing awareness about the need for spending time outdoors, there are a lot of benefits associated with foraging. When you learn to identify, harvest, and prepare wild edibles or medicines using ingredients you foraged, it strengthens your relationship with the ecosystem. Lack of proper information, misinformation, and overzealous behavior harms the environment. Foraging is helpful when done properly. Remember, every function has a limit. This is a basic rule of math we were all taught in school. This is also the universal rule of nature. Foraging can be fun, exciting, interesting, and even therapeutic, provided it is done properly. If you aren't careful, this activity can harm the environment. In this chapter, let's look at some simple tips you should always remember while foraging to ensure it is an ethical practice.

Safe Forage

Of primary importance to anyone interested in foraging must be SAFETY.

1. Positive ID: Before eating ANY wild plant, make sure you identify the plant with 100% accuracy—99% accuracy is not good enough. If you can access a local foraging expert, consult them, but in any case also cross-check the plant ID with at least two edible plant field guides who are specific to your local area. Make sure the field guides, whether in print or online, offer color photos—black and white photos shouldn't be used for plant identification. Some edible plants have poisonous "look-alikes" and it is even more important to go over all of the features of the toxic and non-toxic plants to make sure you can tell them apart in the case of look-alike plants.

2. Taste Test: After 100% positive identification is made, it is best to sample only a small bit of the plant at first. It's not only poisonous plants we must be aware of: allergic reactions can also happen with non-toxic plants. Best to eat a bit and wait, especially when encountering any given plant for the first time.

3. Avoid Polluted Plants: Avoid picking plants from areas that have been sprayed with chemical fertilizers, insecticides or weed control. Although it can be difficult to tell, if you suspect the area you are foraging in is polluted with waste water, it is also best to avoid it. Although roadside stops can be tempting, plants growing alongside busy roads and highways can be contaminated with gasoline and other fossil fuels.

4. Always Wash: Although it can be tempting to take a nibble of a juicy, wild strawberry right away, always bring your treasures home and wash them before consuming. In addition to possible pollution, plants may have come in contact with insects or animal droppings. A quick wash will ensure plants are 100% ready to eat.

5. Personal Safety: Do not forage on private land without permission, or in protected national parks or in any other areas where it would be considered trespassing. You could find yourself ticketed, or even arrested! If you are foraging in areas known for wildlife such as bears, big cats etc. please familiarize yourself with the safest ways to be in those areas. It is always safer to forage in secluded areas with a "buddy" as well.

Beginner Foragers' Guide To Basic Rules

Before you embark on this exciting activity, you need to observe the following guidelines:

Do not forage on the endangered species

Regardless of the rich color or edibility of flowers, weeds, or mushrooms, you shouldn't pick illegal or endangered species. You can check from local authorities or online for rare or protected plants. Be aware that some crops may seem locally abundant but are rare or endangered throughout their ranges.

Be sure of edible plants

An easy way of identifying edible plants is through physical description such as color, texture, feel, and smell. It's quite dangerous to eat plants you aren't sure about as these could be poisonous. Also, take caution as some edible plants have poisonous lookalikes. Thus, you might need to get relevant information from people conversant with these plants.

Do not overharvest plants

The rule of the thumb is only to harvest 10–20 percent of a crop to facilitate continued growth. However, this rule is, overlooked, especially in those popular edible plants, but it's worth cautioning. Thus, if you are interested in making powder from sassafras leaves, ensure you don't uproot its sapling; only pick all you need and leave the rest for the next foraging venture.

You shouldn't harvest the root

If you forage the roots, the chances are that the crop can no longer progress with growth. The most acceptable parts of the plant to pick are the leaves or flowers, though sometimes roots have to be harvested. For instance, when picking the wild ginger leaves, make sure that you harvest a little portion of the edible root.

Confirm the water sources

This rule applies when harvesting the wild water plants when you need to eat the wild plant raw. Find out the water in which plants are grown to avoid taking plants grown in contaminated water. Dirty water and chemically polluted water may contain dangerous compounds that heat might not break down.

Wear protective clothing

Beginners may be faced with numerous challenges, especially when harvesting stinging or crops with odor. The majority of forage food is based on dense parks and forests where there could be dangerous animals. Ensure that you wear long-sleeved clothing, pants, and close-toed shoes. Also, carry along gloves, scissors, a small rake, and a trowel. You might need a raincoat, especially if foraging in the spring.

Try cultivating wild edible crops

Despite the crop being considered wild, some of them are easy to transplant or propagate into your garden. For example, you can cultivate ramps, which are at the risk of getting rare from over-harvesting. Nonetheless, you need to research the best conditions to grow edible wild crops based on your environment. This step is good for preservation and makes your foraging convenient.

Don't forage on toxic places

Its common knowledge to avoid areas like busy roads as the crop might absorb heavy metals from the toxic exhaust, like lead. Most chemicals are in soils and come from exhausts and the use of pesticides or herbicides. To avoid eating contaminated crops, ensure that you only pick plants that appear healthy. This helps reduce the risk of falling sick and boosts your nutrient intake.

Obtain permission

Most forests or parks where edible plants grow are under specific management; thus, you must respect property rights and laws. Courtesy matters and failure to secure permission might lead to legal battles.

Now that you know the basic rules you ought to observe, it is time to know what you can forage.

Foraging Tips

Have a Plan

You should always have a plan. There is no reason why foraging must be an exception. Before you decide to head anywhere, regardless of whether it is only the local park, ensure you are aware of what you are looking for. Not just that, but also select an area or a general area where you should be looking at the plant in question. Once you have both these pieces of information in place, stick to the plan. While you do this if you stumble across something else that interests you, take a picture and document it so you can look it up later. If you have a field guide with you, check it before you decide to forage. This is a great way to ensure you do not misidentify a particular plant variety or harvest something that is at risk or endangered.

Always Identify

Perhaps the most important rule of foraging is to identify. Before you decide to forage, learn to identify the plant you are foraging. The same rule applies to mushrooms as well. Never rely on a single source of identification, such as the stem, leaf, or bloom. Instead, make it a point to look for at least three characteristics before you harvest any plant. The fragrance, life cycle of the plant, location, fruit, bloom, leaf color, the stem, branch, bark, spore print, and soil conditions are some factors you should consider.

Harvest from Clean Areas

The areas you harvest from are as important as what you decide to harvest. If you are harvesting from an area along the roadside, near an industrial area, or even property lines, don't do it. Such areas usually have high levels of contaminants and pollutants. Remember, all the edible plants you harvest must be fit for consumption. If the ingredients are harvested from polluted areas, you are indirectly consuming all the contaminants and pollutants. The best practice is to always look for areas that are unlikely to be traveled on or are even untouched. This is the best bet you have to ensure the harvest is clean and safe for consumption.

Be a Little Conservative

Whenever you're harvesting, ensure you harvest only what you need. Remember, nature is not just for you, but its bounty is meant to be shared with others. If you forage everything, you are depriving your fellow foragers of a good harvest. As a rule of thumb, you should harvest between 1/10th up to 1/3rd of the patch. For instance, if you see a single patch of a specific species, avoid foraging. Walk around and explore your surroundings a little before you forage the first thing you see. Always mark the spot, and you can make your way back to it. This is better than foraging an endangered or at-risk variety.

Apart from this, always consider the life cycle of the plant before foraging. The white blossoms on an elder tree are pretty to look at, and you may be tempted to pluck them. If you do this, there will be no berries in the fall! Always harvest what you need and never harvest because there seems to be plenty available. Be careful and exercise restraint to become an ethical forager.

Do Not Alter the Landscape

While foraging, ensure you leave the area after foraging as good or at least as good as it was before you started. Wouldn't you feel annoyed and disappointed to notice your favorite foraging spot has been ransacked and pillaged? Never litter. If there is any garbage, pick it up, and clean up the mess. Don't ever drastically alter the natural landscape catering to your needs. That means avoid disturbing the natural landscape, such as chopping down trees or their branches, disturbing nests, or deciding to drive off-road. If you notice any unsafe conditions or spots while foraging, don't forget to alert the concerned authorities. A simple practice you can adopt as an ethical forager is to carry an extra bag to pick up any litter you come across while foraging.

Be Prepared

Before you start foraging or heading outdoors, ensure you are prepared with the right clothing and equipment. For instance, wearing flip-flops as you head into a dense forest is a bad idea. When it comes to preparation, ensure you carry a small first aid kit, a couple of field guides, and other requirements to survive in the wilderness. Wearing sturdy shoes, weather-appropriate clothing, and protective gear such as heavy-duty gloves is always a good idea. Whenever possible, wear long sleeves. Apart from that, don't forget to inform others about where you are headed. It's always better to err on the side of caution instead of finding yourself in distress.

The Legal Guidelines

You cannot become an ethical forager until you are a legal one. Before you start foraging plants or even mushrooms, ensure you check the local guidelines and regulations. Certain areas require permits, therefore ensure you have all of them in place before you start foraging. If not, you may end up trespassing or breaking laws. Remember, being unaware of the law is never a defense. To ensure that you do not get into any legal trouble, it's better to check the laws and regulations. Apart from that, be extremely careful about trespassing. If you are foraging on private property or unsure whether the given area is public land or not, please check. Contact the required authorities and always obtain permission before you decide to forage on any private property.

If you are not sure about the legal areas to forage, look at public land records. You can also talk to others in the area to understand if there are any rules involved in this process. Talk to the necessary people and get the required permission before accessing any property. Similarly, you should also check the local hunting season and schedules. This is important to ensure you take all the necessary precautions.

Nature provides us with everything we need. So, it is our responsibility to take care of it as well. We aren't the only living beings around! Foraging isn't an eat-all-you-want-buffet! By following all the different suggestions discussed, you can have a fun and safe foraging experience and ensure everything is legal. Ensure you have the required resources, have properly planned the foraging trip, and show restraint in order to become an ethical forager.

Tools For Foraging

Similar to any endeavor, coming up with the right tools and techniques greatly enhances your chances of being successful. In foraging, other than knowledge and your senses, a good set of tools can assist you in picking not only the right herbs but the best ones too. To get started, here's a quick list of the tools you need to prepare in foraging.

Picking Tools

Although your hands can be enough to pick herbs and plants, it's still a good idea to use the right picking tool particularly if you are harvesting an herb that might potentially cause an injury. Gardening gloves can help prevent irritation and offer protection if you want to pick herbs using your hands. Using plastic mitts is also a good idea particularly if you're targeting a prickly herb.

However, for plants that need to be cut at the lower stem and you don't want to spend a lot of time yanking the needed part off, using a good pair of scissors can really be helpful. If you're aiming high, using a long stick can greatly lengthen your reach. In case you are digging for roots, using a shorter stick or even a trowel can make your work less laborious than using your hands. For a larger area, you might want to keep a spare shovel in your car just in case.

Knives

Knives or shears are important tools in foraging. Aside from harvesting, it's also a helpful tool in cutting branches and vines that hinder your path. You can also use it as a grasping tool and in marking your trail in the woods.

Storage Containers

Another thing you need to prepare beforehand is your transport containers. You may not need any special type of containers when it comes to foraging. Typically, you only need a few covered containers, big plastic shopping bags, or even freezer bags will do.

First Aid Kits

Because you are in the wild and accidents are always possible, it's a wise idea to be ready in case something happens while you are foraging. In setting up your first aid kit, you can add the following:

- Tweezers and even needles are essential first aid tools in cases of splinters and thorns.
- Antiseptic solutions can come in handy while you are foraging. While slips and bruises are fairly common when you are in the wild, bringing an antiseptic solution even if it's just alcohol or povidone iodine can help ward off infection.
- Keep a fresh set of plantain leaves in your first aid kit. It can help you manage insect bites and even poison ivy rashes.

Water and Rags

Walking under the sun for a certain period of time can cause your body a certain degree of dehydration. If you're going to forage, make sure to bring a few bottles of water with you for hydration. You'll also need water to clean up your hands and your tools. A spare rag can also help you clean up berries, plant parts and even your fingers.

Illustrated Books

Bringing a few illustrated books is necessary in making sure you identify plants and herbs correctly. It's not necessary to take all books with you while you walk because they carry a certain weight. Instead, you can just take one and leave the others in your car for easier cross checking when you've collected all needed herbs.

Sun Protection

Being exposed in the sun is never healthy and safe. However, as foraging makes sun exposure inevitable, it's wise if you can bring a hat or a good sunscreen with you. You may need to frequently reapply the product particularly if you'll be spending a good couple of hours walking outside the shade of trees. Aside from sunscreen, you may also want to bring a good bottle of bug spray just to keep insects away.

Magnifying Glass

You may not always need it but bringing a magnifying glass in your foraging can help make sure you get your hands on the right herbs. The glass can allow you to visually inspect small herbs and plants for any discernable features that can set them apart from the rest of their family and species. A difference in hair or even tiny holes in the stem can be all you need to properly identify an herb. As the eyes are limited in terms of what they can see, a good magnifying glass can make the job a lot easier.

Proper Clothing

While there aren't any strict guides on what you can and can't wear while foraging, the idea is to use something that's both protective and comfortable. Clothes that have long sleeves as well as long pants are good choices because they can help prevent insects from biting you and thorny shrubs from irritating your skin. It's also a good idea to wear a scarf for added protection against the sun. For your feet, it's best if you can stick with a pair of socks and boots.

Snacks

You don't need to bring a lot of food particularly if you'll be spending most of your hours looking for herbs and plants. However, because the activity can be tedious and laborious, it's wise to bring a few snacks with you while you forage.

CHAPTER 53:

Wild Edibles

Best Wild Edibles And How To Gather Them In WINTER

Big Leaf Maple

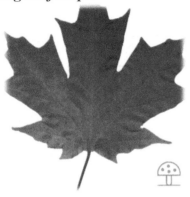

The maple family is most well-known for its syrup. The sugar maple produces the very best syrup, but the big leaf maple can produce earthy-sweet syrup, too!

How to Gather I

The most popular part of the big leaf maple to gather is the flowers. These flowers contain deliciously sweet nectar. They grow in bunches in the spring and are the focus of our recipe for this tree.

This maple can also be tapped for syrup. This takes some hardware but making syrup is a great way to forage, and you can come back to those same trees year after year.

Bittercress

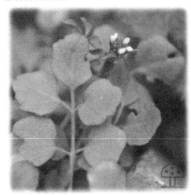

Also known as hairy bittercress, this wild edible got the short end of the stick on the name, but it has a big flavor and is part of a family of mustards filled with character, nutrition, and flavor.

How to Gather

When it comes to harvesting this wild edible, use the forager's shears. They are going to become very handy when trimming the stems of bittercress.

Crab Apples

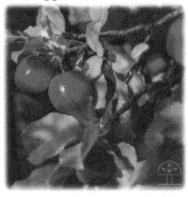

These smaller apples are very prolific and easy to identify. They lend themselves less to raw eating and more to cooked preparations. This is because they have a very tart flavor.

How to Gather

Gathering crab apples is a great opportunity to bring out the tub rugs. You can fill large baskets or other containers with these ripe crab apples.

Grab the fruit and twist. The stem will separate from the tree, and you will have your first crabapple. For taller trees, you are going to need a fruit picker basket to extend into the trees.

Peppergrass

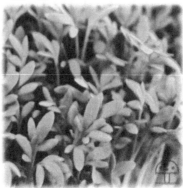

Wild peppergrass or poor man's pepper is a well-documented wild edible used by the Incas and written about by the Roman author Pliny, the Elder. We have been harvesting wild peppergrass for a very long time.

How to Gather

The wonderful thing about gathering peppergrass is that the entire plant is edible. All parts can be consumed, and they can all be consumed raw. It would be a great plant harvest in the same trip as chickweed; they would likely be near one another, too!

Your shears are going to be very useful for harvesting peppergrass.

Siberian Miner's Lettuce

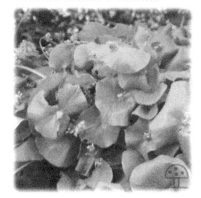

Siberian Miner's Lettuce is easy to find, full of nutrition, and goes by many names: Indian lettuce and clasp leaf miners lettuce.

How to Gather

Siberian Miner's Lettuce is edible in all its forms. Everything from the stems to the roots is edible. It's an easy plant to gather because of that. If you are not interested in gathering roots along with your lettuces, then bring some shears to deal with that.

Best Wild Edibles And How To Gather Them In SPRING

Asparagus

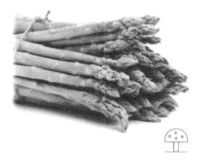

Wild asparagus is a must forage in the spring. There is something magical about finding those pencil-thin stalks popping up from the ground.

How to Gather

Wild asparagus should be treated much like fresh cut flowers. Your sharp knife is the best tool for cutting stalks close to the woody base. When you get them home, store the cut stalks so that water touches the cut parts.

You can keep going back to it when you find a patch of wild asparagus. New stalks will sprout.

Blue Camas

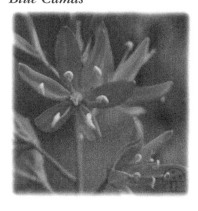

This perennial wild herb grows nearly 2 feet tall in the wild and has a beautiful blue flower.

How to Gather

You are after the bulbs to get the most bang for your buck. These can easily be had using your hori hori to harvest them. Dig around the bulbs, or roots, just underground and pry them loose.

They are sturdy and can be piled atop one another when carrying them.

Catnip

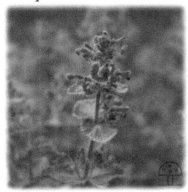

Catnip is a wild herb that is not just for cats. Many parts of the plant are edible and can be used in herbal remedies.

How to Gather

The best tool for gathering catnip will be the forager's shears. They will give you the ability to cut these plants off at the base and gather them.

You could bring your small shovel or hori hori as many people forage wild catnip and then bring it home live, root and all. This plant is great to cultivate and grow on your property.

Common Plantain

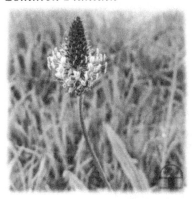

Common plantain is probably the first wild edible you can find as a new forager. There is a good chance you can walk 100 feet from where you are sitting and look down in the grass to find some common plantain.

How to Gather

The trusty shears are going to be your best tool for trimming the leaves of the common plantain. If you find a field that is full of them, you can actually snip some leaves from several plants and never endanger any one plant by taking all its leaves.

Mustard

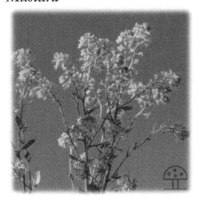

The mustards are a highly opportunistic plant that likes hanging near humans and are packed with nutrition. They are in the brassica family with broccoli and cauliflower.

How to Gather

All parts of this plant are edible. The best time to eat mustard is before the plant bolts or starts to flower. After the flowering begins, mustard can get very bitter.

Your forager's shears are the perfect tool for this wild edible, and some baskets to pile with mustard are great, too.

Wild Ginger

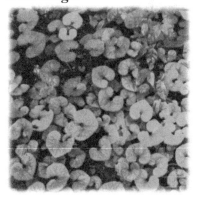

Ginger has been an ingredient and medicine all the way back to the days of Ancient China.

How to Gather

You can gather the flowers and rootstocks. Your hori hori will be great for digging out the roots, and your shears will take the flowers easily.

Wild Strawberry

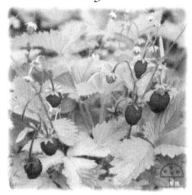

We have all happened to come across these little small wild strawberries snaking through yards and fields in spring.

How to Gather

You can gather the fruit of the wild strawberry, but the flowers and leaves are also nice to have. Wild strawberry is a delicate plant, so your forager's shears should do the job just fine.

Yarrow

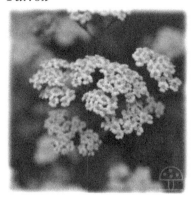

Yarrow is a wild edible plant with a special power. It can help stop bleeding.

How to Gather

All parts of the yarrow plant are edible. The root is a big part of foraging it so bring the hori hori or even a small shovel to help harvest this rhizomatous plant.

Arrowhead

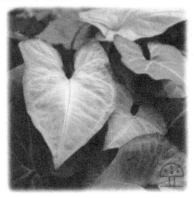

Arrowhead has a very funny nickname. It is also known as duck potato.

How to Gather

If you eat the stalks and leaves, then you should focus on harvesting younger plants. The tubers can be harvested at all times, and they are a good source of carbohydrates.

Black Hawthorn

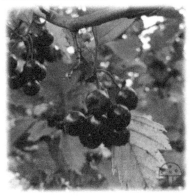

Black hawthorn puts off long and strong spines that can be used as needles or hooks in wilderness survival.

How to Gather

The shoots and bark of this plant have medicinal properties and are worth gathering. Wear strong gloves to deal with the spines.

The berries are delicious and should be gathered at any opportunity.

Bog Cranberry

The bog cranberry is also known as the small cranberry or the swamp cranberry.

How to Gather

The cranberries can be gathered by hand, but because of the nature of their habitat, you will want some waterproof boots to keep your feet and legs dry.

Evergreen Huckleberry

This evergreen species is found in the wild but is also very popular in native landscaping in the Pacific Northwest.

How to Gather

Huckleberries are easy to gather by hand in the late summer and early fall. Just bring gloves as the berries can stain your fingers.

Hazelnut

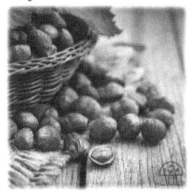

The hazelnut is a luxurious wild edible and is the main flavoring in Nutella.

How to Gather

The nuts are the only edible part of this shrub, so you are just grabbing nuts and gathering them. Bring a bag with you for storage and carrying.

Juniper

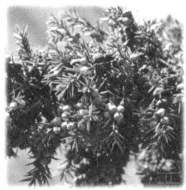

The juniper can live up to 200 years!

How to Gather

The berries are the true edible part of this plant. They are most often used as a flavoring and are the main flavoring ingredient in gin. The berries can be gathered by hand.

Oregon Grape

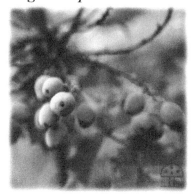

The flower of the Oregon grape is Oregon's state flower.

How to Gather

The grapes themselves are easy to harvest and can be done with some simple gloves and a basket. Pick the whole cluster of berries to be quicker. You can separate them at home.

Milk Thistle

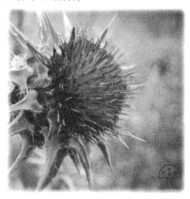

This plant has been in the human diet for over 2,000 years!

How to Gather

You can gather all parts of the milk thistle as it all can be eaten. The leaves are great if you remove the spines. The stems are a great asparagus substitute. Even the seeds can be roasted as a coffee substitute.

Wild Licorice

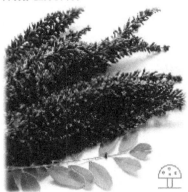

The roots of licorice are very fibrous and can be used as a substitute for a toothbrush.

How to Gather

The roots can be gathered using your hori hori. These have a strong licorice taste and many uses.

Best Wild Edibles And How To Gather Them In SUMMER

Chokecherry

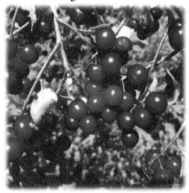

With a name like this, you might not think it's edible, but the chokecherry is delicious.

How to Gather

The chokecherries can be gathered when they are ripe and stacked in baskets or satchels. They are tasty and unique. However, you cannot eat the pit of the fruit as it contains hydrocyanic acid, and this is toxic to humans.

Cloudberry

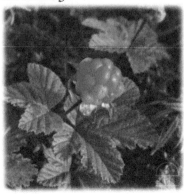

The cloudberry looks like something from a video game or another planet. It's a beautiful orange-yellow berry.

How to Gather

Gathering cloudberries is very simple. You just pluck the berry off the stem and move on to the next one.

Coastal Black Gooseberry

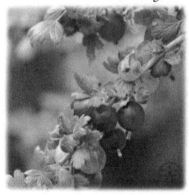

This is the tastiest variety of gooseberry in North America.

How to Gather

The gooseberries can be gathered by hand and plucked. Be sure you wear gloves because the spines hurt!

Oval Leaf Blueberry

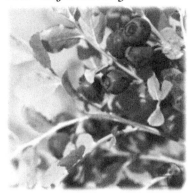

There are many forms of blueberry in the nation, and all of them are edible.

How to Gather

Blueberries can be plucked by hand, but you might want to wear gloves to protect your fingers from staining.

Pipsissewa

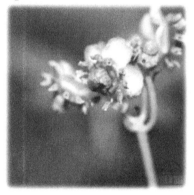

A Native American medicine and flavoring herb.

How to Gather

The plant's leaves can be harvested with shears and used to make medicinal tea or to flavor things like root beer and candy.

Red Currant

This is one of the tastiest members of the gooseberry family.

How to Gather

The ripe red currant berries can be gathered by hand, and they are easy to pick.

Salmonberry

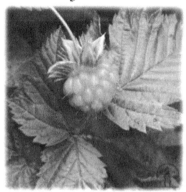

These berries are in the same family as raspberries and blackberries.

How to Gather

These berries are easy to gather and can be done so by hand. Just make sure you have plenty of storage because they are often plentiful. They are delicate, too.

CONCLUSION

Now, you know and have all it takes to begin your incredible journey as a forager. Trust me, it's a very exciting and fun experience as long as you don't go harvesting and eating plants you cannot fully recognize. Before you eat any plant, make sure you try to rub it against your skin or lips and wait for a few minutes to observe your body reaction to it. This may be able to give you an idea of whether you are allergic to the plant or whether it is a poisonous plant.

In addition, it's always better to start out as a group forager. Go on foraging trips with groups of people and learn more about the culture and rules of foraging. Observe how they handle the plants and learn a few recipes from them then you can start your own journey as a forager.

This new path you have chosen will not only help you to stay healthy and fresh, it will also give you a new hobby that you will be proud of and that you may want to share with your friends and family.

Happy foraging!

BOOK 13

ROSEMARY, BASIL, AND THYME BEST RECIPES

70+ Delicious and Simple Recipes for Remedies, Food, and Home using the Most Beneficial Common Herbs

Citali Galwen

INTRODUCTION

This brief introduction about rosemary, basil and thyme plants summarizes their characteristics, kitchen and health benefits, plantation techniques, and how to harvest them.

Rosemary

Rosemary is a famous perennial, woody herb with evergreen needle-like leaves. The scent-like essence of this plant is due to its' characteristic of producing the essential oil. The top surface of the leaves has a dark green color, while the underside is covered with short, dense, and woolly hairs. Depending upon its variety, the flowers of rosemary maybe violet, pink, purple, blue, or white. Flowers of rosemary are fragrant and attractive for birds, butterflies, and bees. The flowers of this plant bloom yearly in warmer areas. The oil that the rosemary plant produces contains rose-marine acid and camphor.

Moreover, rosemary also contains strong antioxidant, antifungal, and antibacterial properties. Its herbs can grow better in warm and humid areas where they can go to the height of several feet, but if they don't get the ideal conditions, it becomes very difficult to manage. It can be grown as an outdoor perennial herb in warm areas, but it should be grown indoors in a pot in cold areas. The germination rate for the rosemary plant is very low. So, it is more favorable to grow the new rosemary plant from the cuttings of already established plants. If the conditions are feasible, then in an outdoor plantation, it can be grown within 8 weeks. There are some specifications to plant the rosemary herb; for example, it should be panted in full sun, given a wide space, and soil should be drained well as rosemary plants cannot tolerate the wet consistency.

Moreover, it should be planted in a garden near beans, carrots, sage, and cabbage. To harvest the rosemary snip off the stem and hang the dried rosemary in the kitchen. To have a fresh taste, harvest the young stems of rosemary. To store the rosemary herb, put it up for air dry and store in an airtight container. Besides having antibacterial capabilities, the rosemary plant is also widely used in the kitchen and garden, and for healing.

Basil

Basil is one of the easiest and most famous herbs to grow. Sweet basil belongs to the mint family. Basil leaves are extremely aromatic and have delightful flavors, from cinnamon to lemony mint and licorice. The color of basil leaves is rich green and sometimes deep purple. Flowers of basil are slightly insignificant but popular with bees. Basil of all types grow very easily in sunny and warm weather. Basil leaves are mostly used in cooking, but its' buds are edible also. It is a fast-growing herb and thrives equally well in containers and gardens. Basil plant gives a bushier growth in warm weather within six weeks. It can grow better in a warm atmosphere, it is better to plant it in greenhouse conditions, but if someone wants to grow the basil from seed, it will be better to grow it indoors. Basil plant gets ready to harvest within 60-90 days. The height of the basil plant depends upon various factors such as weather, growing conditions, seeds, and soil. Sweet basil can get to a maximum height of 6 feet. Basil plant needs sunlight of 6-8 hours daily and moist soil to have fast growth. In short, basil is a heat lover and sensitive to frost. Frozen basil leaves are used for cooking purposes as frozen basil has a strong taste. To freeze the basil, blend it with some olive oil, make small cubes, and store in an airtight container.

Thyme

Thyme is abundantly known as the Mediterranean plant with many medical benefits and culinary addition to the food. Plantation and harvesting of thyme are very easy. Thyme is the best choice as an edible and easy to grow plant as it can grow in versatile climates. Good growth needs well drainage and full sunlight, but if it is to be grown in a pot, it must be placed in an airy place. The thyme plant should not get too much water as it may rot its' roots.

For this reason, it gets the best growth in a warm climate with drained soil. Thyme should be trimmed as one reaches its' wooded area. But it will be better if the residual thyme leaves are crushed to protect them from deep freeze so that they may come back yearly. There are a lot of benefits of using thyme leaves; for example, it lowers blood pressure, is a good cure for cough, boosts the immune system as it is full of vitamin A and C, has excellent antioxidant elements and helps to overcome bad breath; moreover, it can help in reducing the body's inflammation, and is a good source of vitamin K which helps in maintaining bone health. Plant the thyme in a garden with tomatoes, lavender, rosemary, cabbage, and eggplant. Avoid planting the thyme in wet soil. It attracts pollinators and bees to the garden but repels cabbage worms, tomato hornworms, and flea beetles.

Thyme is widely used as a cooking item in soups, stews, and meat seasoning. It gives the bread a better and richer artisan taste. Moreover, it is used in hot water and tea. Planting thyme near lavender provides additional benefits as both demand the same soil and atmospheric conditions to grow. Thyme is used as a common cooking herb in the west. It is used in various savory dishes; fresh and dried thyme can be infused in oil and cooked in soups, stews, and meat. Lemon thyme is a flavorful addition to the seafood. Thyme also has many health benefits; for example, it is used to deal with cold symptoms. It also helps bone health as it has a high consistency of vitamin K, calcium, iron, and manganese.

Moreover, it is also very helpful for digestion and regulates the immune system. Thyme leaves also produce essential oil with antibacterial and anti-inflammatory properties, which helps cure muscle cramping and acne issues. There is no specific season or time to harvest thyme; it usually takes 2.5-3 years to mature, so avoid harvesting the thyme in the 1st year of growth. It depends upon the growth how many times you can harvest the thyme plant in a year. However, if the atmospheric and soil conditions are feasible, they can be harvested in the winter months. To preserve the thyme, wrap it in a plastic bag and refrigerate it. In this way, you can store fresh thyme for at least two weeks.

CHAPTER 54:

ROSEMARY RECIPES

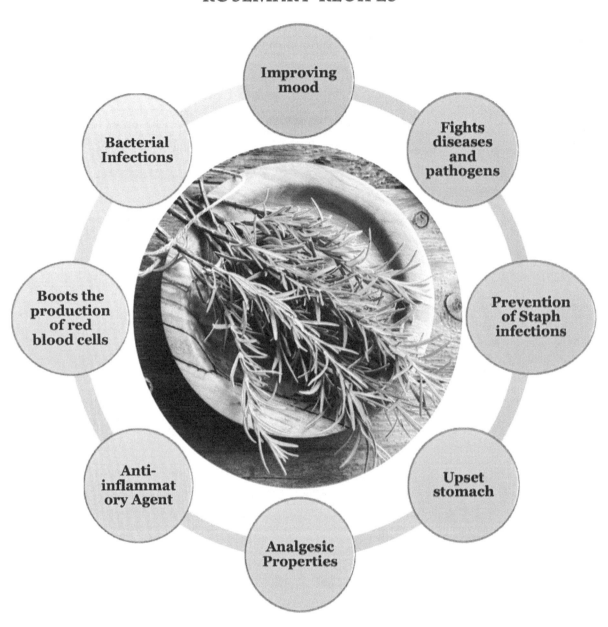

- Improving mood
- Fights diseases and pathogens
- Bacterial Infections
- Prevention of Staph infections
- Boots the production of red blood cells
- Upset stomach
- Anti-inflammatory Agent
- Analgesic Properties

ROSEMARY AS MEDICINE

1. Rosemary Tea

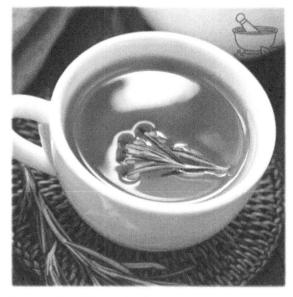

Preparation Time: 1 minute

Cooking Time: 5 minutes

Ingredients:

- 2 cups boiling water
- 2-3 tsp. rosemary leaves

Directions:

1. Put the rosemary in boiling water.
2. Set it aside for five minutes.
3. Strain the rosemary leaves.
4. Enjoy!

2. Rosemary Salve

Preparation Time: 60 minutes

Cooking Time: 3-4 days

Ingredients:

- 8 oz. of almond oil or olive oil
- 8 oz. of dried rosemary herb
- mason jar
- stockpot or crockpot

Directions:

1. Chop the dried rosemary herb and put it in the mason jar.

2. Cover with the oil and gently shake the herb in it.
3. Place the jar in the water bath.
4. Heat the oil and water for 3-5 days and keep the oil temperature around 11 degrees.
5. After 4-5 days, remove the jar from heat and let it cool.
6. Strain the oil.
7. Store in an airtight jar and put it in a dark place.

3. Rosemary Oil

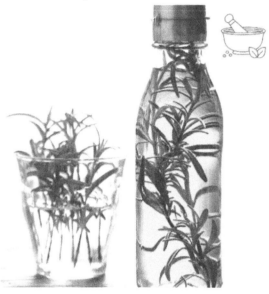

Preparation Time: 30 minutes

Cooking Time: 1 hour

Ingredients:

- 3-4 sprigs of dried rosemary
- 2-3 cups of olive oil

Directions:

1. Wash the rosemary to remove the dust and debris.
2. Take the oil in a saucepan and heat it.
3. Add chopped rosemary to it and cook for 20 minutes at least.
4. Drain the oil and let it cool.
5. Store the rosemary oil in a glass jar.

4. Rosemary Tincture

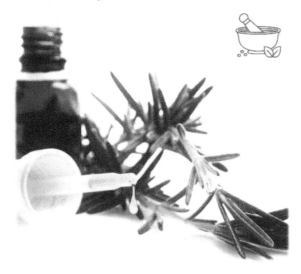

Preparation Time: 20 minutes

Cooking Time: 25 minutes

Ingredients:

- 4-6 sprigs of chopped rosemary
- ¾ cup of vodka

Directions:

1. Bruise the rosemary with the help of a fist.

2. Take the alcohol in a glass bottle.
3. Add the bruised rosemary to it.
4. Cover the glass bottle.
5. Shake it for 60 seconds.
6. Place the bottle in a dark and cool place for 5-8 weeks.
7. Now strain the tincture.
8. Store in a cool place.

5. Orange Rosemary Salt Scrub

Preparation Time: 20 minutes

Cooking Time: 1-2 hours

Ingredients:

- 1 cup of salt
- orange zest
- 1 tsp. of rosemary leaves
- 1/3 cup of olive oil

Directions:

1. Put the rosemary, orange zest, and salt in a food processor.
2. Pulse it until a homogenous mixture is obtained.
3. Add the olive oil and again pulse 3-4 times.
4. Store in a jar.
5. To use, take some scrub and lightly rub it on the skin.

6. Rosemary And Feta Beer Bread Biscuits

Preparation Time: 10 minutes

Cooking Time: 25 minutes

Servings: 12

Ingredients:

- 3 cups whole wheat flour
- 1 tbsp. baking powder
- 1 tbsp. sugar
- 1 can of beer (12 ounces)
- 1 tsp. salt
- ¼ cup of water

Directions:

1. Prepare the oven preheat it to 375 degrees Fahrenheit temperature.
2. Take a bowl, add all the dry ingredients, mix them well, and add cheese and spices, and beer. Mix them well. Add water if the dough looks dry.
3. Take a pan, add dough in, then place in oven. Cook for 45 minutes.
4. Finally, serve and enjoy it!

Nutrition: 119Kcal; Fat: 2g; Carbs: 24g; Protein: 4g

7. Charred Corn With Rosemary Grilled Pizza

Preparation Time: 1 hour

Cooking Time: 30 minutes

Servings: 4

Ingredients:

- Pizza crust
- Fresh mozzarella cheese
- 2 large ears of corn
- 2 cloves garlic
- Gorgonzola
- Salt & pepper

- Fresh rosemary
- Red pepper flakes

Directions:

1. Take corn to remove silks, then take olive oil and brush on its place on grill cook for 7 to 8 minutes then remove the kernels from cooked corn cob.
2. Take pizza, crush olive oil on it, place this on the grill, and cook for a few minutes.
3. Put on the boiler and set its setting on high temperature. Take pizza crust, sprinkle pepper and salt, then add cheese and corn. Take rosemary and gorgonzola and also sprinkle on them. Place in the oven and bake for 4 to 5 minutes or till cheese melts down.
4. Finally, serve and enjoy it!

Nutrition: Calories: 390Kcal; Fat: 34g; Carbs: 144g; Protein: 13g

8. Lemon Rosemary And Olive Oil Shortbread

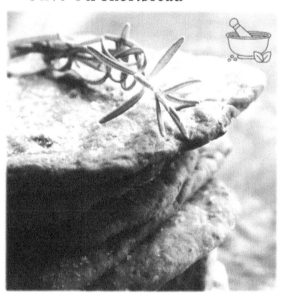

Preparation Time: 15 minutes

Cooking Time: 40 minutes

Servings: 32

Ingredients:

- 3 cups white flour
- 1 ¼ cups sugar powdered
- 1 tsp. salt
- 1 tbsp. rosemary
- Zest of 2 lemons
- 1 cup Olive Oil

Directions:

1. Prepare the oven and preheat it to 325 degrees Fahrenheit temperature.
2. Take a bowl, add sugar, flour, rosemary salt, and lemon zest and mix them well. Then add olive oil and mix them well.
3. Take a pan to add dough to it. Prick the dough surface all over with a fork. Cook it for 45 to 50 minutes.
4. Remove it from the oven, allow it to cool, and then cut it into little pieces.
5. Finally, serve and enjoy it!

Nutrition: Calories: 121Kcal; Fat: 11g; Carbs: 7.2g; Protein: 1.4g

9. Rosemary Tomato Cream Soup

Preparation Time: 15 minutes

Cooking Time: 1 hour 15 minutes

Servings: 6

Ingredients:

- 1 large leek
- 3 sprigs rosemary
- 2 tsp. garlic
- 4 cans tomatoes
- ¼ tsp. cayenne pepper
- 10 leaves basil
- ¼ cup butter
- Cream
- Salt & black pepper

Directions:

1. Take a saucepan, add butter, and heat on medium heat, then rosemary, leek and garlic and cook for approximately 15 to 18 minutes.
2. Then add cayenne pepper and tomatoes, cook them, add basil, and keep it cooking for about 1 hour.
3. Take out half soup and puree in a blender. Add this in saucepan again, then add cream season with pepper and salt.
4. Finally, serve and enjoy it!

Nutrition: Calories: 214Kcal; Fat: 15g; Carbs: 14.2g; Protein: 3.4g

10. Rosemary Parmesan Sweet Potatoes

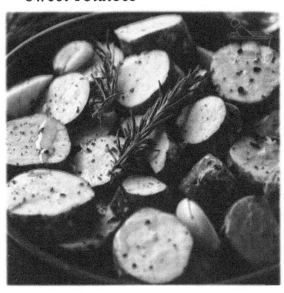

Preparation Time: 15 minutes

Cooking Time: 40 minutes

Servings: 4

Ingredients:

- 1 ½ lb. potatoes
- 3 tbsp. olive oil
- 2 tbsp. Parmesan cheese
- 1 tbsp. fresh rosemary
- Salt and pepper

Directions:

1. Prepare the oven and preheat it to 425 degrees Fahrenheit temperature.
2. Prepare the pan and line it with aluminum foil.
3. Take a bowl, add Parmesan cheese, potatoes, olive oil, and rosemary and mix them well. Add salt and pepper and again mix well. Spread this mixture on a prepared pan
4. Place in oven and cook for 40 minutes.
5. Finally, serve and enjoy it!

Nutrition: Calories: 234Kcal; Fat: 11g; Carbs: 30g; Protein: 5g

11. Baked Roasted Vegetables With Rosemary

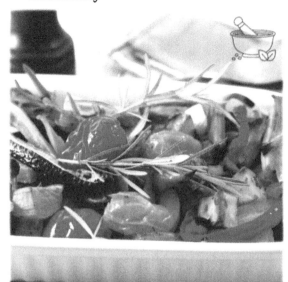

Preparation Time: 10 minutes

Cooking Time: 40 minutes

Servings: 12

Ingredients:

- 1 onion
- 1 yellow squash
- 3 cloves garlic
- 1 red bell pepper
- 1 zucchini
- 1 cup mushrooms
- 1/2 eggplant
- 1 asparagus bunch
- 1/2 cup olive oil
- 1 cup butternut
- 1 cup potatoes
- 1 cup carrots
- salt & pepper
- Fresh rosemary

Directions:

1. Prepare the oven and preheat the oven to 425 degrees Fahrenheit temperature.
2. Take a dish and add all veggies to it. Pour olive oil on it, and mix all ingredients well. Then sprinkle pepper and salt toss until combined.
3. Place in oven and cook for 35 to 40 minutes.

4. Finally, top with rosemary, serve and enjoy it!

Nutrition: Calories: 381Kcal; Fat: 21g; Carbs: 20g; Protein: 27g

12. Vegan Lemon Rosemary Pasta With Mushrooms And Kale

Preparation Time: 10 minutes

Cooking Time: 20 minutes

Servings: 6

Ingredients:

- 12 oz. pasta
- Red pepper flakes
- 2 tbsp. olive oil
- 1 large shallot
- lemon wedges
- 7 garlic cloves
- Salt & pepper
- 2 lbs. sliced mushrooms
- 5 oz. pack baby kale
- ½ heaping tsp. thyme
- 1 ½ cups vegetable

Directions:

1. Take the paste and cook it.
2. Take a pot, add oil and heat it, then add onions and cook for 4 to 5 minutes; add herbs, mushrooms, garlic, and red pepper flakes, salt and pepper, mix them well and cook for 5 to 6 minutes or till properly cooked. Then finally, add kale and cook it.
3. Take cooked pasta, add in broth, mushroom mixture and cook them well.
4. Take a bowl, serve the pasta top with pepper and lemon juice, and enjoy it!

Nutrition: Calories: 692Kcal; Fat: 17g; Carbs: 114g; Protein: 24g

13. Mini Citrus Rosemary Upside-Down Cake

Preparation Time: 10 minutes

Cooking Time: 30 minutes

Servings: 5

Ingredients:

- 1 cup almonds
- 1 cup all-purpose flour

- 1 1/2 tsp. fresh rosemary
- 1/2 tsp. baking soda
- 1 1/2 tsp. baking powder
- 1 tsp. salt
- 1 1/2 cups milk cheese
- 1/2 cup sugar
- 2/3 cup olive oil
- 1 Cara orange zest
- 1 sprig rosemary
- 1 1/2 cups sugar
- 3 eggs
- 3g blood oranges
- 1/2 cup water

Directions:

1. Preheat the oven to 350 degrees Fahrenheit. Spot the sugar on the bottom of the pans.
2. Spot the rosemary and almond in the blender and blend well until completely ground.
3. Transfer the mixture to the bowl, put in baking powder, baking soda, and all-purpose flour, and stir well to combine.
4. Spot the sugar, ricotta cheese, orange zest, and olive oil in a blender and blend for five minutes to mix them completely.
5. Put in the egg and again shake to mix.
6. Blend well half of the flour mixture properly, transfer the other half to the blender, and pulse.
7. With the help of a knife, cut citrus fruit into pieces and spot them in the bottom of the tray.
8. Fill the muffin cavity with the batter a little below the top.
9. Spot the muffin cavity tray in the oven.
10. Cook it for 25 minutes by rotating the tray.
11. Once done, insert a toothpick in the cake to check its doneness.
12. Take a pan on the heat and put rosemary, water, and sugar in it.
13. Boil the water for 2 minutes by shaking it to dissolve the sugar.
14. Set the mixture to simmer and cook for 5 minutes.
15. Remove the cake from the wire rack and allow it to cool for 10 minutes.
16. Apply the rosemary syrup over the cake as its topping.
17. Put it in the freezer for a few minutes and serve.
18. Enjoy.

Nutrition: Calories: 404Kcal; Fat: 21g; Carbs: 49g; Protein: 6g

14. Baked Brie With Apricot Preserves

Preparation Time: 5 minutes

Cooking Time: 35 minutes

Servings: 6

Ingredients:

- 8 oz. brie
- 1 egg
- 1 sheet thawed puff pastry
- 3 tbsp. apricot preserves

Directions:

1. Preheat the oven to 400 degrees Fahrenheit.
2. Remove the sheet from the pastry and spread it evenly on the sheet.
3. Spot the brie over it in the center and apply apricot preserve on the top of the brie.
4. Fold the brie up and whisk the egg well in the bowl.
5. Coat the pastry with egg completely.
6. Spot pastry on the baking sheet and spot in the oven.
7. Cook for 35 minutes. Once done, allow it to rest for ten minutes.
8. Serve and enjoy.

Nutrition: Calories: 129Kcal; Fat: 9g; Carbs: 5g; Protein: 6g

15. Rosemary, Watermelon, And Strawberry Smoothie

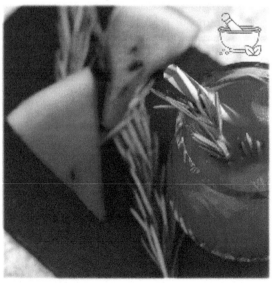

Preparation Time: 5 minutes

Cooking Time: 0 minutes

Servings: 2

Ingredients:

- 2 oranges
- 1 tsp. fresh rosemary
- 2 cups watermelon
- 2 cups strawberries
-

Directions:

1. Take a blender and put in all ingredients.
2. Shake well for sixty seconds until tender.
3. Once done, transfer to the serving glass and serve.
4. Enjoy.

Nutrition: Calories: 210Kcal; Fat: 1.7g; Carbs: 21g; Protein: 1.9g

16. Socca

Preparation Time: 10 minutes

Cooking Time: 25 minutes

Servings: 6

Ingredients:

- 1 tsp. salt
- 1 medium yellow onion
- Extra olive oil for brushing
- 1 cup garbanzo bean flour
- 3 ½ tbsp. extra virgin olive oil
- Extra pepper for sprinkling
- 1 cup water
- 2 tsp. chopped fresh rosemary
- 1 tsp. black pepper

Directions:

1. Take a large bowl: mix salt, garbanzo bean, pepper, and flour in it.
2. Add water and mix thoroughly.
3. Pour 1 ½ tbsp. of olive oil. Mix and set it aside for twenty minutes.
4. Set the oven. Allow it to preheat at 450 degrees Fahrenheit.
5. Take a pan. Add olive oil and heat.
6. Add onion to the pan and let them fry. Add sugar for caramelization.
7. Add rosemary and cook for one minute. Set it aside.
8. Take chickpea batter and add it to the pan containing the onion mixture.
9. Put it in the oven for fifteen minutes.
10. Remove from oven. Cut into slices and serve.

Nutrition: Calories: 158Kcal; Fat: 10g; Carbs: 13g; Protein: 5g

17. Chickpea And Rosemary Soup

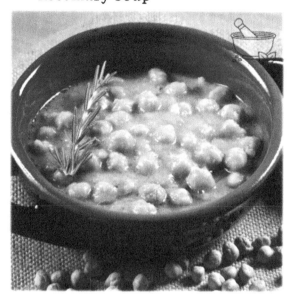

Preparation Time: 5 minutes

Cooking Time: 10 minutes

Servings: 3

Ingredients:

- Olive oil
- 1/3 lb. pasta
- 2 tbsp. parsley
- 15 oz. chickpeas
- 2 tbsp. tomato sauce
- 2 leeks
- 3 tbsp. olive oil
- Salt and pepper
- 6 cups chicken broth
- 2 tbsp. basil
- 1 tbsp. rosemary
- 1 tomato
- 2 tbsp. minced garlic

Directions:

1. Take a saucepan. Add olive oil to it and heat.
2. Add leeks and garlic to it.
3. Once the garlic is golden brown, add rosemary, tomato, and tomato sauce. Let it simmer for four minutes.
4. Then add parsley, chickpeas, broth, and basil. Allow it to boil.
5. Add pasta and cook for seven more minutes.

6. Turn off the heat. Transfer it to a bowl and season with salt and pepper.

Nutrition: Calories: 640Kcal; Fat: 21g; Carbs: 85g; Protein: 28g

18. Dukan Tofu Bread Sticks

Preparation Time: 10 minutes

Cooking Time: 20 minutes

Servings: 4

Ingredients:

- Flavoring
- Salt
- 125 g tofu
- 1 egg

- Fresh rosemary
- 1 tsp. yeast

Directions:

1. Set the oven. Allow it to preheat at 180 degrees Fahrenheit.
2. In the blender, add yeast, tofu, rosemary, egg, and salt. Blend them.
3. Divide the dough into two. Add pizza flavoring to one dough and bacon flavoring to the second.
4. Cover a baking pan with parchment paper.
5. Put the dough in the pan.
6. Put the pan in the oven for twenty minutes.
7. Take it out of the oven and slice it into breadsticks.
8. Serve and enjoy!

Nutrition: Calories: 50Kcal; Fat: 2.8g; Carbs: 10g; Protein: 4g

19. Focaccia With Feta, Red Onion, And Rosemary

Preparation Time: 10 minutes

Cooking Time: 40 minutes

Servings: 8

Ingredients:

- 4 garlic cloves
- 2 tbsp. olive oil
- ¾ tsp. salt
- ½ cup whole wheat flour
- 1 ½ tsp. honey
- 1 cup warm water
- ¼ oz. fast-rising yeast
- 2 ½ cups all-purpose flour
- ½ cup feta cheese
- 1 tbsp. olive oil
- 3 tbsp. fresh rosemary
- 1 cup thinly sliced onion

Directions:

1. Take a bowl. Add yeast, 1 cup flour, salt, and whole wheat flour.
2. Add honey, water, garlic, and olive oil.
3. Knead the dough for five minutes.
4. Cover the dough and set it aside.
5. Take a pan. Add olive oil to it and heat.
6. Fry onions in it and set aside.
7. Take the dough and put it in the pan.
8. Put onions over it and add cheese and rosemary. Let the dough rise.
9. Put it in the oven for thirty minutes at 350 degrees Fahrenheit.

Nutrition: Calories: 253Kcal; Fat: 69g; Carbs: 39g; Protein: 6.8g

20. Figs With Zabaglione

Preparation Time: 5 minutes

Cooking Time: 15 minutes

Servings: 8

Ingredients:

- 1 sprig of fresh mint
- 4 cups quartered fresh figs, red raspberries, blueberries, blackberries, and halve strawberries
- ½ cup light dairy sour cream
- 1 ½ cups milk
- 1 tsp. rosemary
- ¼ cup sugar1 pinch ground cinnamon
- ¼ cup dry Marsala
- 2 eggs
- 4 tsp. cornstarch

Directions:

1. Take a saucepan and add milk, sugar, rosemary, and cornstarch.
2. Cook for two minutes until it thickens.
3. Turn off the heat.
4. Add eggs into the pan. Again, cook for two minutes.

5. Place the custard in a bowl and add Marsala and sour cream. Put it in the refrigerator for twenty-four hours.
6. Once properly chilled, take it out, top with fruit, mint, and cinnamon.
7. Serve and enjoy!

Nutrition: Calories: 113Kcal; Fat: 3g; Carbs: 15g; Protein: 5g

21. Chicken And Veggie Rosemary Skewers

Preparation Time: 10 minutes

Cooking Time: 15 minutes

Servings:6

Ingredients:

- ½ cup Italian salad dressing
- 1 large onion
- 2 boneless, skinless chicken breasts
- 1 tsp. rosemary
- 24 cherry tomatoes
- 2 small zucchini
- Cooking spray

Directions:

1. Allow the boiler to preheat.
2. Spray a baking sheet with cooking spray.
3. Take a bowl and add dressing, chicken breasts, rosemary, onion, tomatoes, and zucchini. Mix well.
4. Take skewers and thread chicken and vegetables onto skewers.
5. Put them on the baking sheet.
6. Let them boil for fifteen minutes on high heat.
7. Transfer to a plate and serve.

Nutrition: Calories: 191Kcal; Fat: 5g; Carbs: 10g; Protein: 25g

22. Rosemary Shampoo Bar

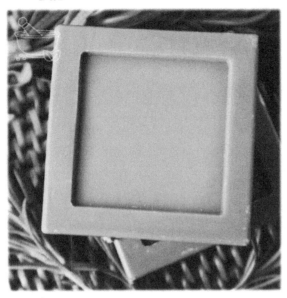

Preparation Time: 20 minutes

Cooking Time: 1 hour

Ingredients:

- 1 lb. Of glycerin of goat milk
- 1 tsp. of mango butter
- 2 tsp. of castor oil
- 16 drops of rosemary oil
- 16 drops of cedar wood oil
- 1 tsp. rosemary, chopped
- Boiler
- 1 soap mold
- 1 spray bottle

Directions:

1. Melt the soap base over low heat.
2. Add mango butter to it. Let the mango butter melt.
3. Remove it from the heat and add castor oil.
4. Mix well.
5. Now mix the rosemary and ceda rwood oil in it.

6. Add the chopped rosemary to it.
7. Now pour the mixture in the mold.
8. To avoid air bubbles, spray some rubbing alcohol.
9. Let it cool for 3-4 hours.
10. Remove it from mold and store it in a container.

23. Rosemary Pest Deterrent

Preparation Time: 10 minutes

Cooking Time: 25-30 minutes

Ingredients:

- 1 cup of dried rosemary
- Quarter of water

Directions:

1. Take the rosemary leaves and water in a pot and boil for 5-10 minutes.
2. Strain the rosemary water in a container and pour the blend in the squirt bottles to spray the water directly on the skins and pits.
3. It can also be stored in the refrigerator.

24. Rosemary Tooth Paste

Preparation Time: 20 minutes

Cooking Time: 1 hour

Ingredients:

- 3 tbsp. of coconut oil
- 16-18 drops of rosemary oil
- 2 tbsp. of baking soda
- ¼ Tsp of stevia powder

Directions:

1. Take a small bowl and mix the baking soda and coconut oil in it.
2. Add the essential oils in it along with the stevia powder.
3. Mix well until everything is combined well.
4. Store the paste in a container.

CHAPTER 55:

BASIL RECIPES

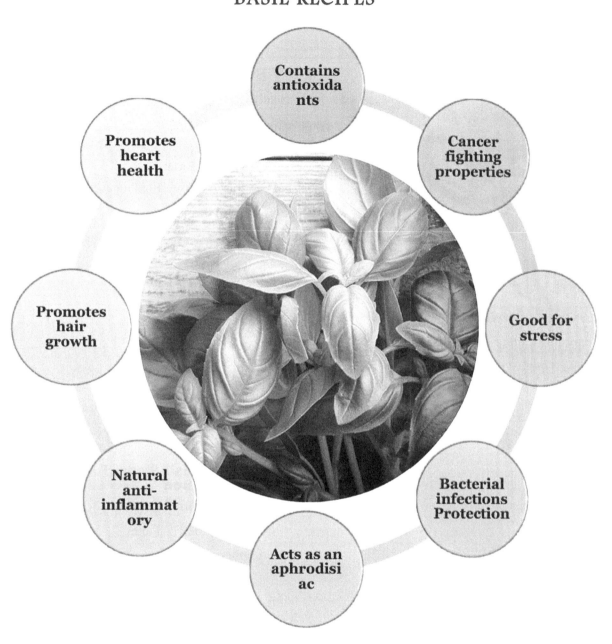

Contains antioxidants

Cancer fighting properties

Promotes heart health

Good for stress

Promotes hair growth

Bacterial infections Protection

Natural anti-inflammatory

Acts as an aphrodisiac

25. Basil And Honey Tea For Digestion

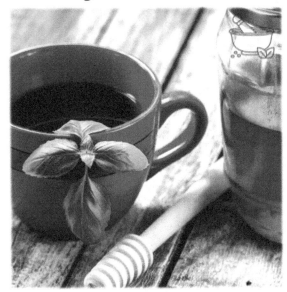

Preparation Time: 5 minutes

Cooking Time: 2 minutes

Ingredients:

- 1-quart water
- 3 leaves mint
- 1 tbsp. honey
- 1 tsp. lemon juice
- 1 tsp. cumin
- 1 tsp. lime zest
- 1 tsp. ginger

Directions:

1. Place the pot over medium heat.
2. Put in water and boil.
3. Shake in lime juice, cumin, honey, lime zest, mint, and ginger.
4. to infuse the flavor, shake well and cook for two minutes.

26. Simple Basil Tea For Cough

Preparation Time: 5 minutes

Cooking Time: 0 minutes

Ingredients:

- 1 black tea bag
- ½ lemon slice
- 6 basil leaves

Directions:

1. Boil the water into the pot.
2. Mix well lemon and basil leaves in the glass.
3. Put the teabag in the cup and pour the boiled water into it.
4. Soak it for 5 minutes to infuse the flavor.
5. Drink and enjoy.

27. Basil Vinegar For Warm Bath

Preparation Time: 10 minutes

Cooking Time: 0 minutes

Ingredients:

- 1 cup basil
- 1/8 tsp. pepper
- ½ cup olive oil
- ½ cup shallot
- 3 tbsp. red wine vinegar
- ½ tsp. salt

Directions:

1. Put all the ingredients in a blender.
2. Bled well for 1 minute until mixture is completely mixed.

28. Fresh Basil Steam For Congestion

Preparation Time: 5 minutes

Cooking Time: 5 minutes

Ingredients:

2 quarts water

Basil leaves

Directions:

1. Take a pot and pour water into it
2. Boil water over medium heat.
3. Add basil leaves in water and soak for 5 minutes.
4. Make a tent with a towel over your head.
5. Inhale the steam for five to ten minutes.

29. Basil Essential Oil

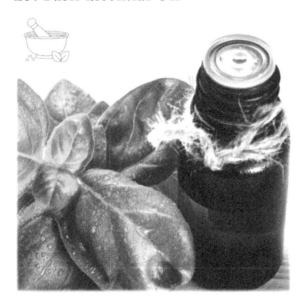

Preparation Time: 5 minutes

Cooking Time: 0 minutes

Ingredients:

- 2 oz. basil
- 12 oz. olive oil

Directions:

1. From the stem, discard the basil leaves.
2. Put the oil in the jar and fill basil into it with a shut top.
3. Place the jar in sunlight for one day.
4. Stain the oil and, with a spoon, mash it.
5. Remove the basil leaves and move them to another jar.
6. Freeze it for one week.

30. Basil And Tomato Pasta

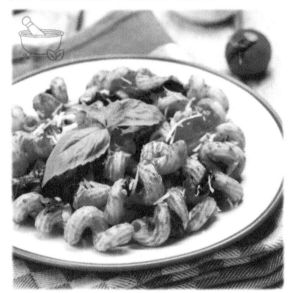

Preparation Time: 10 minutes

Cooking Time: 45 minutes

Servings: 6

Ingredients:

- ½ cup olive oil
- Salt
- 2 garlic cloves
- Pepper
- ½ cup fresh basil
- ¾ tsp. salt
- 1 lb. pasta
- Cherry tomatoes

Directions:

1. Mix salt, olive oil, and garlic in a bowl properly.
2. On the cutting board, chop tomatoes and move to the bowl.
3. Shake the mixture, allow it to rest, and cook the pasta according to the direction written on the package.
4. Strain the pasta and store some of the pasta water aside.
5. Stir in the pasta in the tomatoes mixture.
6. Put in some pasta water in tomato mixture and shake well.
7. Put in basil and more pasta water to make the mixture tender.

8. Sprinkle pepper and salt and put basil over it for garnishing.
9. Serve.

Nutrition: Calories: 448Kcal; Fat: 19g; Carbs: 58g; Protein: 10g

31. Basil Pesto Minestrone

Preparation Time: 20 minutes

Cooking Time: 40 minutes

Servings: 4

Ingredients:

- 1 tbsp. olive oil
- 400g borlotti beans
- 1 brown onion
- 80 g frozen beans
- 1 carrot
- ½ cup penne rigate
- 1 celery stick
- 1 zucchini
- 400g tomatoes
- 1 cup basil leaves
- 4 cups chicken like liquid stock
- 25g parmesan
- ¼ cup pine nuts
- ¼ cup olive oil
- 1 garlic clove

Directions:

1. Pour the oil into the saucepan and heat on medium heat.
2. Stir in carrot, onion, and celery, and cook until onion tender for five minutes.
3. Put in zucchini, stock, and tomato and set it to simmer. Decrease the heat and shake and cook for 20 minutes to make the soup thicker.
4. Put in pasta and cook for 10 minutes until softened.
5. Stir in borlotti beans and peas and cook for five minutes.
6. Chop pine nuts, basil, and garlic with a knife on the cutting board and move to a bowl.
7. Shake in parmesan and oil and coat with pepper and salt.
8. Distribute the soup in bowls equally and Put basil pesto over it.

9. Serve and enjoy.

Nutrition: Calories: 468Kcal; Fat: 31g; Carbs: 27g; Protein: 16g

32. Mozzarella Stuffed Basil Turkey Burger

Preparation Time: 10 minutes

Cooking Time: 15 minutes

Servings: 4

Ingredients:

- 1 lb. turkey
- Black pepper and salt
- 1 egg
- ¼ tsp. garlic powder
- 15 oz. black beans
- ½ cup mozzarella cheese
- ½ red bell pepper

Directions:

1. Take a bowl and mix garlic powder, egg, mozzarella cheese, ground turkey, salt, red bell pepper, and black pepper until completely incorporated.
2. Prepare 4 patties from the above mixture.
3. Put the skillet over medium heat and put it in turkey patties.
4. Cook for seven to ten minutes from all the sides until no pink appears.
5. Once completely cooked, move to the serving plate and serve.

Nutrition: Calories: 225Kcal; Fat: 12g; Carbs: 2g; Protein: 28g

33. Garlic Basil Ravioli With Alfredo Sauce

Preparation Time: 15 minutes

Cooking Time: 30 minutes

Servings: 6

Ingredients:

- 2 lb. chicken
- Spaghetti noodles
- 5 tbsp. olive oil
- 10 oz. alfredo sauce
- 1 tbsp. white wine vinegar
- 1/8 tsp. Pepper
- ¼ cup basil
- ¼ tsp. salt
- 5 garlic cloves
- 1 shallot

Directions:

1. With the help of a knife, cut the chicken into cubes and spot it in a sealed container.
2. Take a bowl and mix white wine vinegar, garlic cloves, pepper, salt, olive oil, shallot, and basil properly.
3. Spot the mixture in the sealed container of chicken and shake the bag to coat the chicken with the mixture completely.
4. Spot the container in the refrigerator and aloe it to refrigerate for 24 hours.
5. Remove the chicken from the refrigerator and sprinkle olive oil on it.
6. Place the pan on medium heat and put in the marinated chicken.
7. Cook the chicken for about twenty minutes until the pink color disappear.
8. Cook the spaghetti according to the direction written on the package.
9. Discard the water from the spaghetti and transfer it to a bowl.
10. Spot alfredo sauce and cooked chicken over it and mix to rub the chicken completely.
11. Serve and enjoy it.

Nutrition: Calories: 692Kcal; Fat: 39g; Carbs: 49g; Protein: 23g

34. Basil Roasted Vegetables Panzanella

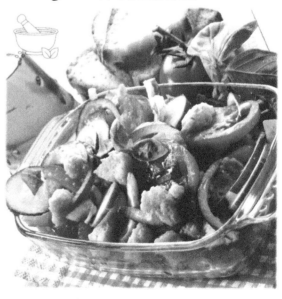

Preparation Time: 20 minutes

Cooking Time: 15 minutes

Servings: 8

Ingredients:

- 5 cups wheat bread
- ½ cup black olives
- ½ cup cucumber, chopped
- ½ cup olive oil
- 1 red onion
- ¼ cup red wine vinegar
- ½ cup basil
- 6 tomatoes
- ¼ cup lemon juice
- ½ tsp. salt
- ¼ cup parsley
- ½ cup parmesan cheese

Directions:

1. Preheat the oven to over 350 degrees Fahrenheit.
2. Place cubes of the bread on the baking sheet.
3. Toss and cook the bread for fifteen minutes until browned.
4. Take a bowl and put in lemon juice, vinegar, salt, and parsley.
5. The vinegar is evenly distributed in the parmesan cheese, onion, olives, cucumber, basil, and toasted bread.
6. Serve and enjoy.

Nutrition: Calories: 268Kcal; Fat: 17.6g; Carbs: 21.5g; Protein: 7.4g

35. Basil Lettuce Wraps

Preparation Time: 10 minutes

Cooking Time: 5 minutes

Servings:4

Ingredients:

- 1 lb. chicken
- Lettuce leaves
- Diced Jalapeno
- 2 cups rice
- 1 tsp. soy sauce
- Fresh basil
- 1 tsp. hoisin sauce
- 2 tbsp. white sugar
- 1 tbsp. water

Directions:

1. Mix all the ingredients with brown chicken.
2. Put in torn basil to wilt.
3. Now put in cooked rice in the mixture and cook.

4. Put over the lettuce leaves and apply fresh herbs and extra basil on the top.
5. Serve and enjoy.

Nutrition: Calories: 582Kcal; Fat: 16g; Carbs: 83g; Protein: 28g

36. Basil Mint Yellow Squash Spiralized Salad

Preparation Time: 10 minutes

Cooking Time: 11 minutes

Servings: 2

Ingredients:

- 2 yellow summer squash
- Sea salt
- 1 celery stalk
- Black pepper
- 1 tbsp. fresh basil
- Red pepper flakes
- 2 tsp. olive oil
- ¼ tsp. cumin
- 2 tsp. lemon juice
- ½ tsp. lemon zest
- 1 tsp. fresh mint

Directions:

1. Mix all the ingredients in a bowl.
2. Shake well to rub properly.
3. Put mint or basil leaves and pepper over it for garnishing.
4. Serve and enjoy.

Nutrition: Calories: 143Kcal; Fat: 1.9g; Carbs: 26g; Protein: 7.5g

37. Loaded Spinach Avocado And Basil Salad

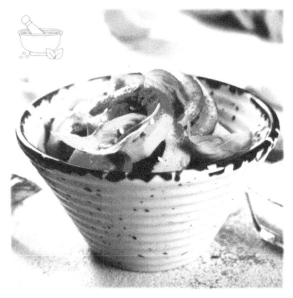

Preparation Time: 10 minutes

Cooking Time: 15 minutes

Servings:4

Ingredients:

- ½ cup dry quinoa
- 1 tomato
- 1 cup water
- 5 oz. spinach leaves
- 15 oz. chickpeas
- ½ tbsp. coarse salt
- 1 tbsp. olive oil
- 1 avocado
- Water
- 5 basil leaves
- Salt
- 1 garlic clove
- 2 tbsp. lemon juice

Directions:

1. Take a saucepan and boil water and quinoa in it.
2. Cook for 15 minutes with cover top by decreasing the heat.
3. Pour the oil into the oil and heat over medium heat. Put in salt and chickpeas.
4. Cook for fifteen minutes until browned.
5. Put water, lemon juice, avocado, basil leaves, garlic, and salt in the blender and shake well to prepare the dressing.
6. Put the spinach in the bowl and add tomato chunks, quinoa, chickpeas, and dressing over it.

7. Rub the salad completely and coat with pepper and salt.
8. Serve and enjoy.

Nutrition: Calories: 354Kcal; Fat: 15g; Carbs: 45g; Protein: 13g

38. White Fish With Burst Cherry Tomato And Basil

Preparation Time:5 minutes

Cooking Time:25 minutes

Servings:4

Ingredients:

- 2 cherry tomatoes
- ¼ lb. white fish
- 1 tbsp. olive oil
- ½ cup basil leaves
- 15 garlic cloves
- Black pepper
- Coarse salt

Directions:

1. Preheat the oven to 425 Fahrenheit.
2. Take a pan and mix salt, garlic, pepper, salt, and tomatoes, and basil; cook for fifteen minutes.
3. Shake well and move from the oven.
4. Roast fish with tomatoes for ten minutes in the oven.
5. Once done, distribute the fish in serving plates equally.
6. Garnish with basil and tomatoes.
7. Serve and enjoy.

Nutrition: Calories: 396Kcal; Fat: 6g; Carbs: 3g; Protein: 16g

39. Basil Quinoa Pizza Pie

Preparation Time: 10 minutes

Cooking Time: 45 minutes

Servings: 2

Ingredients:

- ¾ cup quinoa
- Red pepper flakes
- ¼ cup water
- Fresh basil
- ½ tsp. baking powder
- 1 cup shredded goat cheese
- ½ tsp. salt

- ½ cup tomato sauce
- 1 tbsp. olive oil

Directions:

1. Steep the quinoa in water for eight hours.
2. Preheat the oven to 425 degrees Fahrenheit and cover the baking sheet with parchment paper.
3. Wash the soaked quinoa.
4. Take a lender and put in olive oil, water, quinoa, salt, and baking powder.
5. Blend completely to make the mixture tender.
6. Spread the prepared batter over the baking pan evenly.
7. Cook the pizza crust by flipping for twenty minutes from each side until brown and crispy.
8. Remove from the oven and apply the toppings with cheese and sauce.
9. Spot again in the oven and bake for more than 15 minutes.
10. Once done, transfer to the serving plate and allow it to cool.
11. Spot pepper flakes, cheese, and herbs over it for garnishing.
12. Serve and enjoy.

Nutrition: Calories: 297Kcal; Fat: 11g; Carbs: 41g; Protein: 9g

40. Peanut Noodles With Cabbage And Basil

Preparation Time: 15 minutes

Cooking Time: 10 minutes

Servings: 14

Ingredients:

- 16 oz. penne pasta
- ½ cup peanuts
- ½ cup peanut butter
- ½ cup chopped basil
- 2 tbsp. maple syrup
- 1 cup carrots
- 2 tbsp. soy sauce
- 1 cup chopped scallions
- 4 tsp. white vinegar
- 2 cups red cabbage
- One garlic clove
- ½ tsp. salt
- 1 tsp. ginger
- 2 tsp. hot sauce

Directions:

1. Over medium-high heat, in a pot, boil the water.
2. Cook pasta according to the instruction written on the package.
3. Strain the pasta and put some of the pasta water aside.
4. Sprinkle cold water over the pasta.
5. Take a bowl and put in hot water and peanut butter. Stir well.
6. Put in hot sauce, salt, ginger, maple syrup, tamari, garlic, and vinegar.
7. Sir, in the paste, to season properly.
8. Now put in scallions, basil, cabbage, peanuts, and carrots and shake well to rub completely.
9. Once done, serve and enjoy.

Nutrition: Calories: 345Kcal; Fat: 2g; Carbs: 50g; Protein: 13g

41. Melon Sorbet With Basil

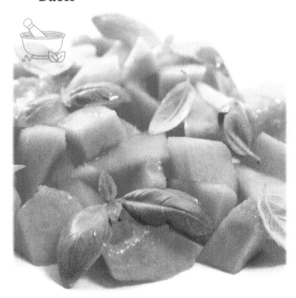

Preparation Time: 10 minutes

Cooking Time: 6 hours

Servings: 4

Ingredients:

- 30 basil leaves
- 1 ripe melon

Directions:

1. Take a food processor and put in basil leaves and frozen melon pieces.
2. Chopped properly and shake until consistency become thick and creamy.
3. Move the mixture to the sealed container and place it in the freezer.
4. Freeze it for 3 hours and serve.

Nutrition: Calories: 30Kcal; Fat: 0.1g; Carbs: 10.3g; Protein: 0.6g

42. Bruschetta's With Tomato And Basil

Preparation Time: 15 minutes

Cooking Time: 8 minutes

Servings: 6

Ingredients:

- 2 tomatoes
- 4 tbsp. parmesan cheese
- ½ onion
- 225 g bread
- 2 tbsp. olive oil
- 1 tsp. parsley
- 1 tbsp. oregano
- 1 tsp. basil

Directions:

1. Preheat the oven.
2. Take a bowl and mix olive oil, oregano, tomatoes, parsley, and onion properly.
3. Spot the bread on the baking sheet and apply the tomato mixture to it.
4. Drizzle with parmesan.
5. Cook in the preheated oven for eight to ten minutes until lightly browned.
6. Once done, allow it to cool and serve.

Nutrition: Calories: 178Kcal; Fat: 1.9g; Carbs: 22.8g; Protein: 5.7g

43. Ricotta Mango Basil Parfait

Preparation Time: 25 minutes

Cooking Time: 5 minutes

Servings: 6

Ingredients:

- 14 sweet potatoes and grain cracker
- 4 oz. mason
- 15 oz. ricotta cheese
- 3 strawberries
- 1 mango
- 6 basil leaves
- ¼ tsp. cinnamon

Directions:

1. Put the crackers in the food processor, blend to make the crumbs, and move to a bowl.
2. Put in the cinnamon, basil leaves, ricotta cheese, and diced mango and shake to make a smooth mixture.
3. In the bottom of the jar, place the crumbs and apply the topping with a prepared ricotta mixture.
4. Again, put in the crumbs to make another layer.
5. Spot the chopped basil, cracker crumbs, and strawberry half on the top of each parfait.
6. Once done, serve and enjoy.

Nutrition: Calories: 270Kcal; Fat: 9g; Carbs: 14g; Protein: 10g

44. Basil Hair Oil

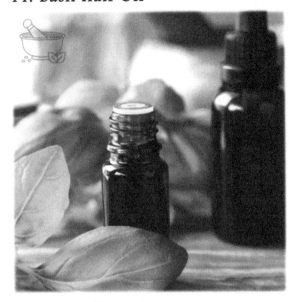

Preparation Time: 5 minutes

Cooking Time: 10 minutes

Ingredients:

- 30-gram basil leaves
- ¾ cup olive oil

Directions:

1. Take a pot and boil the water over medium heat.
2. Put in the basil leaves and boil.
3. Strain the water and discard the basil leaves.
4. Now dry basil leaves with a towel.
5. Take a blender and put in the olive oil and leaves.
6. Blend the mixture completely until the mixture is smooth.
7. Now move the oil to cover the top container.
8. Place the oil in the refrigerator.
9. Use oil within two to four days.

45. Basil Perfume

Preparation Time: 6 weeks

Cooking Time: 0 minutes

Ingredients:

- 1 lemon zest
- 8 oz. vodka
- 1 grapefruit zest
- Basil oil

Directions:

1. Take a glass and mix citrus zest in it.
2. Put in vodka and stir until liquid appears above the zest.
3. Cover it tightly and stir well once or more than one time every day.
4. Strain the mixture after 6 weeks and discard the peel from the cologne.
5. Transfer the cologne to a decorated bottle with a diffuse top.
6. Now put in few drops of basil oil in it.
7. Increase the quantity of oil to want the strong cologne.

46. Basil Based Insect Repellent

Preparation Time: 4 hours

Cooking Time: 0 minutes

Ingredients:

- Basil leaves
- ¼ tsp. basil oil
- ½ cup boiling water
- ½ cup vodka

Directions:

1. Take a cup and pour water into it. Soak the basil leaves in it for two to four hours.
2. Take the liquid from the leaves by compressing the leaves.
3. Take a spray bottle put it in the infused liquid.
4. To increase the potency, put in basil oil.
5. Shake in the vodka to mix all the content completely.
6. Spray on the skin to repel the mosquitoes.

CHAPTER 56:

THYME RECIPES

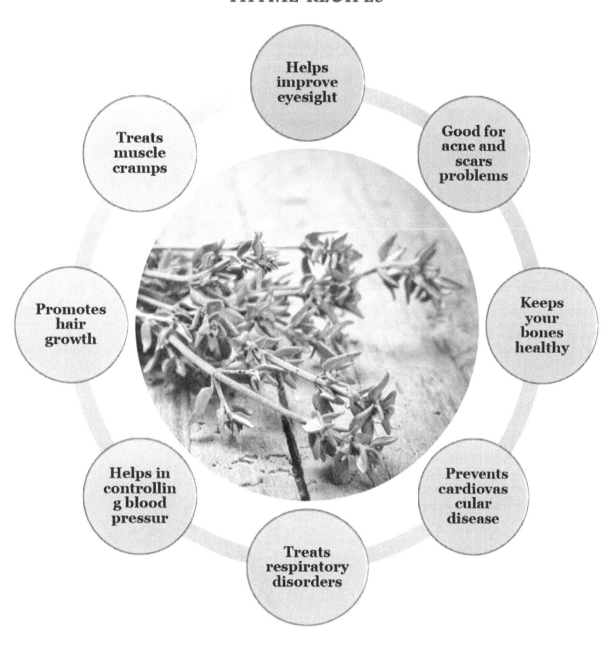

Helps improve eyesight

Good for acne and scars problems

Treats muscle cramps

Keeps your bones healthy

Promotes hair growth

Prevents cardiovas cular disease

Helps in controllin g blood pressur

Treats respiratory disorders

THYME AS MEDICINE

47. Thyme Tea

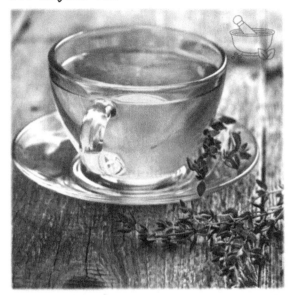

Preparation Time: 1 minute

Cooking Time: 5 minutes

Ingredients:

- 1 ½ cup boiling water
- Three sprigs of fresh thyme

Directions:

1. Take a teacup. Put thyme sprigs in it.
2. Add boiling water into the cup and cover it.
3. Set it aside for five minutes.
4. Uncover it and remove the sprigs.
5. Enjoy!

48. Homey Thyme Cough Syrup

Preparation Time: 5 minutes

Cooking Time: 10 minutes

Ingredients:

- 1 cup organic raw honey
- 2 cups water
- 3 tbsp organic fresh thyme

Directions:

1. Take a saucepan. Add water into a saucepan and let it boil.
2. Remove the pan and add thyme to it.

3. Cover the pan and set it aside for ten minutes.
4. Strain it and mix honey in it.
5. Put the mixture in the refrigerator.
6. Take 1 or 2 tsp. whenever needed.

49. Thyme Tincture

Preparation Time: 15 minutes

Cooking Time: 0 minutes

Ingredients:

- 300 ml vodka
- One hand dried thyme

Directions:

1. Take a glass jar. Add herbs to it.
2. Put vodka in it.
3. Set the jar aside after covering. Don't expose it to direct sunlight.
4. Set the jar aside for forty days. Shake it from time to time.
5. Drain the mixture after forty days.
6. The tincture is ready; now, just store it in a jar in a dark place.

50. Thyme Essential Oil

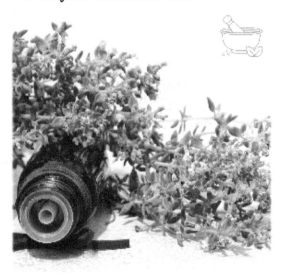

Preparation Time: 10 minutes

Cooking Time: 3 hours

Ingredients:

- 50 g thyme
- 1 L vegetable oil

Directions:

1. In a vacuum, the pouch adds thyme and oil.

2. Cook sous vide at 131 degrees Fahrenheit for three hours.
3. Transfer it to an ice bath. Allow it to cool.
4. Strain the oil and remove thyme.

51. Thyme, Ginger, Garlic, And Mint Tea For Tonsillitis

Preparation Time: 2 minutes

Cooking Time: 5 minutes

Ingredients:

- One glass water
- Two branches of fresh mint
- One piece of fresh ginger
- Five sprigs of thyme
- Two garlic cloves

Directions:

1. Take a pan. Fill it with water.
2. Take ginger chunks and put them in the pan. Boil it for five minutes.
3. Rinse the herbs.
4. Chop garlic cloves. Add the garlic along with herbs to the pan.
5. Let it steep for eight minutes.
6. Serve with honey.

THYME AS FOOD

52. White Bean Hummus With Thyme

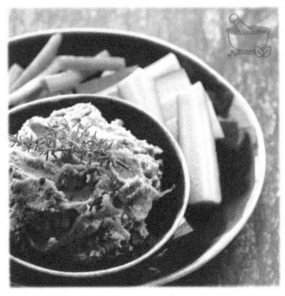

Preparation Time: 15 minutes

Cooking Time: 0 minutes

Servings: 6

Ingredients:

- Freshly ground black pepper
- 1 tbsp. freshly squeezed lemon
- ¼ cup fresh basil
- ½ tbsp. Dijon mustard
- One small garlic clove
- 2 cups cooked cannellini beans
- 1-2 tbsp. water
- 2-3 tsp. fresh thyme
- 2 tbsp. red wine vinegar
- 2 tbsp. tahini
- ½ tsp. salt

Directions:

1. Take all the ingredients, excluding basil, thyme, and water.
2. Blend them in a food processor until smooth, adding water occasionally.
3. Transfer the pasta to a bowl and garnish with thyme and basil.
4. Serve and enjoy!

Nutrition: Calories: 125Kcal; Fat: 5g; Carbs: 16g; Protein: 5g

53. Parsnip "Rice" With Fresh Thyme And Sage

Preparation Time: 10 minutes

Cooking Time: 15 minutes

Servings: 6

Ingredients:

- Fine sea salt
- Ten leaves of fresh minced sage
- Four large parsnips
- Freshly ground black pepper
- Five sprigs of fresh thyme
- 2 tbsp. of unrefined coconut oil
- 1-inch piece of freshly grated ginger

Directions:

1. First, wash the parsnips.
2. Peel the parsnips and cut them in spirals.
3. Put them in the food processor and blend for twenty seconds or until it looks like rice
4. Take a large pan—heat coconut oil in it over medium heat.
5. Add parsnip "rice" to the pan and cook for five minutes.
6. Add black pepper, thyme, sage, and sea salt.
7. Stir continuously and cook for ten minutes.
8. Transfer to a bowl and serve.

Nutrition: Calories: 524Kcal; Fat: 42g; Carbs: 28.5g; Protein: 10.8g

54. Roasted Grape Crostini With Brie And Thyme

Preparation Time: 10 minutes

Cooking Time: 20 minutes

Servings: 4

Ingredients:

- Freshly ground black pepper
- ¼ lb. wedge of brie
- 1 lb. seedless red grapes
- Salt
- 1 to 2 sprigs of fresh thyme
- 3 tbsp. olive oil
- One small loaf of crusty whole-grain bread

Directions:

1. Set the oven. Allow it to preheat at 400 degrees Fahrenheit temperature.
2. Line two baking trays with parchment paper.
3. Take grapes and remove stems. Season them with olive oil, salt, and pepper. Transfer to the small baking trays.
4. Likewise, take the large baking sheet and place bread slices in it. Brush the slices with olive oil as well.
5. Put both dishes in the oven for twenty minutes.
6. Meanwhile, take brie and cut it into strips.
7. Remove toasts and grapes from the oven.
8. Put the brie and grapes on the toast and spread some pepper and fresh thyme.
9. Serve and enjoy!

Nutrition: Calories: 562Kcal; Fat: 18.5g; Carbs: 78.8g; Protein: 16.4g

55. Potato And Kale Soup With Thyme

Preparation Time: 10 minutes

Cooking Time: 30 minutes

Servings: 8

Ingredients:

- 1 tbsp. white vinegar
- 32 oz. vegetable broth
- 1 tsp. dried sage
- 1 cup sliced celery
- 2 tbsp. olive oil
- Parmesan cheese
- Fresh cracked pepper
- 4-5 cups chopped kale
- 1.5 lb. baby red potatoes
- Homemade croutons
- Kosher salt
- 13.5 oz. full-fat coconut milk
- 2 tsp. dried oregano
- 1 cup sliced carrot
- Fresh chopped parsley
- 2 tsp. dried thyme
- Five garlic cloves
- One yellow onion

Directions:

1. Take a large pot. Put olive oil in it and heat over medium heat.
2. Put celery, carrots, and onion in it.

3. Season with salt and pepper.
4. After some time, add sage, oregano, garlic, and thyme.
5. After about one minute, add coconut milk and veggie broth to it. Add some salt and pepper.
6. Allow it to cook for twelve minutes.
7. Add kale and white vinegar to it and season with salt and pepper.
8. Serve and enjoy!

Nutrition: Calories: 294Kcal; Fat: 19.5g; Carbs: 29g; Protein: 4.8g

56. Smoky Lentil And Quinoa Soup

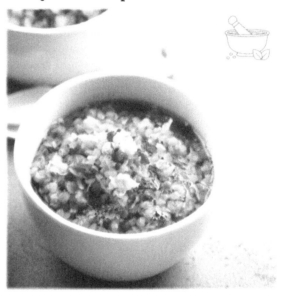

Preparation Time: 15 minutes

Cooking Time: 40 minutes

Servings: 6

Ingredients:

- Chopped parsley
- Salt and pepper
- 2-3 bay leaves
- ½ cup dried quinoa
- 1/8 tsp. nutmeg
- 1 tsp. dried thyme
- 1 tsp. smoked paprika
- One small onion
- Two large carrots
- 1-2 tbsp. balsamic vinegar
- 6-7 cups vegetable broth
- 15 oz. diced tomatoes
- 1 cup dried lentils

- 1 tsp. dried basil
- 1 tsp. cumin
- Two garlic cloves
- Two ribs of celery
- ¼ cup water

Directions:

1. Take lentils and quinoa. Rinse well.
2. Take a pot. Put garlic, celery, onions, and carrots in it. Cook for five minutes, then add nutmeg, paprika, thyme, cumin, and basil. Cook for one more minute.
3. Next, add tomatoes, broth, quinoa, lentils, and bay leaf to the pot—season with salt and pepper.
4. Cook for forty minutes.
5. Remove the pot and transfer soup to a bowl. Remove bay leaves. Add balsamic vinegar and serve.

Nutrition: Calories: 305Kcal; Fat: 2.6g; Carbs: 56.5g; Protein: 16.8g

57. Thyme Infused Vegetables

Preparation Time: 10 minutes

Cooking Time: 40 minutes

Servings: 8

Ingredients:

- 1 tbsp. fresh thyme, chopped
- Two medium red skin potatoes
- ¼ cup olive oil
- One small rutabaga
- Eight medium shallots
- Two medium parsnips
- Two garlic cloves
- Four medium carrots
- Two medium turnips

Directions:

1. Set the oven. Allow it to preheat at 450 degrees Fahrenheit.
2. Take a large bowl: mix vegetables, oil, thyme, and garlic.
3. Season with salt and pepper.
4. Take a baking dish. Put the veggie mixture in the baking dish.
5. Put it in preheated oven for about forty minutes.
6. Serve and enjoy!

Nutrition: Calories: 137Kcal; Fat: 7g; Carbs: 17g; Protein: 2g

58. Creamy Lemon Garlic Chicken With Thyme

Preparation Time: 5 minutes

Cooking Time: 25 minutes

Servings: 4

Ingredients:

- ½ tsp. dried thyme
- ½ cup milk
- 1 tbsp butter
- 1 tsp. salt
- 1 tsp. garlic
- 1 tbsp olive oil
- ½ tsp. lemon zest
- 1 tsp. all-purpose flour
- ½ tsp. pepper
- 1 tbsp lemon juice
- Four boneless chicken breasts

Directions:

1. Marinate the boneless chicken breasts with salt, lemon juice, pepper, and garlic. Set it aside for twenty minutes.
2. Take a large pan. Put chicken breasts in it and cook for five minutes on each side.
3. Transfer the chicken breasts to the plate.
4. Now heat some butter in the pan. Add flour and start adding milk. Stir continuously.
5. Cook till it is thick. Then add some thyme, salt, and lemon zest to it.
6. Put chicken breasts in the pan containing sauce and cook for two minutes.
7. Serve and enjoy!

Nutrition: Calories: 292Kcal; Fat: 18g; Carbs: 6g; Protein: 27g

59. Sautéed Carrot With Thyme

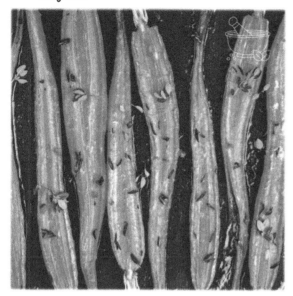

Preparation Time: 10 minutes

Cooking Time: 15 minutes

Servings: 4

Ingredients:

- Kosher salt
- One garlic clove
- 2 tbsp. unsalted butter
- 1 lb. carrot
- Freshly ground black pepper
- Four thyme sprigs
- Two scallions
- ½ cup unsalted chicken stock
- 2 tbsp. canola oil

Directions:

1. Chop the carrots and sliced scallions.
2. Take a pan and pour some oil into it. Heat the oil and melt some butter.
3. Add chicken stock along with garlic, onions, thyme, and carrots. Sprinkle some salt and pepper.
4. Let the mixture cook for about eight minutes while keeping the lid closed.
5. Remove the lid and let the liquid evaporate.
6. Serve and enjoy!

Nutrition: Calories: 167Kcal; Fat: 13.16g; Carbs: 12.6g; Protein: 1.9g

60. Mushroom Pasta With Goat Cheese And Thyme

Preparation Time: 5 minutes

Cooking Time: 15 minutes

Servings: 2

Ingredients:

- 2 tbsp. spreadable goat cheese
- ½ tsp. crushed red pepper flakes
- 2 tbsp. tomato paste
- 3 tbsp. Panko breadcrumbs
- 1 oz. pea greens
- 4 oz. Cremini mushrooms
- ½ lb. Lumaca Rigato Pasta
- ¼ cup grated Parmesan cheese
- One shallot
- 2 tbsp. butter
- One bunch thyme
- Two garlic cloves
- 6 oz spinach

Directions:

1. Take a large pot. Boil water and add salt.
2. Meanwhile, chop garlic, pea greens, and slice shallot and mushrooms.
3. Boil pasta in the pot containing boiling water.
4. Heat olive oil in another pan, and add thyme sprigs, garlic, and breadcrumbs. Sprinkle salt and pepper.
5. Transfer them to a plate and remove thyme sprigs.
6. In the same pan, add olive oil, mushrooms, shallot, thyme, and garlic.
7. Add salt and pepper and allow it to cook for two to three minutes.
8. Add tomato paste in the pan along with red pepper.
9. Add water, salt, and pepper—Cook for three more minutes.
10. In the pan containing pasta, add mushrooms, butter, goat cheese, pea greens, sauce, and spinach—Cook for two minutes.
11. Transfer to a dish, season with salt and pepper, and decorate with parmesan cheese and garlic-thyme breadcrumbs.
12. Serve and enjoy!

Nutrition: Calories: 820Kcal; Fat: 21g; Carbs: 117g; Protein: 28g

61. Spaghetti And Italian Vegan Thyme Meatball

Preparation Time: 10 minutes

Cooking Time: 40 minutes

Servings: 6

Ingredients:

- Sea salt
- ½ tsp. garlic powder
- 2 tsp. dried thyme
- 1 cup of oats
- ½ cup walnuts
- One small yellow onion
- 1 tbsp. olive oil
- Pepper
- Red pepper flakes
- 1 tbsp. Italian seasonings
- 15 oz. beans
- Two garlic cloves
- 8 oz. mushrooms

Directions:

1. Take a pan and add oil, garlic, mushrooms, and onion to it. Cook for five minutes and add herbs.
2. In the food processor, blend nuts, beans, and veggies and adjust seasoning.
3. Shape the mixture into balls with the dried thyme
4. Transfer the balls to the baking sheet.
5. Bake the balls into the oven for half an hour at 400 degrees Fahrenheit.
6. Remove and let it cool.
7. Cook the meatballs and sauce together for ten minutes.
8. Cook pasta separately.
9. Transfer the spaghetti to a bowl. Add sauce, vegan meatballs, salt, and pepper to it.
10. Garnish with fresh parsley and basil.
11. Serve and enjoy!

Nutrition: Calories: 475Kcal; Fat: 6g; Carbs: 88g; Protein: 9g

62. Thyme Winter Salad

Preparation Time: 10 minutes

Cooking Time: 0 minutes

Servings: 8

Ingredients:

- 2 cups torn kale
- 6 cups torn romaine lettuce
- ½ cup extra virgin olive oil
- 1 tbsp. sliced green onion
- 3 tbsp. fresh lemon juice
- 3 cups sliced Bok Choy
- Salt
- 1 tsp. chopped fresh thyme
- 1 tsp. grated lemon peel
- Freshly ground pepper

Directions:

1. First, prepare the dressing.
2. Take green onion, thyme, lemon peel, and lemon juice in the blender. Add oil and blend them.
3. Sprinkle salt and pepper.
4. Take a large bowl. Add bok choy, kale, and lettuce to it.
5. Pour the dressing over it and toss to combine. Serve and enjoy!

Nutrition: Calories: 132Kcal; Fat: 13.7g; Carbs: 2.6g; Protein: 1g

63. Thyme Mini Salsa With White Beans Loaves

Preparation Time: 10 minutes

Cooking Time: 30 minutes

Servings: 6

Ingredients:

- 1 tsp. fresh thyme
- ½ tsp. garlic salt
- Three garlic cloves
- Six green onions
- One whole egg
- 1 cup salsa
- 1 tsp. fresh thyme
- ½ tsp. black pepper
- 1 tbsp. Italian seasoning
- ¾ cup shredded cheddar cheese
- ¼ cup rolled oats
- ¾ cup breadcrumbs
- 15 oz. white beans

Directions:

1. Set the oven. Allow it to preheat at 400 degrees Fahrenheit.
2. Take white beans. Rinse them and put them in a bowl. Mash them using a fork.
3. Add fresh herbs, thyme, minced garlic, pepper, Italian seasonings, garlic salt, beaten

eggs, breadcrumbs, rolled oats, shredded cheese, salsa, and green onions to the same bowl. Mix well.
4. Make mini loaves with the mixture.
5. Take a large baking sheet. Line it with parchment paper
6. Place the loaves on the baking sheet and bake for half an hour.
7. Transfer to a plate and serve.

Nutrition: Calories: 151Kcal; Fat: 4g; Carbs: 23g; Protein: 8g

64. Lemon Thyme Salad Dressing

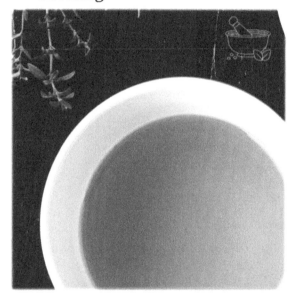

Preparation Time: 15 minutes

Cooking Time: 0 minutes

Servings: 16

Ingredients:

- ½ cup extra virgin olive oil
- ½ tsp. freshly ground black pepper
- Two medium garlic cloves
- ¼ cup fresh lemon juice
- 1 tsp. fresh thyme leaves
- 1 tsp. kosher salt
- 1 tsp. honey
- One small lemon

Directions:

1. Take the lemon and cut it into thin slices.
2. Chop the lemon slices and place them in a lemon jar.
3. Mix all the other ingredients in a jar as well.
4. Serve and enjoy!

Nutrition: Calories: 64Kcal; Fat: 6g; Carbs: 1g; Protein: 0g

65. Pumpkin Orzo Pasta With Thyme

Preparation Time: 5 minutes

Cooking Time: 30 minutes

Servings: 5

Ingredients:

- Salt
- 6-7 sprigs of thyme
- 2 cup vegetable broth
- 1 cup Orzo pasta
- Olive oil
- Two garlic cloves
- 1 cup pumpkin puree
- Pepper

Directions:

1. Take a skillet. Heat olive oil in it and add thyme and garlic. Fry for one minute, then add orzo pasta and mix well.
2. Add pumpkin puree, vegetable broth, and season with salt and pepper. Let the mixture boil.
3. Transfer the pasta to a dish. Garnish with herbs, shaved Romano cheese, and pistachios.
4. Serve and enjoy!

Nutrition: Calories: 230Kcal; Fat: 3g; Carbs: 44g; Protein: 8g

66. Sautéed Mushrooms And Hen With Thyme And Garlic

Preparation Time: 10 minutes

Cooking Time: 15 minutes

Servings: 4

Ingredients:

- Hen of woods mushrooms
- Garlic
- Flaky sea salt
- King trumpet mushrooms
- Olive oil
- Fresh thyme
- Freshly ground black pepper

Directions:

1. Take trumpet mushrooms, wipe them, and then cut them into thin slices.
2. Take a large pan and add olive oil to it. Add garlic to it and cook for one minute.
3. Put mushrooms in the pan and season them with salt and pepper and add thyme.
4. Cook for two or three minutes.
5. Transfer to a plate and serve with fried crispy garlic and thyme.

Nutrition: Calories: 365Kcal; Fat: 35g; Carbs: 10g; Protein: 7g

67. Thyme Based Cantaloupe Coastal Breeze Cocktail

Preparation Time: 5 minutes

Cooking Time: 60 minutes

Servings: 1

Ingredients:

- Melon balls
- Ice cubes
- 1 oz. melon
- 0.5 oz. London dry gin
- ½ cantaloupe
- ½ cup water
- One sprig of fresh thyme
- One pinch salt
- 0.75 oz. syrup
- 1.5 oz. dry sherry
- 12 sprigs fresh thyme
- ½ cup sugar

Directions:

1. Take a saucepan. Add water and sugar to it. Dissolve the sugar and add fresh thyme. Cook for half an hour.
2. Pour the syrup into the cup and place it in a bowl containing ice water. Let it cool.
3. Take cantaloupe. Peel the cantaloupe and remove the seeds.
4. In the blender, put melon chunks and blend until smooth. Strain the juice.
5. Add ice cubes, 1 oz. melon puree, 0.75 oz. thyme syrup, sherry gin, salt, and lemon juice in a cocktail shaker.
6. Strain the cocktail in a cocktail glass. Spread thyme and pierce lemon balls, and set them over the glass.
7. Serve and enjoy!

Nutrition: Calories: 610Kcal; Fat: 3g; Carbs: 20g; Protein: 1.5g

68. Thyme Stuffed Acorn Squash With Wild Rice

Preparation Time: 15 minutes

Cooking Time: 45 minutes

Servings: 8

Ingredients:

- ½ tsp. black pepper
- 2 tbsp. chopped fresh flat-leaf parsley
- 1 tsp. fresh thyme leaves
- 3 oz. fresh shiitake mushrooms
- 1 cup chopped yellow onion
- ¾ tsp. kosher salt
- 1 tsp. olive oil
- 1 tbsp. fresh lemon juice
- 6 oz. fresh spinach
- 1 tbsp. minced garlic
- ½ cup chopped celery
- 3 oz. sweet Italian turkey sausage
- 1 lb. acorn squashes
- 2/3 cup uncooked wild rice

Directions:

1. Set the oven. Allow it to preheat at 425 degrees Fahrenheit.
2. Take rice and cook as directed on the package.
3. Take squashes and coat them with oil. Sprinkle salt over them.
4. Take a baking tray and line it with parchment paper.
5. Place squashes in the baking sheet and bake for twenty minutes.
6. Take a pan and heat olive oil.
7. Put sausages in the pan, cook for three minutes, add onion, mushrooms, spinach, garlic, celery, and thyme, and cook for ten minutes.
8. Add rice to the mixture and season with salt and pepper. Add parsley and juice as well.
9. Take baked squashes and add ½ cup rice mixture to each squash.
10. Again, bake for ten minutes.
11. Remove from the pan and transfer to a plate.
12. Serve and enjoy!

Nutrition: Calories: 197Kcal; Fat: 3g; Carbs: 38g; Protein: 9g

69. Thyme-Based Repellent For Mosquitoes

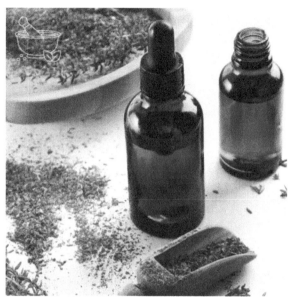

Preparation Time: 5 minutes

Cooking Time: 0 minutes

Ingredients:

- 10-15 drops citronella essential oil
- 1 tbsp. extra virgin olive oil
- 1 tbsp. dried thyme
- 2 tbsp. neem seed oil
- 1 tbsp. coconut oil

Directions:

1. Start by melting coconut oil.
2. Take a jar and mix all the ingredients in it.
3. The jar should contain an eyedropper.
4. The repellent is ready to use.

70. Thyme Based Mouthwash

Preparation Time: 30 minutes

Cooking Time: 0 minutes

Ingredients:

- One drop of lemon essential oil
- 4 drops thyme essential oil
- 1 tbsp. sodium bicarbonate
- 3 drops peppermint essential oil
- 1 tsp. salt
- 250 ml distilled water

Directions:

1. Take a glass jar. Add sodium bicarbonate and distilled water in it. Mix well.
2. Put all the ingredients in the jar as well.
3. Mix well by shaking the jar.
4. Put the mixture in the refrigerator for one week.
5. Mouthwash is ready to use.

71. Thyme Disinfectant

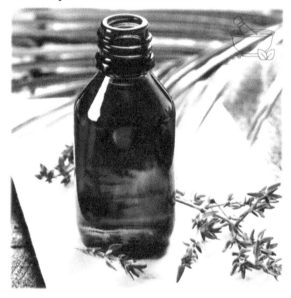

Preparation Time: 5 minutes

Cooking Time: 20 minutes

Ingredients:

- 5 drops tea tree oil
- 1 tsp. lemon essential oil
- 1 tsp. baking soda
- 1 tbsp. thyme extract
- A bunch of garden-fresh thyme
- 2 cups water
- ¼ tsp. thyme essential oils
- 2 tsp. castile soap
- 2 tsp. borax
- 2 cups lemon verbena hydrosol
- One lemon

Directions:

1. Take a small pot, put thyme, lemon, and water in it. Allow it to simmer over medium heat.
2. Turn off the heat and set it aside for one hour.

3. Strain the mixture.
4. To the strained liquid, add borax and baking soda and mix well.
5. Add other ingredients as well.

6. Transfer the mixture to a spray bottle.
7. Don't forget to label the bottle.

CONCLUSION

If we go back to the stone era of mankind, we will come to know that, at that time, the main source of what we call medicine was herbs. This is because they knew natural drugs are rich in antioxidants, anti-inflammation, anti-microbial, and much more such pharmaceutical agents. Plant-based medicines' pharmaceutical properties make them perfect, cost-effective, and easily available treatment options to cure many chronic diseases.

Along with being used in medicines, herbs are also commonly used in the kitchen because of their excellent scent and flavor. You must have noticed that in almost all the recipes, after the main ingredient, usually meat or vegetable, the other main ingredient that is specially added to the dish after salt and pepper is herbs. Moreover, if you watch or read the recipe book of any known chef, you come across the word of the magical or secret word at the end of the recipe, which is mostly any herb. Herbs are so important for any chef because, besides their health benefits, the chefs know that herbs can take your dish to another level of taste because of the aura and flavor they give to your dish; three such herbs, rosemary, basil, and thyme, are discussed in this book.

These three herbs were discussed in terms of their basic features and harvesting tips followed by recipes for food, medicine, and home. Rosemary is rich in vitamins and calcium and is native to the Mediterranean region. It adds scent and flavor to the food and gains health benefits while eating it with food. Basil having a pungent flavor is the most commonly culinary herb which enhances the taste of curries. It is originally from Asia and is a member of the mint family. Thyme has a minty or lemon-like flavor and adds taste to marinades, teas, soups, braised vegetables, or meat.

Made in the USA
Monee, IL
03 December 2022

19474523R00168